Current Progress and Future Directions of Spine Surgery

Current Progress and Future Directions of Spine Surgery

Guest Editors

Dong-Gune Chang
Sam Yeol Chang

MDPI

Basel • Beijing • Wuhan • Barcelona • Belgrade • Novi Sad • Cluj • Manchester

Guest Editors

Dong-Gune Chang
Department of Orthopedic Surgery
Inje Univeristy Sanggye Paik Hospital
Seoul
Republic of Korea

Sam Yeol Chang
Department of Orthopedic Surgery
Seoul National University Hospital
Seoul
Republic of Korea

Editorial Office
MDPI AG
Grosspeteranlage 5
4052 Basel, Switzerland

This is a reprint of the Special Issue, published open access by the journal *Journal of Clinical Medicine* (ISSN 2077-0383), freely accessible at: https://www.mdpi.com/journal/jcm/special_issues/822B95NCZ6.

For citation purposes, cite each article independently as indicated on the article page online and as indicated below:

Lastname, A.A.; Lastname, B.B. Article Title. *Journal Name* **Year**, *Volume Number*, Page Range.

ISBN 978-3-7258-6155-2 (Hbk)
ISBN 978-3-7258-6156-9 (PDF)
https://doi.org/10.3390/books978-3-7258-6156-9

Contents

About the Editors

Dong-Gune Chang

Dong-Gune Chang is an academic researcher from the Department of Orthopedic Surgery, Inje University Sanggye Paik Hospital, College of Medicine, Inje University, and was previously affiliated with the Catholic University of Korea. In his professional life, he has contributed to research on the topics of medicine and scoliosis, with his primary clinical and research interests being pediatric spine deformity, and he has published a vast number of articles in peer-reviewed journals. He is currently an active member of the Scoliosis Research Society (SRS), participating in numerous international and intersociety collaborations.

Sam Yeol Chang

Sam Yeol Chang is an established spine surgeon at the Department of Orthopedic Surgery, Seoul National University Hospital, Korea. He is a graduate of Seoul National University Medical School, where he obtained his medical degree. He completed his residency at the Department of Orthopedic Surgery, Seoul National University Hospital, where he also finished his fellowship in spine surgery. He specializes in pediatric spine deformities, spinal tumors, and minimally invasive fusion techniques. He has a special interest in the correction of complex pediatric spinal deformities using novel technologies, such as stereotactic navigation and robotics.

Journal of
Clinical Medicine

MDPI

Article

Multidisciplinary Digital Therapeutics for Chronic Low Back Pain Versus In-Person Therapeutic Exercise with Education: A Randomized Controlled Pilot Study

Dong-Ho Kang [1,2,†], Jae Hyeon Park [3,†], Chan Yoon [4], Chi-Hyun Choi [4], Sanghee Lee [4], Tae Hyun Park [4], Sam Yeol Chang [2,5,*] and Seong-Ho Jang [3,*]

1 Department of Orthopedic Surgery, Samsung Medical Center, Seoul 06351, Republic of Korea
2 Department of Orthopedic Surgery, Seoul National University College of Medicine, Seoul 03080, Republic of Korea
3 Department of Rehabilitation Medicine, Hanyang University College of Medicine, Guri-si 11923, Republic of Korea; jhpark3.md@gmail.com
4 EverEx, Seoul 06641, Republic of Korea; chan.yoon@everex.co.kr (C.Y.); leo@everex.co.kr (C.-H.C.); ellie@everex.co.kr (S.L.); bill@everex.co.kr (T.H.P.)
5 Department of Orthopedic Surgery, Seoul National University Hospital, Seoul 03080, Republic of Korea
* Correspondence: hewl3102@gmail.com (S.Y.C.); systole@hanyang.ac.kr (S.-H.J.); Tel.: +82-2-2072-7607 (S.Y.C.); +82-031-560-2415 (S.-H.J.)
† These authors contributed equally to this work.

Abstract: Background: Chronic lower back pain (CLBP) is a global health issue leading to significant disability and socioeconomic burden. Traditional treatments, including exercise and cognitive behavioral therapy (CBT), are often limited by physical and temporal constraints. This study aimed to evaluate the efficacy of multidisciplinary digital therapeutics (MORA Cure LBP) compared to conventional treatments. **Methods:** This multicenter, randomized, controlled pilot study enrolled 46 participants. Participants were randomly assigned in a 1:1 ratio to either a MORA Cure LBP group or control group, which received conventional treatment. **Results:** At eight weeks, both groups demonstrated improvements compared to baseline. No statistically significant differences were observed between the MORA Cure LBP and control groups in reductions in usual pain intensity (MORA Cure LBP: 3.1 ± 1.9 vs. control: 3.0 ± 1.5, $p = 0.809$), worst pain intensity (MORA Cure LBP: 5.00 ± 2.18 vs. control: 4.27 ± 1.83, $p = 0.247$), and functional disability (ODI, MORA Cure LBP: 15.6 ± 9.6 vs. control: 15.6 ± 10.0, $p > 0.999$). Compliance was significantly higher in the MORA Cure LBP group during the first 4 weeks (MORA Cure LBP: 74.7% ± 27.4 vs. control: 53.1% ± 28.6, $p < 0.001$). **Conclusions:** Both multidisciplinary digital therapeutics (MORA Cure LBP) and conventional treatments were effective in reducing pain and functional disability in patients with CLBP, with no significant differences between the two groups. Digital therapeutics, particularly those that integrate CBT and exercise, offer promising alternatives to conventional therapies by improving accessibility and potentially enhancing patient engagement.

Keywords: chronic low back pain; digital therapeutics; cognitive behavioral therapy; exercise therapy; multidisciplinary treatment; randomized controlled trial

1. Introduction

Chronic low back pain (CLBP) is a significant global health concern, with a lifetime prevalence exceeding 70% in industrialized countries and worldwide prevalence of 84% [1,2]. It imposes a substantial socioeconomic burden [3,4] and is the leading cause of disability worldwide [5]. Although acute low back pain often resolves within 4–6 weeks [6], chronic cases have a poorer prognosis, with up to 65% of patients experiencing persistent pain for 12 months or longer [7]. Several biological, psychological, social, and occupational factors are associated with poor clinical outcomes in patients with CLBP. These factors include severe disability, sciatica, advanced age, poor overall health, increased psychological or psychosocial distress, negative cognitive characteristics, poor relationships with colleagues, excessive physical labor demands, and secondary compensation [8]. Although many clinical guidelines have focused on pharmacological treatments, physical therapy, and appropriate management of patients with radicular pain [9], a recent study suggests that moderate-to-severe CLBP is associated with reduced health-related quality of life, health status, increased absenteeism, and increased healthcare utilization, regardless of whether patients use prescription medications [10,11].

For chronic low back pain, pharmacological interventions alone are limited to short-term benefits (<3 months) and are associated with increased adverse effects compared to placebo, according to a recent meta-analysis [12]. Therefore, emerging clinical guidelines recommend a multidisciplinary approach or collective back pain treatment that combines pharmacological interventions with psychological interventions, exercise therapy, and invasive treatments [9,11,13,14]. Among psychological interventions, cognitive behavioral therapy (CBT) has shown well-established effectiveness in improving CLBP outcomes [15–19]. A recent meta-analysis reported that these psychological interventions are more effective for pain relief and physical function enhancement when provided in combination with physical or exercise therapy rather than as standalone treatments [20]. However, traditional face-to-face CBT and physical or exercise therapy face challenges related to physical and time constraints, potentially leading to low adherence to such collective back pain treatments. Therefore, to improve treatment effectiveness, there is a need to increase the accessibility of cognitive–behavioral and exercise therapies, which can be achieved through the development of digital therapeutic devices utilizing artificial intelligence (AI), portable devices, and applications.

Based on this background, we developed the MORA Cure LBP, which is a digital therapeutic device for managing and treating CLBP. This study aimed to evaluate the efficacy of MORA Cure LBP compared to conventional therapy, including in-person therapeutic exercise with education in patients with CLBP. We hypothesized that the MORA Cure LBP group would show greater improvements in pain intensity, overall treatment effect, lumbar function, quality of life, muscle strength, and psychological state than the in-person therapeutic exercise with education group. The primary outcomes of this randomized controlled pilot study were usual pain intensity, worst pain intensity, and functional disability (as measured using the Oswestry Disability Index [ODI]) at eight weeks post-baseline. In this study, we assessed the potential of MORA Cure LBP as an accessible and effective digital therapeutic option for CLBP management, potentially addressing the limitations of traditional face-to-face therapies and improving treatment adherence.

2. Materials and Methods

2.1. Study Design and Ethical Considerations

This study was a multicenter, prospective, randomized controlled trial conducted at the Seoul National University Hospital and Hanyang University Guri Hospital. This trial aimed to evaluate the efficacy of multidisciplinary digital therapeutics (MORA Cure LBP) compared to conventional treatment, which includes in-person therapeutic exercise with education for CLBP. The study protocol was approved by the Institutional Review Boards of Seoul National University Hospital (IRB number: 2211-148-1381) and Hanyang University Guri Hospital (IRB number: 2022-12-049). All procedures were conducted in accordance with the ethical standards of the responsible committees on human experimentation (institutional and national) and the Declaration of Helsinki of 1975, as revised in 2000.

2.2. Participants

Eligibility criteria included adults aged 18–65 years with CLBP persisting for >12 weeks and a minimum average pain score of 3 on the 11-point Numeric Pain Rating Scale (NPRS). The participants were required to be capable of using a smartphone application for treatment and provide voluntary informed consent. Exclusion criteria included any history of previous spinal surgery, spinal injection therapy within one month prior to enrollment, or spinal trauma within three months. Participants were also excluded if they presented with radicular pain with sensory or motor deficits, leg muscle strength of grade $\leq$3 on manual muscle testing, or structural spinal abnormalities, such as spondylolisthesis or scoliosis with a Cobb angle >10°. Those exhibiting red flag signs, such as unexplained weight loss or bowel/bladder dysfunction, or those with tumors, infections, metabolic bone diseases, cognitive disorders, fibromyalgia, or systemic inflammatory diseases, were also excluded. Further exclusion criteria included pregnancy or breastfeeding, current use of opioids stronger than tramadol, a history of substance abuse or psychiatric conditions affecting pain perception, and an inability to communicate or follow instructions.

2.3. *Randomization and Blinding*

The participants were randomly assigned in a 1:1 ratio to either a DTx group (MORA Cure LBP digital therapeutics) or a control group (conventional treatment) using a stratified randomization method. Stratification was based on the study site, Seoul National University Hospital or Hanyang University Guri Hospital. Randomization was performed using a web-based program provided by the Seoul National University Medical Research Collaboration Center. This study was open-label; however, allocation concealment was maintained by independent study staff who were not involved in the data collection or analysis.

2.4. *Interventions*

Participants in the DTx group underwent an eight-week program using the MORACure LBP digital therapeutic device, which included a smartphone application delivering CBT and exercise therapy (Figure 1). The program comprised one CBT session at the beginning of each week, followed by daily exercise sessions for the remaining six days. These CBT sessions addressed the identification and management of negative emotions and thoughts associated with pain, fostering positive coping skills and applying relaxation techniques. The program was designed to enhance the participants' pain management self-efficacy through cognitive restructuring, positive self-talk, and strategies for handling setbacks. Patients underwent patient-tailored exercise therapy, education, and behavioral therapy. Evaluation using AI pose estimation and the results of subjective symptom evaluation were used to create a patient-tailored treatment curriculum. The exercises focused on core and lower extremity strengthening and incorporated stretching, with adjustments based on pain scales, following the principles of progressive overload. Participants in the control group received conventional treatment, including exercise therapy with controlled exercise intensity, which included up to four face-to-face sessions with a physician experienced in musculoskeletal disorders. They also engaged in self-directed exercises based on educational materials provided at baseline, with a treatment duration of eight weeks, mirroring that of the DTx group. Additionally, the last exercise therapy session was repeated for the remaining four weeks after the eight-week course.

2.5. *Outcome Measures and Data Collection*

The primary outcomes of this study included changes in usual pain intensity, as assessed by the NPRS, at baseline and after eight weeks. Additionally, the worst pain intensity, measured using the NPRS at these time points, and functional disability, assessed using the ODI [21], constituted the primary outcomes. Secondary outcomes included health-related quality of life assessed using the EQ-5D at baseline and at 4, 8, and 12 weeks [22]. Psychological status was measured using the Patient Health Questionnaire-9 (PHQ-9) [23], Pain Catastrophizing Scale (PCS) [24], and Fear-Avoidance Beliefs Questionnaire (FABQ) at baseline and 8 and 12 weeks [25]. Higher ODI scores indicate greater levels of functional disability, while higher NPRS scores reflect more intense pain. Conversely, lower EQ-5D scores represent poorer health-related quality of life. For psychological measures, higher

PHQ-9, PCS, and FABQ scores denote greater levels of depression, pain catastrophizing, and fear-avoidance beliefs, respectively. Spinal alignment was evaluated using radiographic assessment at baseline and eight weeks, while muscle endurance and balance were assessed using the Prone Bridge Test and Single-Limb Stance Test at baseline and 4, 8, and 12 weeks [26,27]. Data were collected at baseline and at 4, 8, and 12 weeks (four weeks post-intervention) through a combination of in-person visits and telephone follow-ups. The participants were instructed to refrain from using rescue medication for 24 h prior to the assessment visits to minimize its effect on the outcome measures. Treatment compliance was assessed at 4, 8, and 12 weeks after the baseline. Compliance was calculated as the percentage of sessions completed relative to the total number of prescribed sessions. The DTx group automatically collected compliance data as time data from the application, whereas the control group wrote their own logs. Comparisons between the intervention and control groups were made at each time point to evaluate adherence to the treatment protocol.

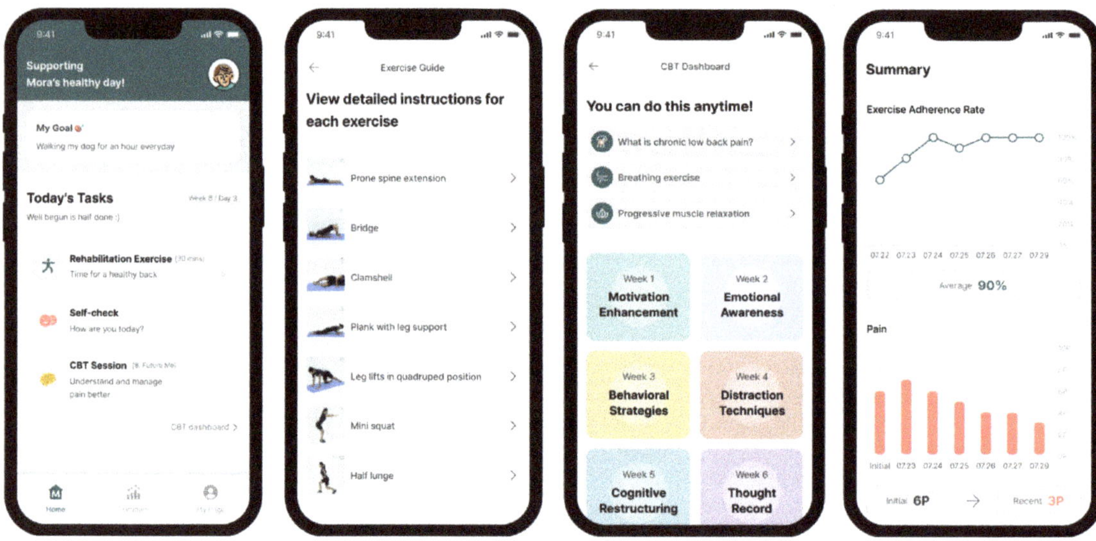

Figure 1. Example of the patient user interface of MORA Cure LBP. After pose estimation, real-time feedback was provided to assist patients in adopting correct postures during exercise sessions. Additionally, CBT sessions and worksheet records are displayed for patient reference and progress tracking.

2.6. Statistical Analysis

Continuous variables are summarized as mean ± standard deviation, while categorical variables are presented as frequencies and percentages. Between-group comparisons were conducted using two-sample *t*-tests for continuous variables and the Pearson's chi-squared tests for categorical variables. Wilcoxon's rank-sum tests were performed for non-normally distributed data. Primary outcomes were analyzed using repeated-measures analysis of variance, and changes over time within each group were assessed using paired *t*-tests. All statistical analyses were performed using SAS software (version 9.4), with the significance level set at $p < 0.05$.

3. Results

3.1. Participant Characteristics

In total, 46 participants were randomized, with 45 included in the safety analysis set (22 in the DTx group and 23 in the control group). The full analysis set comprised 43 participants (20 in the DTx group and 23 in the control group) (Figure 2). There were no statistically significant differences between the groups in terms of baseline demographic characteristics or clinical features, except for sacral slope (SS) (Table 1). The sacral slope was significantly higher in the control group than that in the DTx group (38.6° vs. 34.0°, $p = 0.035$). The mean age was 38.1 ± 10.0 years in the DTx group and 38.5 ± 7.4 years in the control group ($p = 0.930$). Most of the participants were female (80.0% in the DTx group and 81.8% in the control group, $p = 0.594$). For baseline usual pain intensity (NPRS), the DTx group reported a mean score of 4.3 ± 1.4, while the control group reported 4.3 ± 1.3 ($p = 0.910$). For worst pain intensity (NPRS), the DTx group reported a mean score of 6.0 ± 1.6, while the control group reported 6.0 ± 1.7 ($p = 0.990$). For baseline functional disability measured by the ODI, the DTx group had a mean score of 19.7 ± 8.3, while the control group scored 19.6 ± 8.7 ($p = 0.949$)

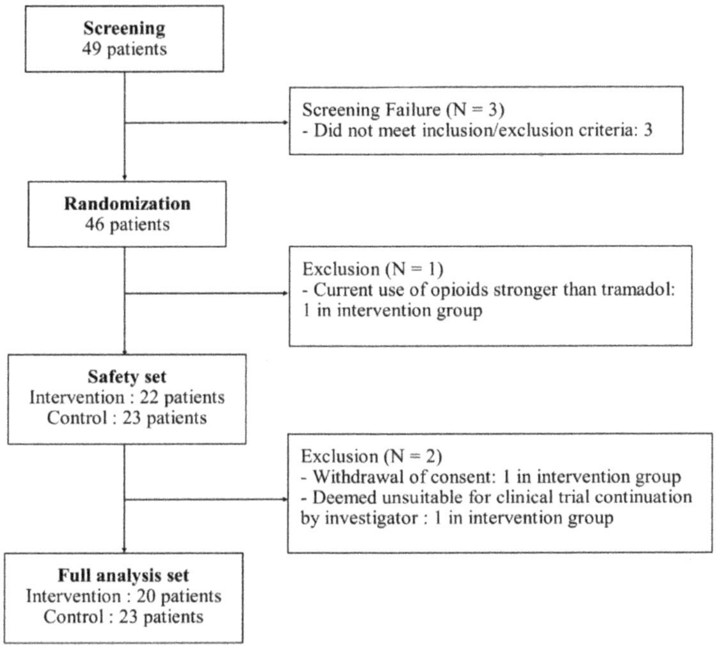

Figure 2. Flowchart of participants.

Table 1. Baseline characteristics of study participants (full analysis set).

	Intervention (n = 20)	Control (n = 23)	*p* Value
Age (years)	38.1 ± 10.0	38.5 ± 7.4	0.930
Female (n [%])	16 [80.0]	18 [81.8]	0.594
Body mass index (kg/m^2)	22.6 ± 4.4	23.4 ± 3.3	0.399
Prior pain medication use (n [%])	5 [25.0]	4 [17.4]	0.711
Onset of backpain (months)	88.9 ± 55.5	58.7 ± 52.6	0.078
Usual pain (NPRS)	4.4 ± 1.4	4.2 ± 1.1	0.792
Worst pain (NPRS)	6.1 ± 1.6	5.9 ± 1.7	0.679
Functional disability (ODI)	19.9 ± 8.4	18.9 ± 8.3	0.724
QoL (EQ-5D)	8.0 ± 2.2	7.8 ± 2.5	0.600
Depression (PHQ-9)	3.9 ± 4.1	3.8 ± 3.6	0.961
Pain catastrophizing (PCS)	8.5 ± 7.8	11.9 ± 13.4	0.654
Fear-avoidance beliefs (FABQ)	32.5 ± 20.4	29.4 ± 20.2	0.689
Muscle endurance (Prone Bridge, s)	63.2 ± 39.2	46.9 ± 32.6	0.161

Table 1. *Cont.*

	Intervention (n = 20)	Control (n = 23)	p Value
Balance ability (Single Limb Stance)	4.3 ± 2.0	4.3 ± 2.4	0.897
Pelvic incidence (°)	48.3 ± 9.5	49.5 ± 7.1	0.649
Lumbar lordosis (°)	46.3 ± 12.3	49.8 ± 10.5	0.335
Sacral slope (°)	34.0 ± 8.0	38.6 ± 6.1	0.035
Pelvic tilt (°)	14.2 ± 8.5	10.9 ± 6.8	0.150
Sagittal vertical axis (mm)	5.3 ± 29.6	−3.7 ± 23.6	0.265
Cobb's angle (°)	3.3 ± 2.3	2.8 ± 2.6	0.350

NPRS, Numeric Pain Rating Scale; ODI, Oswestry Disability Index; QoL, quality of life.

3.2. Primary Outcomes

At eight weeks, no statistically significant differences in usual pain intensity were observed between the intervention and control groups in usual pain intensity (NPRS). The DTx group reported a mean score of 3.1 ± 1.9, while the control group reported 3.0 ± 1.5 (p = 0.809). Similarly, no significant differences were found in terms of worst pain intensity (NPRS) or ODI scores. The mean worst pain score was 5.00 ± 2.18 in the DTx group and 4.27 ± 1.83 in the control group (p = 0.247). The mean ODI score was 15.6 ± 9.6 for the DTx group and 15.6 ± 10.0 for the control group (p > 0.999).

3.3. Secondary Outcomes

Both the DTx and control groups showed significant reductions in usual and worst pain over time compared with baseline (Figure 3). In the DTx group, the usual pain decreased significantly from baseline at 4, 8, and 12 weeks (p < 0.0167). Worst pain showed significant reductions at 4 and 12 weeks compared to baseline. In the control group, the usual and worst pain (NRS) scores significantly decrease at 4, 8, and 12 weeks. Although not statistically significant, improvements in ODI and quality of life EQ-5D were observed in both the DTx and control groups over time. No significant differences in secondary outcomes were observed between the groups at 4, 8, or 12 weeks. At 12 weeks, the mean usual pain intensity showed no significant difference, with the DTx group reporting 2.9 ± 1.8 compared to 2.6 ± 1.7 in the control group (p = 0.653). For worst pain intensity, there was also no significant difference, with scores of 4.7 ± 2.5 in the DTx group and 4.0 ± 2.5 in the control group (p = 0.406). Functional disability, measured by the ODI, showed no significant difference at 12 weeks, with the DTx group scoring 15.2 ± 9.2 and the control group scoring 14.6 ± 10.3 (p = 0.821). Similarly, quality of life, as measured by the EQ-5D, yielded no significant differences between the groups at any time point; at 12 weeks, the DTx group scored 7.0 ± 1.7, compared to 7.5 ± 2.2 for the control group (p = 0.610). Psychological measures, including depression (PHQ-9), pain catastrophizing (PCS), and fear-avoidance beliefs (FABQ), showed no significant differences between the groups at 8 or 12 weeks. Specifically, the PHQ-9 scores at 12 weeks were 3.4 ± 3.8 for the DTx group and 2.8 ± 3.0 for the control group (p = 0.704); the PCS scores were 8.7 ± 10.1 and 6.4 ± 8.4, respectively (p = 0.482); and the FABQ scores were 32.5 ± 20.4 and 29.4 ± 20.2, respectively (p = 0.689). Both the DTx and control groups showed no significant improvements in the PHQ-9, PCS, or FABQ scores compared with baseline at 8 or 12 weeks (Figure 4). The radiographic spinal alignment parameters generally showed no significant differences between the groups, except for the SS measured by the whole spine standing lateral radiograph at eight weeks, where the DTx group recorded 34.0 ± 8.0° compared to 38.6 ± 6.1° in the control group, indicating a significant difference (p = 0.035). Finally, no significant differences were observed between the groups in the Prone Bridge Test or Single Limb Stance Test at any time point. Between-group comparisons revealed a statistically significant difference in treatment compliance during the 1–4-week period (p < 0.001), with the DTx group showing a mean compliance of 74.7% ± 27.4, compared to 53.1% ± 28.6 in the control group. However, no significant differences were observed from

1 to 8 weeks ($p = 0.145$), as the intervention and control groups reported 64.7% ± 34.6 and 61.5% ± 29.2, respectively.

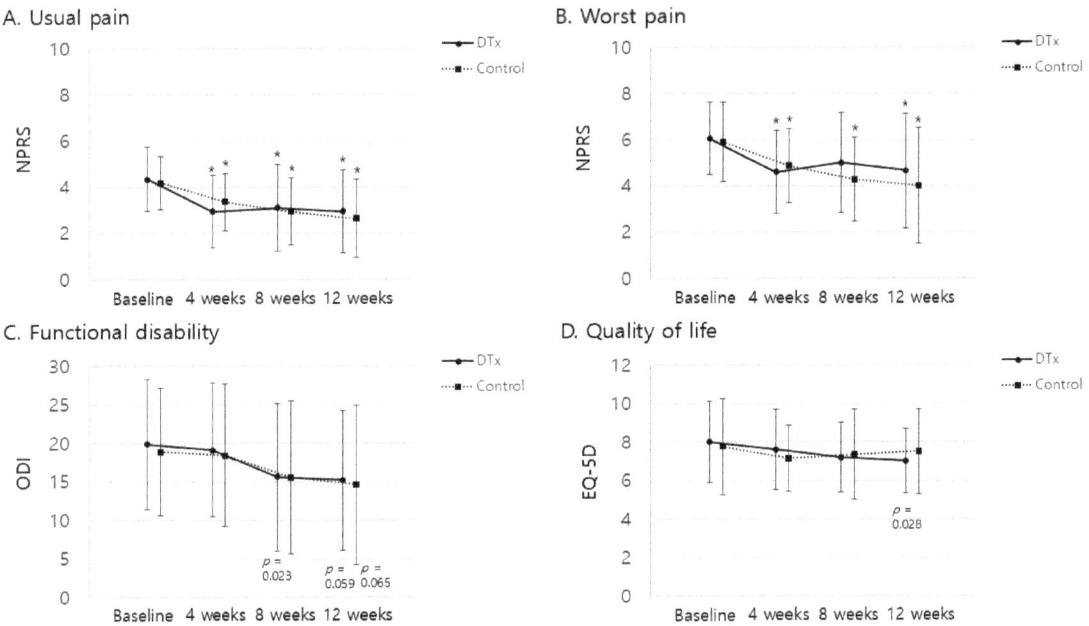

Figure 3. Changes in pain intensity, functional disability, and quality of life over time in the DTx and control groups. (**A**) Usual pain intensity measured by the Numeric Pain Rating Scale (NPRS) at baseline, 4 weeks, 8 weeks, and 12 weeks. (**B**) Worst pain intensity measured by NPRS over the same time points. (**C**) Functional disability, assessed by the Oswestry Disability Index (ODI), at baseline, 4 weeks, 8 weeks, and 12 weeks. (**D**) Quality of life, evaluated using the EQ-5D, at the same time intervals. * $p < 0.05/3$ compared with baseline.

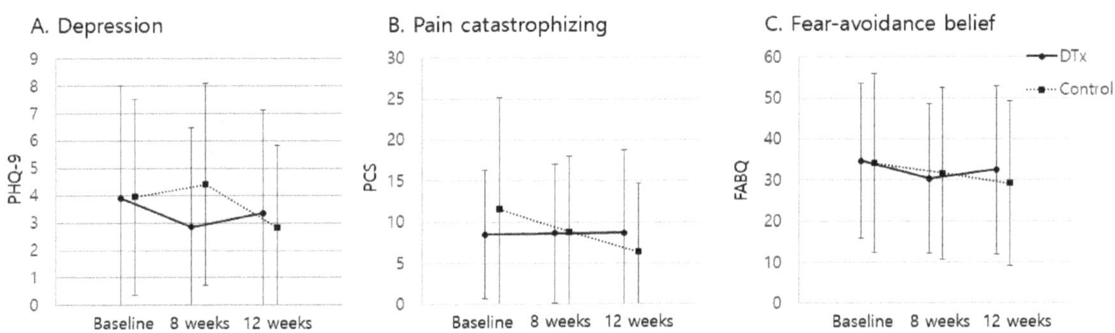

Figure 4. Changes in psychological outcomes over time in the DTx and control groups. (**A**) Depression levels measured by the Patient Health Questionnaire-9 (PHQ-9) at baseline, 8 weeks, and 12 weeks. (**B**) Pain catastrophizing, assessed by the Pain Catastrophizing Scale (PCS), at the same time points. (**C**) Fear-avoidance beliefs, measured by the Fear-Avoidance Beliefs Questionnaire (FABQ), over the same period. * $p < 0.05/3$ compared with baseline.

3.4. Safety Outcomes

The incidence of adverse events was similar between the intervention and control groups, with 77.27% (17/22) of the participants in the DTx group and 60.87% (14/23) in the control group experiencing at least one adverse event (p = 0.2348). The majority of adverse events were unexpected adverse device effects, whereas device-related adverse events (ADEs) were relatively infrequent, occurring in 18.18% (4/22) of the patients in the DTx group and none in the control group (p = 0.0490). The specific ADEs reported in the DTx group included musculoskeletal disorders (three participants, 13.64%), arthralgia (two participants, 9.09%), back pain (two participants, 9.09%), and neck pain (one participant, 4.55%). No serious adverse events were reported in the DTx group, and no unexpected device-related adverse events were reported in either group. Overall, the safety profiles were similar between the two groups, with most adverse events being mild to moderate in severity. No major safety concerns were observed in either group, suggesting that the MORA Cure LBP digital therapeutic device was generally well tolerated.

4. Discussion

This randomized controlled pilot study showed significant reductions in usual pain intensity, worst pain intensity, and functional disability over time with both multidisciplinary digital therapeutics (MORA Cure LBP) and conventional treatment groups. No statistically significant differences were observed between the two interventions for CLBP across various outcome measures. Although a statistically significant difference in sacral slope was noted between the groups (intervention group: 34.0°; control group: 38.6°; p = 0.035), the 4.6° difference likely falls within the range of measurement error and is unlikely to have clinical significance. Both treatments were safe and well tolerated, with MORA curing LBP demonstrating no serious adverse events and a safety profile comparable to that of conventional treatments.

When compared to similar studies, our results align with several previous findings in which digital therapeutics demonstrated improvements in pain management over time, although often with no significant differences between groups. Toelle et al. also found significant pain reduction using the Kaia App for back pain management, with no substantial differences between the digital and conventional therapy groups [28]. Similarly, Shi et al. demonstrated the non-inferiority of telerehabilitation compared to outpatient-based exercise, with both groups improving in terms of pain and disability [29]. Rughani et al. and Shebib et al. observed significant reductions in pain outcomes in both app-based interventions and control groups receiving conventional care [30,31]. In a study of 93 patients with low-back-pain-related disabilities, Chhabra et al. found that recovery rates were higher after 12 weeks of smartphone-based treatment (54.79%) than those after conventional treatment (51.52%) [32]. Almhdawi et al. also reported greater improvement in back-pain-related disability after six weeks of app-based intervention (35.70%) than that after conventional intervention (2.86%) in a study of 40 office workers with CLBP [33]. In our study, both the DTx and control groups showed improvements. The lack of a significant difference between the two groups may be due to the greater intensive care provided to the control group compared to that in previous studies. Unlike studies where the control group received only medication or verbal encouragement to exercise, our control group underwent monthly one-on-one supervised exercise sessions, up to four times in eight weeks, each time for >30 min, guided by an orthopedic surgeon or rehabilitation medicine specialist, which likely provided more comprehensive care.

Most other studies focused on exercise-based digital interventions without a significant CBT component. Our study included a comprehensive CBT component therapy combined with a structured exercise regimen. Shebib et al. demonstrated that a 12-week digital care program (DCP) combining CBT, exercise, and education significantly reduced pain intensity and functional disability in patients with CLBP compared to a control group receiving only educational materials [30]. Pain improved by 52–64%, and disability by 31–55% in the DCP group, with high weekly engagement (90%) and reduced surgical interest. Similarly,

Chiauzzi et al. employed a self-management program featuring CBT alongside goal setting and wellness activities, demonstrating a significant improvement in disability outcomes but not in pain intensity [34].

Traditional CBT and exercise therapy, when conducted in regular face-to-face sessions, often pose financial burdens and constraints related to the time and location of patients. Psychological interventions conducted in humans have the same limitations. Enhancing the physical and time-related barriers, it is essential to overcome the accessibility of CBT and time-related barriers. Application-based (app-based) treatment is an excellent solution for addressing these challenges. Many studies have shown that the use of app-based interventions improves patient compliance [30–32,35–38]. In our study, the DTx group demonstrated a mean compliance of 74.7%, which was significantly higher than that of the control group (53.1% during the 1–4-week period ($p < 0.001$)). Shebib et al. reported a high weekly engagement rate of 90% in their digital care program [30]. Our study expressed engagement as an hour of rehabilitation, whereas Shebib's study expressed the percentage of patients who completed treatment without dropping off for a certain period of time, making a direct comparison difficult; however, both studies showed good engagement. In a survey conducted with 127 healthcare professionals specializing in musculoskeletal disorders, 95.3% acknowledged the need for app-based treatment in clinical practice, and the majority expressed positive views toward its use [39]. Thus, integrating digital therapeutics for exercise and CBT could help improve treatment accessibility, reduce healthcare costs, and minimize inconvenience in patients with CLBP.

In our study, initial compliance to the intervention showed significant differences between the DTx and control groups during the first four weeks ($p < 0.001$), with DTx participants showing higher compliance (74.7% vs. 53.1%). However, from 1 to 8 weeks, the compliance rates were similar in both groups (64.7% vs. 61.5, $p = 0.145$). To optimize compliance and increase patient engagement, it is essential to explore the methods used in similar studies. For example, several app-based interventions aimed at chronic CLBP reported that enhancing user engagement through gamification and personalized feedback significantly improved adherence [30,32]. In a study by Shebib et al., the use of biofeedback and peer support within the app led to adherence rates as high as 90% in the first four weeks, although this decreased slightly over time [30]. In our study, the incorporation of CBT alongside exercise therapy was unique and could positively influence compliance; however, further improvement strategies, such as adding reward systems and more interactive features, might be beneficial [32]. Implementing real-time progress tracking, regular reminders, and personalized milestones could help maintain engagement to further increase compliance. Moreover, enhancing the usability of the application and ensuring that exercise routines are adaptable to the patient's daily life are crucial steps for minimizing dropout rates [32]. By focusing on these aspects, we could potentially achieve higher adherence rates, as observed in other digital therapeutic studies.

Although no statistically significant differences were observed in secondary psychological outcomes (e.g., PHQ-9, PCS, FABQ) between the intervention and control groups, it is noteworthy that these measures also did not show significant improvement within either group at 8 or 12 weeks. This was unexpected, particularly given the inclusion of CBT in the intervention group. However, significant reductions in usual pain, worst pain, and functional disability were observed in both groups, suggesting that the mechanisms driving pain reduction may not be directly linked to changes in psychological measures. Further research is needed to elucidate the relationship between improvements in pain and functional outcomes and psychological measures, potentially identifying mediators that could enhance the effectiveness of digital therapeutics

The safety profile of the DTx group was comparable with that of the control group, and no significant safety concerns were observed throughout this study. Although the incidence of adverse events was slightly higher in the DTx group (77.27%) than that in the control group (60.87%), the difference was not statistically significant ($p = 0.235$). Most adverse events were mild or moderate in nature, and device-related adverse events were relatively infrequent (18.18% in the DTx group). These findings align with those of similar studies on digital therapeutics for chronic pain management, where adverse events were often mild and device-related incidents were infrequent. For example, a study involving AI-based self-management applications for musculoskeletal conditions reported a low incidence of adverse events, mostly attributable to normal fluctuations in pain during treatment [30,40]. In our study, arthralgia, back pain, and neck pain were the most commonly reported adverse events in the DTx group. Similar safety profiles were observed in related trials, such as those by Hartmann et al. and Shebib et al., who documented mild adverse events without serious risks associated with app-based therapies [30,41].

In our study, both groups showed significant pain improvements from the 4-week mark, consistent with previous studies indicating that chronic low back pain treatments yield benefits within the first month [42]. Although this pilot study demonstrates promising improvements in adherence and accessibility through digital therapeutics, the long-term efficacy and clinical relevance of such interventions remain to be fully established. Sustained adherence to digital platforms is likely to play a pivotal role in maintaining therapeutic benefits over time [43]. Evidence from prior studies indicates that higher initial compliance is often associated with better long-term outcomes in pain and disability management [44]. However, future large-scale, longitudinal studies are necessary to confirm whether these short-term benefits translate into lasting clinical improvements.

Our study has several limitations. First, the relatively short follow-up period restricts our ability to assess the long-term effects of the intervention. Second, although compliance was generally good, adherence tracking was not as detailed as that in the control group, limiting our understanding of comparative adherence. Third, the sample size was small, which may have affected the generalizability of our findings. Fourth, although our intervention combined CBT and exercise, we could not isolate the specific components that contributed the most to the observed outcomes. Future studies could employ a factorial design, including separate groups for CBT-only, exercise-only, and combined interventions, to better understand the individual and synergistic effects of these components. Such an approach would help refine the intervention and optimize its efficacy.

5. Conclusions

This pilot study demonstrated that multidisciplinary digital therapeutics (MORA Cure LBP) are safe and effective options for managing CLBP, resulting in significant improvements in pain, disability, and quality of life over time. The digital and conventional treatment groups achieved similar outcomes, with higher early compliance in the MORA Cure LBP group.

Author Contributions: Conceptualization, C.Y., J.H.P. and S.Y.C.; methodology, C.Y., J.H.P., S.Y.C. and D.-H.K.; software, C.-H.C., S.L. and T.H.P.; validation, C.-H.C., S.L. and T.H.P.; formal analysis, C.-H.C., S.L. and T.H.P.; resources, C.-H.C., S.L. and T.H.P.; data curation, C.-H.C., S.L., T.H.P. and D.-H.K.; writing—original draft preparation, D.-H.K.; writing—review and editing, D.-H.K., J.H.P., C.Y. and S.Y.C.; visualization, D.-H.K. and J.H.P.; supervision, S.Y.C. and S.-H.J.; project administration, C.Y., J.H.P., S.Y.C., D.-H.K. and S.-H.J. All authors have read and agreed to the published version of the manuscript.

Funding: This study was partially funded by the Daegu-Gyeongbuk Medical Innovation Foundation.

Institutional Review Board Statement: This study was conducted in accordance with the Declaration of Helsinki. The study protocol was approved by the Institutional Review Boards of Seoul National University Hospital (IRB number: 2211-148-1381) and Hanyang University Guri Hospital (IRB number: 2022-12-049).

Informed Consent Statement: Informed consent was obtained from all the participants involved in this study.

Data Availability Statement: Data underlying this article cannot be shared publicly because of the privacy of individuals who participated in the study. The data may be shared with the corresponding authors upon reasonable request.

Conflicts of Interest: Authors Chan Yoon, Chi-Hyun Choi, Sanghee Lee and Tae Hyun Park were employed by the company EverEx, The remaining authors declare that the research was conducted in the absence of any commercial or financial relationships that could be construed as a potential conflict of interest.

References

1. van Tulder, M.; Becker, A.; Bekkering, T.; Breen, A.; del Real, M.T.G.; Hutchinson, A.; Koes, B.; Laerum, E.; Malmivaara, A.; COST B13 Working Group on Guidelines for the Management of Acute Low Back Pain in Primary Care. European guidelines for the management of acute nonspecific low back pain in primary care. *Eur. Spine J.* **2006**, *15* (Suppl. 2), S169–S191. [CrossRef]
2. van Dieën, J.H.; Kuijer, P.P.; Burdorf, A.; Marras, W.S.; Adams, M.A. Non-specific low back pain. *Lancet* **2012**, *379*, 1874–1875. [CrossRef] [PubMed]
3. Hartvigsen, J.; Hancock, M.J.; Kongsted, A.; Louw, Q.; Ferreira, M.L.; Genevay, S.; Hoy, D.; Karppinen, J.; Pransky, G.; Sieper, J.; et al. What low back pain is and why we need to pay attention. *Lancet* **2018**, *391*, 2356–2367. [CrossRef] [PubMed]
4. Foster, N.E.; Anema, J.R.; Cherkin, D.; Chou, R.; Cohen, S.P.; Gross, D.P.; Ferreira, P.H.; Fritz, J.M.; Koes, B.W.; Peul, W.; et al. Prevention and treatment of low back pain: Evidence, challenges, and promising directions. *Lancet* **2018**, *391*, 2368–2383. [CrossRef] [PubMed]
5. Abbafati, C.; Abbas, K.M.; Abbasi, M.; Abbasifard, M.; Abbasi-Kangevari, M.; Abbastabar, H.; Abd-Allah, F.; Abdelalim, A.; Abdollahi, M.; Abdollahpour, I. Global burden of 369 diseases and injuries in 204 countries and territories, 1990–2019: A systematic analysis for the Global Burden of Disease Study 2019. *Lancet* **2020**, *396*, 1204–1222. [CrossRef]
6. Maher, C.; Underwood, M.; Buchbinder, R. Non-specific low back pain. *Lancet* **2017**, *389*, 736–747. [CrossRef]
7. Costa, L.D.M.; Henschke, N.; Maher, C.G.; Refshauge, K.M.; Herbert, D.R.; McAuley, J.H.; Das, A.; Costa, L.O.P. Prognosis of chronic low back pain: Design of an inception cohort study. *BMC Musculoskelet. Disord.* **2007**, *8*, 4. [CrossRef]
8. Hayden, J.A.; Chou, R.; Hogg-Johnson, S.; Bombardier, C. Systematic reviews of low back pain prognosis had variable methods and results: Guidance for future prognosis reviews. *J. Clin. Epidemiol.* **2009**, *62*, 781–796.e1. [CrossRef]
9. Hong, J.Y.; Song, K.S.; Cho, J.H.; Lee, J.H.; Kim, N.H. An updated overview of low back pain management. *Asian Spine J.* **2022**, *16*, 968–982. [CrossRef]
10. Perrot, S.; Doane, M.J.; Jaffe, D.H.; Dragon, E.; Abraham, L.; Viktrup, L.; Bushmakin, A.G.; Cappelleri, J.C.; Conaghan, P.G. Burden of chronic low back pain: Association with pain severity and prescription medication use in five large European countries. *Pain Pract.* **2022**, *22*, 359–371. [CrossRef]
11. Baroncini, A.; Maffulli, N.; Schäfer, L.; Manocchio, N.; Bossa, M.; Foti, C.; Klimuch, A.; Migliorini, F. Physiotherapeutic and non-conventional approaches in patients with chronic low-back pain: A level I Bayesian network meta-analysis. *Sci. Rep.* **2024**, *14*, 11546. [CrossRef] [PubMed]
12. Kuijpers, T.; van Middelkoop, M.; Rubinstein, S.M.; Ostelo, R.; Verhagen, A.; Koes, B.W.; van Tulder, M.W. A systematic review on the effectiveness of pharmacological interventions for chronic non-specific low-back pain. *Eur. Spine J.* **2011**, *20*, 40–50. [CrossRef] [PubMed]
13. Kreiner, D.S.; Matz, P.; Bono, C.M.; Cho, C.H.; Easa, J.E.; Ghiselli, G.; Ghogawala, Z.; Reitman, C.A.; Resnick, D.K.; Watters, W.C.; et al. Guideline summary review: An evidence -based clinical guideline for the diagnosis and treatment of low back pain. *Spine J.* **2020**, *20*, 998–1024. [CrossRef] [PubMed]
14. O'Sullivan, K.; O'Keeffe, M.; O'Sullivan, P. NICE low back pain guidelines: Opportunities and obstacles to change practice. *Br. J. Sports Med.* **2017**, *51*, 1632–1633. [CrossRef] [PubMed]
15. Nalamachu, S.; Rauck, R.L.; Hale, M.E.; Florete, O.G.; Robinson, C.Y.; Farr, S.J. A long-term, open-label safety study of single-entity hydrocodone bitartrate extended release for the treatment of moderate to severe chronic pain. *J. Pain Res.* **2014**, *7*, 669–678. [CrossRef]
16. Kumar, S.; Negi, M.P.S.; Sharma, V.P.; Shukla, R.; Dev, R.; Mishra, U.K. Efficacy of two multimodal treatments on physical strength of occupationally subgrouped male with low back pain. *J. Back Musculoskelet. Rehabil.* **2009**, *22*, 179–188. [CrossRef]
17. Ferreira, M.L.; Ferreira, P.H.; Latimer, J.; Herbert, R.D.; Hodges, P.W.; Jennings, M.D.; Maher, C.G.; Refshauge, K.M. Comparison of general exercise, motor control exercise and spinal manipulative therapy for chronic low back pain: A randomized trial. *Pain* **2007**, *131*, 31–37. [CrossRef]
18. Koldaş Doğan, S.; Sonel Tur, B.; Kurtaiş, Y.; Atay, M.B. Comparison of three different approaches in the treatment of chronic low back pain. *Clin. Rheumatol.* **2008**, *27*, 873–881. [CrossRef]
19. Clarke, J.; van Tulder, M.; Blomberg, S.; de Vet, H.; van der Heijden, G.; Bronfort, G. Traction for low back pain with or without sciatica: An updated systematic review within the framework of the Cochrane Collaboration. *Spine* **2006**, *31*, 1591–1599. [CrossRef]

20. Ho, E.; Ferreira, M.; Chen, L.X.; Simic, M.; Ashton-James, C.; Comachio, J.; Hayden, J.; Ferreira, P.; Wang, D.X.M.; Ferreira, P.H. Psychological interventions for chronic, non-specific low back pain: Systematic review with network meta-analysis. *Br. Med. J.* **2022**, *376*, 24. [CrossRef]
21. Fairbank, J.C.; Pynsent, P.B. The Oswestry disability index. *Spine* **2000**, *25*, 2940–2952; discussion 2952. [CrossRef] [PubMed]
22. Rabin, R.; de Charro, F. EQ-5D: A measure of health status from the EuroQol Group. *Ann. Med.* **2001**, *33*, 337–343. [CrossRef] [PubMed]
23. Kroenke, K.; Spitzer, R.L.; Williams, J.B. The PHQ-9: Validity of a brief depression severity measure. *J. Gen. Intern. Med.* **2001**, *16*, 606–613. [CrossRef] [PubMed]
24. Darnall, B.D.; Sturgeon, J.A.; Cook, K.F.; Taub, C.J.; Roy, A.; Burns, J.W.; Sullivan, M.; Mackey, S.C. Development and validation of a daily pain catastrophizing scale. *J. Pain* **2017**, *18*, 1139–1149. [CrossRef] [PubMed]
25. Waddell, G.; Newton, M.; Henderson, I.; Somerville, D.; Main, C.J. A Fear-Avoidance Beliefs Questionnaire (FABQ) and the role of fear-avoidance beliefs in chronic low back pain and disability. *Pain* **1993**, *52*, 157–168. [CrossRef]
26. Bohannon, R.W.; Steffl, M.; Glenney, S.S.; Green, M.; Cashwell, L.; Prajerova, K.; Bunn, J. The prone bridge test: Performance, validity, and reliability among older and younger adults. *J. Bodyw. Mov. Ther.* **2018**, *22*, 385–389. [CrossRef]
27. Balogun, J.A.; Ajayi, L.O.; Alawale, F. Determinants of single limb stance balance performance. *Afr. J. Med. Med. Sci.* **1997**, *26*, 153–157.
28. Toelle, T.R.; Utpadel-Fischler, D.A.; Haas, K.K.; Priebe, J.A. App-based multidisciplinary back pain treatment versus combined physiotherapy plus online education: A randomized controlled trial. *npj Digit. Med.* **2019**, *2*, 34. [CrossRef]
29. Shi, W.; Zhang, Y.; Bian, Y.; Chen, L.; Yuan, W.; Zhang, H.; Feng, Q.; Zhang, H.; Liu, D.; Lin, Y. The physical and psychological effects of telerehabilitation-based exercise for patients with nonspecific low back pain: Prospective randomized controlled trial. *JMIR mHealth uHealth* **2024**, *12*, e56580. [CrossRef]
30. Shebib, R.; Bailey, J.F.; Smittenaar, P.; Perez, D.A.; Mecklenburg, G.; Hunter, S. Randomized controlled trial of a 12-week digital care program in improving low back pain. *npj Digit. Med.* **2019**, *2*, 1. [CrossRef]
31. Rughani, G.; Nilsen, T.I.L.; Wood, K.; Mair, F.S.; Hartvigsen, J.; Mork, P.J.; Nicholl, B.I. The selfBACK artificial intelligence-based smartphone app can improve low back pain outcome even in patients with high levels of depression or stress. *Eur. J. Pain* **2023**, *27*, 568–579. [CrossRef] [PubMed]
32. Chhabra, H.S.; Sharma, S.; Verma, S. Smartphone app in self-management of chronic low back pain: A randomized controlled trial. *Eur. Spine J.* **2018**, *27*, 2862–2874. [CrossRef] [PubMed]
33. Almhdawi, K.A.; Obeidat, D.S.; Kanaan, S.F.; Oteir, A.O.; Mansour, Z.M.; Alrabbaei, H. Efficacy of an innovative smartphone application for office workers with chronic non-specific low back pain: A pilot randomized controlled trial. *Clin. Rehabil.* **2020**, *34*, 1282–1291. [CrossRef] [PubMed]
34. Chiauzzi, E.; Pujol, L.A.; Wood, M.; Bond, K.; Black, R.; Yiu, E.; Zacharoff, K. painACTION-back pain: A self-management Website for people with chronic back pain. *Pain Med.* **2010**, *11*, 1044–1058. [CrossRef]
35. Yang, J.Y.; Wei, Q.; Ge, Y.L.; Meng, L.J.; Zhao, M.D. Smartphone-based remote self-management of chronic low back pain: A preliminary study. *J. Healthc. Eng.* **2019**, *2019*, 4632946. [CrossRef]
36. Nordstoga, A.L.; Bach, K.; Sani, S.; Wiratunga, N.; Mork, P.J.; Villumsen, M.; Cooper, K. Usability and acceptability of an app (SELFBACK) to support self-management of low back pain: Mixed methods study. *JMIR Rehabil. Assist. Technol.* **2020**, *7*, e18729. [CrossRef]
37. Sitges, C.; Terrasa, J.L.; García-Dopico, N.; Segur-Ferrer, J.; Velasco-Roldán, O.; Crespí-Palmer, J.; González-Roldán, A.M.; Montoya, P. An educational and exercise mobile phone-based intervention to elicit electrophysiological changes and to improve psychological functioning in adults with nonspecific chronic low back pain (BackFit app): Nonrandomized clinical trial. *JMIR mHealth uHealth* **2022**, *10*, e29171. [CrossRef]
38. Vad, V.B.; Madrazo-Ibarra, A.; Estrin, D.; Pollak, J.P.; Carroll, K.M.; Vojta, D.; Vad, A.; Trapness, C. Back Rx, a personalized mobile phone application for discogenic chronic low back pain: A prospective pilot study. *BMC Musculoskelet. Disord.* **2022**, *23*, 923. [CrossRef]
39. Biebl, J.T.; Rykala, M.; Strobel, M.; Kaur Bollinger, P.K.; Ulm, B.; Kraft, E.; Huber, S.; Lorenz, A. App-based feedback for rehabilitation exercise correction in patients with knee or hip osteoarthritis: Prospective cohort study. *J. Med. Internet Res.* **2021**, *23*, e26658. [CrossRef]
40. Marcuzzi, A.; Nordstoga, A.L.; Bach, K.; Aasdahl, L.; Nilsen, T.I.L.; Bardal, E.M.; Boldermo, N.Ø.; Falkener Bertheussen, G.; Marchand, G.H.; Gismervik, S.; et al. Effect of an Artificial Intelligence-Based Self-Management App on musculoskeletal Health in Patients with Neck and/or Low Back Pain Referred to Specialist Care: A Randomized Clinical Trial. *JAMA Netw. Open* **2023**, *6*, e2320400. [CrossRef]
41. Hartmann, R.; Avermann, F.; Zalpour, C.; Griefahn, A. Impact of an AI app-based exercise program for people with low back pain compared to standard care: A longitudinal cohort-study. *Health Sci. Rep.* **2023**, *6*, e1060. [CrossRef] [PubMed]
42. Dillingham, T.; Kenia, J.; Popescu, A.; Plastaras, C.; Becker, S.; Shofer, F. Pain outcomes with an elliptical regimen (POWER) study: Identifying the proper dosage of exercise for therapeutic effect in persons with chronic back pain. *J. Phys. Med. Rehabil.* **2020**, *2*, 23–28. [PubMed]

43. Li, Y.; Gong, Y.; Zheng, B.; Fan, F.; Yi, T.; Zheng, Y.; He, P.; Fang, J.; Jia, J.; Zhu, Q.; et al. Effects on adherence to a mobile app-based self-management digital therapeutics among patients with coronary heart disease: Pilot randomized controlled trial. *JMIR mHealth uHealth* **2022**, *10*, e32251. [CrossRef] [PubMed]
44. Areias, A.C.; Costa, F.; Janela, D.; Molinos, M.; Moulder, R.G.; Lains, J.; Scheer, J.K.; Bento, V.; Yanamadala, V.; Correia, F.D. Long-term clinical outcomes of a remote digital musculoskeletal program: An ad hoc analysis from a longitudinal study with a non-participant comparison group. *Healthcare* **2022**, *10*, 2349. [CrossRef] [PubMed]

Journal of
Clinical Medicine

MDPI

Article

Comparative Evaluation of Large Language and Multimodal Models in Detecting Spinal Stabilization Systems on X-Ray Images

Bartosz Polis [1,†], Agnieszka Zawadzka-Fabijan [2,†], Robert Fabijan [3], Róża Kosińska [1], Emilia Nowosławska [1] and Artur Fabijan [1,*]

1 Department of Neurosurgery, Polish-Mother's Memorial Hospital Research Institute, 93-338 Lodz, Poland; jezza@post.pl (B.P.); roza.w.kosinska@gmail.com (R.K.); emilia.nowoslawska@iczmp.edu.pl (E.N.)
2 Department of Rehabilitation Medicine, Faculty of Health Sciences, Medical University of Lodz, 90-419 Lodz, Poland; agnieszka.zawadzka@umed.lodz.pl
3 Independent Researcher, Luton LU2 0GS, UK; robert.f.fabijan@gmail.com
* Correspondence: artur8944@wp.pl
† These authors contributed equally to this work.

Abstract: Background/Objectives: Open-source AI models are increasingly applied in medical imaging, yet their effectiveness in detecting and classifying spinal stabilization systems remains underexplored. This study compares ChatGPT-4o (a large language model) and BiomedCLIP (a multimodal model) in their analysis of posturographic X-ray images (AP projection) to assess their accuracy in identifying the presence, type (growing vs. non-growing), and specific system (MCGR vs. PSF). **Methods:** A dataset of 270 X-ray images (93 without stabilization, 80 with MCGR, and 97 with PSF) was analyzed manually by neurosurgeons and evaluated using a three-stage AI-based questioning approach. Performance was assessed via classification accuracy, Gwet's Agreement Coefficient (AC1) for inter-rater reliability, and a two-tailed z-test for statistical significance ($p < 0.05$). **Results:** The results indicate that GPT-4o demonstrates high accuracy in detecting spinal stabilization systems, achieving near-perfect recognition (97–100%) for the presence or absence of stabilization. However, its consistency is reduced when distinguishing complex growing-rod (MCGR) configurations, with agreement scores dropping significantly (AC1 = 0.32–0.50). In contrast, BiomedCLIP displays greater response consistency (AC1 = 1.00) but struggles with detailed classification, particularly in recognizing PSF (11% accuracy) and MCGR (4.16% accuracy). Sensitivity analysis revealed GPT-4o's superior stability in hierarchical classification tasks, while BiomedCLIP excelled in binary detection but showed performance deterioration as the classification complexity increased. **Conclusions:** These findings highlight GPT-4o's robustness in clinical AI-assisted diagnostics, particularly for detailed differentiation of spinal stabilization systems, whereas BiomedCLIP's precision may require further optimization to enhance its applicability in complex radiographic evaluations.

Keywords: scoliosis; artificial intelligence; BiomedCLIP; ChatGPT-4o; medical image analysis; machine learning in healthcare

1. Introduction

Open-source artificial intelligence models (OSAIM) are freely available, publicly accessible tools that have found extensive applications in both computer science and medicine, significantly contributing to advancements in diagnostics and treatment planning [1–6].

While these models offer advanced capabilities for processing and interpreting visual data, most are not specifically designed for the analysis of medical images, such as X-ray scans. To address this gap, specialized models like BiomedCLIP have been developed, integrating natural language processing with medical image analysis, thereby opening new possibilities for diagnostic support and treatment selection [7]. Increasing research on the clinical applications of OSAIM underscores their potential in radiology and other fields of medicine.

In the past year, there has been a growing global interest in open-source AI models, exemplified by the development of advanced language models such as ChatGPT by OpenAI. One of the key products of this organization is Contrastive Language–Image Pretraining (CLIP), which enables zero-shot image classification, image captioning, and visual question answering [8]. Trained on extensive image-text datasets, CLIP serves as the foundation for specialized models such as SDA-CLIP, designed for surgical activity analysis, and SleepCLIP, which supports the diagnosis of sleep disorders [9,10]. One of the most advanced CLIP-based models is BiomedCLIP (Bio-med-CLIP-PubMedBERT_256-vit_base_patch16_224), which integrates natural language processing with medical image interpretation. Trained on the PMC-15M dataset, comprising 15 million image−caption pairs from PubMed Central, BiomedCLIP utilizes PubMedBERT for medical text analysis and Vision Transformer for biomedical imaging. As a result, BiomedCLIP demonstrates high efficacy in image classification, cross-modal retrieval, and question−answering, making it a valuable tool for diagnostics, research, and medical education [11].

In our previous study, we evaluated BiomedCLIP in detecting and classifying scoliosis in pediatric posturographic X-ray images. The analysis revealed that the model performed well in identifying advanced cases of scoliosis, particularly in severe stages. However, its accuracy was limited when detecting milder forms and distinguishing between single-curve and double-curve scoliosis. These findings highlight BiomedCLIP's potential in medical image analysis, while also indicating the need for further refinement of the model and expansion of the training dataset to enhance its clinical applicability [7].

ChatGPT, as an advanced language model, has also been explored for medical diagnostics and biomedical data analysis, although its effectiveness remains under investigation. Suthar et al. reported that ChatGPT-4 achieved a diagnostic accuracy of 57.86%, highlighting both its potential and limitations [12]. Lee et al. compared its ability to analyze chest X-ray images with the KARA-CXR algorithm, demonstrating that dedicated AI systems outperformed ChatGPT in medical image interpretation [13]. Additionally, Sohail examined ChatGPT's early impact on medical sciences and biomedical engineering, emphasizing both its diagnostic potential and the challenges related to accuracy and interpretability [14].

In our studies, we assessed the ability of AI models, including ChatGPT and Microsoft Bing, to diagnose single-curve scoliosis from posturographic X-ray images. ChatGPT demonstrated 100% accuracy in scoliosis detection, but its Cobb angle assessment accuracy was only 43.5%, showing significant discrepancies compared to expert evaluations. Moreover, the model struggled with determining curve direction, scoliosis classification, and vertebral rotation detection, while Microsoft Bing failed to detect scoliosis in any case. These findings suggest that while AI holds promise in scoliosis identification, significant improvements in image analysis and precise diagnostic assessment are required before these models can be reliably implemented in clinical practice [15].

Scoliosis is defined as a three-dimensional spinal deformity in which the coronal plane curvature exceeds 10 degrees, measured using the Cobb method, which serves as the clinical diagnostic standard [16]. The gold standard for scoliosis diagnosis is X-ray imaging of the spine in two projections: anteroposterior (AP) and lateral. This imaging approach enables precise assessment of spinal curvature severity, vertebral rotation, and deformity progression, facilitating the planning of appropriate therapeutic procedures [17,18]. Scoliosis can be classified based on various criteria, including patient age, etiology, curve location, and severity measured by the Cobb angle [19].

The management of scoliosis is highly individualized but generally follows established clinical guidelines. According to AO Spine recommendations, mild scoliosis (10–20 degrees) is typically managed through regular monitoring and physiotherapy, while moderate scoliosis (20–40 degrees) may require orthotic bracing. In severe cases (>40 degrees), surgical intervention is often indicated [19]. In adolescent idiopathic scoliosis (AIS), the most common form of spinal deformity in children, treatment options range from conservative therapy (e.g., physiotherapy) to surgical interventions, such as dynamic fixation or posterior spinal fusion (PSF) [20].

For early-onset scoliosis (EOS), occurring before the age of 10, growth-friendly surgical techniques such as magnetically controlled growing rods (MCGR) are frequently used to facilitate spinal and thoracic development while maintaining deformity correction. Traditional approaches, such as posterior spinal fusion (PSF), may lead to complications, including thoracic insufficiency syndrome, growth restriction, and respiratory issues, if performed too early. MCGR systems offer a promising alternative by reducing the need for repeated surgical lengthening procedures, thereby minimizing complications and psychosocial burden on young patients [21] (Figure 1).

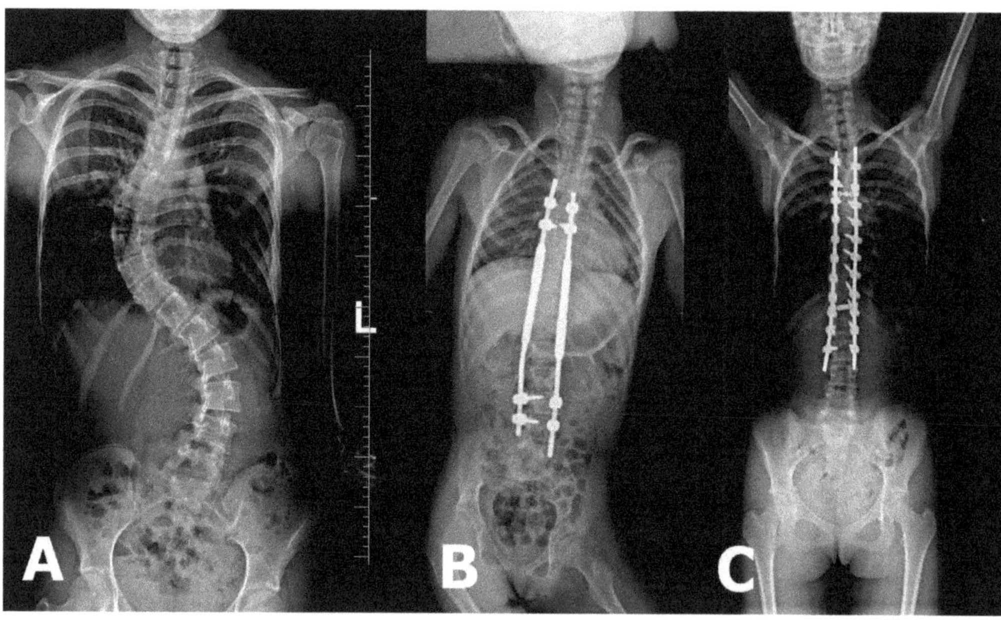

Figure 1. (**A**) X-ray image depicting severe double-curve scoliosis with Cobb angle measurements of 62° between L4/L5 and Th11/Th12 and 77° between Th11/Th12 and Th6/Th5. (**B**) X-ray image showing the magnetically controlled growing-rod (MCGR) system used for spinal stabilization. (**C**) X-ray image illustrating the final spinal stabilization procedure.

The primary objective of this study is to compare two types of artificial intelligence models—large language models (LLLM), such as ChatGPT-4o (Omni), and the multimodal model BiomedCLIP—in terms of their ability to detect and classify spinal stabilization systems in posturographic X-ray images in the anteroposterior (AP) projection.

1.1. Justification

The selection of LLLM (ChatGPT-4o) and BiomedCLIP for comparison is based on their differing approaches to data analysis and their specific applications in medical imaging diagnostics:

ChatGPT-4o:

- ○ Although primarily a language model, ChatGPT-4o demonstrates strong capabilities in image analysis, particularly in recognizing detailed objects and structures.
- ○ With its image-processing functionality, it can be applied to detect complex structures, such as spinal stabilization systems, especially when they are clearly visible on X-ray images.
- ○ Its primary advantage lies in its ability to generate precise descriptions and interpret results, making it valuable in medical applications where detailed descriptions are essential.

BiomedCLIP:

- ○ BiomedCLIP is a multimodal model that integrates images and text, enabling it to compare visual features of an image with textual descriptions.
- ○ Its performance depends on the quality of the provided textual descriptions and the accuracy of image−text associations.
- ○ This model is particularly useful for tasks where textual context aids in recognizing and classifying objects in medical images.
- ○ However, its efficacy may be limited in more complex scenarios, such as distinguishing subtle details in medical imaging.

This study aims to determine which of these models is more suitable for medical diagnostics, particularly in the radiographic assessment of spinal stabilization systems in surgical applications. A comparative analysis of these two AI approaches can provide valuable insights into the effectiveness of artificial intelligence in medicine, especially in automating diagnostic processes.

1.2. Research Hypotheses

Accuracy in detecting spinal stabilization systems:

H1. *BiomedCLIP will demonstrate significantly higher accuracy in detecting the presence of spinal stabilization systems on posturographic anterior–posterior (AP) X-ray images compared to ChatGPT-4o.*

Consistency of model responses:

H2. *BiomedCLIP will exhibit greater consistency (i.e., reproducibility of results) in classifying X-ray images regarding the presence and type of spinal stabilization systems than ChatGPT-4o.*

Effectiveness in classifying the type and nature of the stabilization system:

H3. *While ChatGPT-4o may be more effective in recognizing the general presence of spinal stabilization systems, BiomedCLIP will outperform in the precise classification of the system type (growing vs. non-growing) and specific system (MCGR vs. PSF).*

2. Materials and Methods

The study was conducted at the Polish Mother's Memorial Hospital Research Institute as part of scientific research activities. The bioethics committee determined that the analysis of the obtained radiological images did not require formal approval. This study, conducted between January 2024 and December 2024, focused on analyzing radiological images in the anterior–posterior (AP) projection in patients aged 3 to 17 years. The X-ray images were collected from January 2022 to December 2024, and out of 590 available images, a total of 270 images were selected, including:

- 93 posturographic AP images without a visible stabilization system,
- 80 images with a visible growing rod system (MCGR),
- 97 images showing the final stabilization (PSF).

Consent for the use of X-ray images was obtained from the legal guardians of the patients. In accordance with data protection principles, all personal information was anonymized.

Inclusion and Exclusion Criteria:

The inclusion criteria required technically correct images. For images without a stabilization system, only cases of severe scoliosis (>40° Cobb angle) were included, in line with AO Spine guidelines, which qualify curves exceeding 40° for surgical correction. Additionally, images with a visible MCGR system and final stabilization (PSF) were selected. Image quality was assessed to exclude illegible images, errors in image stitching, or improper framing.

The exclusion criteria included:

- Images that were improperly stitched,
- X-rays covering an incomplete view of the spine,
- Scoliosis cases with additional bone defects, such as hyperkyphosis,
- Images featuring additional implants unrelated to the studied stabilization systems.

Imaging and Analysis:

All of the tests were performed using the same radiological equipment, and the X-ray images were not modified in any way. They were saved in JPEG format with a resolution of 2663 × 1277 px.

The dataset was evaluated by two independent neurosurgery specialists (B.P. and E.N.), who focused on 270 AP posturographic images, including 93 cases of severe scoliosis, with curvatures ranging from 45° to 96°. The analysis aimed to develop baseline scoliosis descriptions, detailing key parameters such as:

- Degree of deformation (Cobb method),
- Precise identification of the affected spine segment.

These descriptions were later used to evaluate the capabilities and classification accuracy of open AI systems in scoliosis assessment.

2.1. Manual Measurement

The evaluation of posturographic X-ray images was carried out independently by two neurosurgery specialists. For image analysis and Cobb angle measurements, RadiAnt software (version 2023.1) was utilized.

2.2. AI System Evaluation Methodology

As part of this study, an analysis of artificial intelligence models was conducted, including ChatGPT-4o (OpenAI, San Francisco, CA, USA). The experiments took place between 1 January and 30 January 2025, following a three-stage methodology designed to assess the model's ability to interpret posturographic X-ray images.

Three-Stage Questioning Approach

1. General Image Interpretation

Question: *'What do you see in the image?'*

This open-ended question allowed the model to describe the X-ray without any prior hints, such as the presence or absence of a spinal stabilization system.

2. Detection of a Stabilization System

Question: *'Do you observe any spinal stabilization system in the image?'*

If the model answered 'no' for an image without a stabilization system, it confirmed correct recognition.

If it answered 'yes' incorrectly, it indicated a misinterpretation of bone structures or artifacts as a stabilization system.

3. Identification of the Stabilization System Type

Question: *'If yes, what type of stabilization system is visible?'*

For images without a stabilization system, the correct response was 'none' or 'not applicable'. If the model identified a system where none was present, it was considered a misclassification.

For images with stabilization, the model was expected to specify whether the system was growing (MCGR) or non-growing (PSF).

Evaluation Criteria

Each image was processed individually, and the model was asked the three questions in sequence. Only three key pieces of information were extracted from its responses:

- Presence of a stabilization system (if applicable),
- Type of stabilization system (growing vs. non-growing),
- Specific system identification (MCGR or PSF, if applicable).

Scoring System

For images without a stabilization system:

- Correctly identifying the absence of a system → 1 point
- Incorrectly identifying a system → 0 points
- Correctly stating no type/system was present → 1 point
- Incorrectly specifying a type/system → 0 points

For images with a stabilization system:

- Correctly detecting the presence of a system → 1 point
- Failing to detect a system → 0 points
- Correctly identifying the type (growing/non-growing) → 1 point
- Incorrectly classifying the type or failing to specify it → 0 points
- Correctly recognizing the specific system (MCGR or PSF) → 1 point
- Incorrectly identifying the system (e.g., misclassifying MCGR as VEPTR) or failing to specify → 0 points

To assess the model's consistency and reliability, the entire study was repeated three times to evaluate whether the AI provided repeatable and stable responses.

The classification of scoliosis followed the AO Spine criteria, and the therapeutic approach was determined based on AO Spine qualifications for surgical intervention (Figure 2).

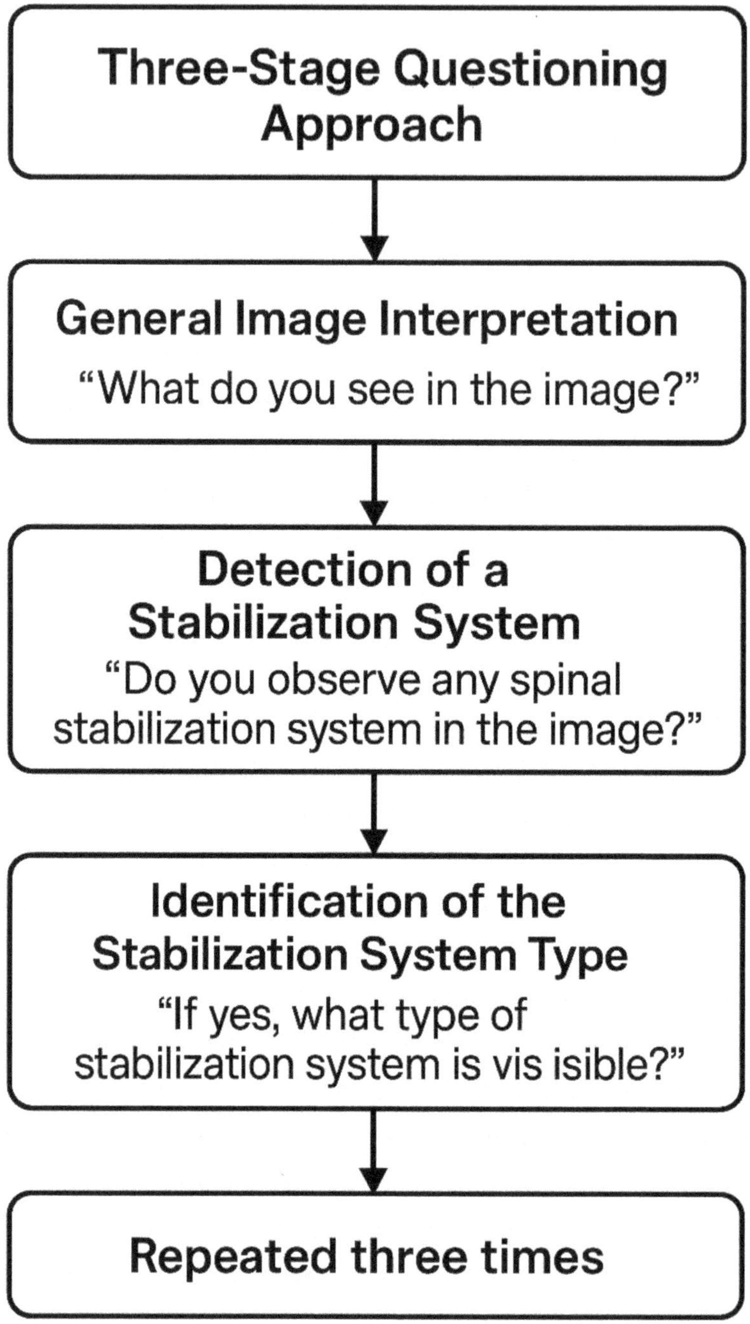

Figure 2. Flowchart illustrating the standardized three-stage questioning approach used to evaluate AI model performance. For each X-ray image, the model was asked: (1) to describe the image freely, (2) to determine the presence of spinal stabilization hardware, and (3) to identify the type of system if applicable. This sequence was repeated across three independent trials to assess consistency and diagnostic accuracy.

2.3. *BiomedCLIP Methodology*

2.3.1. Model Selection and Adaptation

Pediatric spine X-ray images were classified across three conditions—pre-treatment, post-targeted stabilization system, and post-MAGEC system application—utilizing the Biomed CLIP model. Biomed CLIP, a refined variant of the Contrastive Language–Image Pretraining (CLIP) model, was selected due to its demonstrated superior performance in zero-shot classification of complex biomedical imagery, surpassing alternatives such as DALL-E, MedCLIP, and PubMedCLIP. Its open-source accessibility further facilitated its adoption for this research. To augment its specialization in pediatric spinal image analysis, Biomed CLIP underwent fine-tuning on the PMC-15 dataset. This comprehensive dataset comprises 15 million biomedical image−text pairs derived from 4.4 million scientific articles, encompassing a diverse array of medical specialties, thereby providing a robust foundation for model training.

2.3.2. Hyperparameters

The fine-tuning of Biomed CLIP followed the same hyperparameters as those used for training the original CLIP ViT-B/16 model (Table 1).

Table 1. Hyperparameters used for fine-tuning BioMed CLIP, following the same setup as the original CLIP ViT-B/16 model.

Hyperparameter	Value
Learning Rate	4×10^{-4}
Weight Decay	0.2
Adam β1	0.9
Adam β2	0.98
Adam ε	1.00×10^{-6}
Batch size	32,768
Training epochs	32
Warm-up iterations	2000
Gradient clipping	Max temperature of 100

2.3.3. Computational Infrastructure

Computational tasks were executed on the RunPod platform, employing two NVIDIA L40S GPUs, 16 vCPUs, 124 GB of RAM, and 96 GB VRAM. A standardized software environment was instantiated via a Docker image (pytorch:2.1.0-py3.10-cuda11.8.0-devel-ubuntu22.04), pre-configured with requisite CUDA and PyTorch modules to facilitate model training and subsequent evaluation.

2.3.4. Model Architecture and Training Protocol

The Biomed CLIP architecture incorporates a Vision Transformer (ViT-B/16) as its vision encoder and PubMedBERT for text encoding. The ViT-B/16, selected for its superior efficiency relative to smaller variants, segments input images into 16 × 16 pixel patches, natively supporting a 224 × 224 pixel image size. While experimentation with a 384 × 384 pixel resolution indicated enhanced retrieval capabilities, this was accompanied by a commensurate increase in pre-training duration. The text encoder's context window was extended to 256 tokens, from the conventional 77, to accommodate the verbose nature of biomedical image annotations. The ViT-B/16 vision encoder comprises 86 million trainable parameters. Model training was conducted on a cluster of 16 NVIDIA A100 or V100 GPUs, incorporating techniques such as gradient checkpointing and automatic mixed precision to optimize memory utilization and enhance computational throughput.

2.3.5. Data and Performance Evaluation

Model performance was directly evaluated against a curated database of anonymized pediatric X-ray images. This approach enabled iterative assessment across various treatment stages and hardware configurations. The evaluation protocol prioritized the model's classification accuracy and generalization capacity to unseen medical image data, thus providing a rigorous assessment of both the robustness and clinical applicability of Biomed CLIP.

The evaluation was conducted by interfacing directly with a database of anonymized X-ray images. This setup allowed for an iterative assessment of the model's performance across different stages of treatment and varying hardware configurations. The evaluation focused on the model's accuracy in image classification and its ability to generalize across unseen medical image data. This methodology not only tests the robustness of Biomed CLIP, but also its applicability to real-world medical diagnostics. For this task, descriptive text labels were prepared to represent the classification of each category:

1. First Category:
    - 'This is an image of spine with stabilization system'
    - 'This is an image of spine without stabilization system'
2. Second Category:
    - 'This is an image of spine with growing stabilization system'
    - 'This is an image of spine with non-growing stabilization system'
    - 'This is an image of spine without stabilization system'
3. Third Category:
    - 'This is an image of spine with magnetic control growing rod system (MCGR)'
    - 'This is an image of spine with posterior spinal fusion system (PSF)'
    - 'This is an image of spine without stabilization system'

Each X-ray image was preprocessed through normalization before being input into the model. The model then computed the probability of the image belonging to each scoliosis category, with a confidence score ranging from 0 to 1. This score was used as a quantitative measure of the model's certainty in its predictions.

The evaluation emphasized accuracy in image classification and the ability to generalize across unseen medical image data, testing both the robustness and real-world applicability of Biomed CLIP in clinical diagnostics.

2.4. Statistical Analysis

The detection rates of spinal stabilization systems were reported as count (n) and percentage (5) for binary classification tasks and as mean (M) and standard error (SE) for proportion-based analyses.

2.4.1. Agreement Assessment

The assessment of inter-rater reliability for binary variables with multiple measurements was conducted using Gwet's Agreement Coefficient 1 (AC1), due to its robustness in handling imbalanced category distributions and its reduced sensitivity to high agreement levels [22–24]. Gwet's AC1 was then computed using Formula (1):

$$AC1 = \frac{pa - pe}{1 - pe} \tag{1}$$

where pa is the observed agreement estimated by (2):

$$pa = \frac{number\ of\ agreements}{total\ number\ of\ ratings} \tag{2}$$

The expected agreement by chance *pe* was conducted using (3):

$$pe = \sum_{k=1}^{C} \left(\frac{1}{C}\right)^2 \tag{3}$$

where C is the number of categories.

Described by (1)–(3), AC1 remains robust and interpretable, not artificially deflated by the prevalence effect, thereby providing a more accurate reflection of inter-rater reliability, making it the optimal choice for the current analysis [25].

2.4.2. Estimation Difference in Identification Rates Between AIs

To evaluate the significance of differences in detection proportions between GPT-4o and BiomedCLIP AI, a two-tailed z-test for the difference in proportions was conducted.

The standard error (SE) of the difference between the two means was computed using Formula (4):

$$SE = \sqrt{SE_1^2 + SE_2^2}, \tag{4}$$

where SE_1 and SE_2 represent the standard errors of the detection rates for GPT-4o and BiomedClip, respectively.

To determine the statistical significance of the difference, a z-score was calculated by (5):

$$z = \frac{M1 - M2}{SE}, \tag{5}$$

where M_1 and M_2 are the mean detection rates of GPT-4o and BiomedClip, respectively.

Finally, the *p*-value was derived from the standard normal distribution based on the calculated z-score. As a two-tailed test was used, the *p*-value was obtained according to (6):

$$p = 2 \times P(Z > |z|), \tag{6}$$

where $P(Z > |z|)$ represents the probability that a standard normal variable (Z) takes a value greater than the absolute value of the calculated z-score.

A significance threshold of $\alpha = 0.05$ was applied to determine whether the observed differences were statistically significant.

2.4.3. Statistical Tool

Analyses were conducted using the R Statistical language (version 4.3.3; [26]) on Windows 11 Pro 64 bit (build 22631), using the packages irrCAC (version 1.0; [27]) report (version 0.5.8; [28]), patchwork (version 1.2.0; [29]), gtsummary (version 1.7.2; [30]), ggplot2 (version 3.5.0; [31]), and dplyr (version 1.1.4; [32]).

3. Results

3.1. Comparative Sensitivity and Consistency in Detecting Spinal Stabilization Systems

The performance of GPT-4o and BiomedCLIP in detecting and classifying spinal stabilization systems (SSS) in 270 posturographic X-ray images (93 No Stabilization, 97 PSF, 80 MCGR) was evaluated using sensitivity (proportion of correct responses), Gwet's AC1 for inter-rater agreement, and Cohen's h for effect size (Table 2). A summary of findings aligned with the research hypotheses (H1: accuracy, H2: consistency, H3: classification) is presented in Table 3.

Table 2. Comparative sensitivity and inter-rater agreement for GPT-4o and BiomedCLIP in detecting spinal stabilization systems (SSS) in advanced scoliosis (≥40°) using posturographic radiographic images.

SSS Type	Classification Task	GPT-4o Sensitivity, % (95% CI)	BiomedCLIP Sensitivity, % (95% CI)	GPT-4o Gwet's AC1 (95% CI)
No Stabilization	Presence	97.0 (94.0–100.0)	99.6 (99.6–99.6)	0.97 (0.94–1.00)
	Type	97.0 (94.0–100.0)	66.9 (63.0–70.8)	0.97 (0.94–1.00)
	Kind	97.0 (94.0–100.0)	30.2 (23.9–36.5)	0.97 (0.94–1.00)
PSF	Presence	100.0 (100.0–100.0)	5.1 (3.9–6.3)	1.00 (1.00–1.00)
	Type (Non-growing)	98.0 (96.0–100.0)	0.6 (0.4–0.8)	0.99 (0.97–1.00)
	Kind (PSF)	84.0 (78.8–89.2)	11.0 (7.8–14.2)	0.87 (0.80–0.94)
MCGR	Presence	100.0 (100.0–100.0)	6.6 (5.5–7.7)	1.00 (1.00–1.00)
	Type (Growing)	70.0 (51.2–88.8)	66.3 (62.8–69.8)	0.32 (0.16–0.49)
	Kind (MCGR)	18.0 (4.6–31.4)	4.2 (0.9–7.5)	0.50 (0.36–0.64)

Notes: Gwet's AC1 for BiomedCLIP is 1.00 (perfect agreement) for all tasks and is not tabulated to avoid redundancy but is noted in the caption. Individual rater percentages and detailed agreement statistics (pa, pe, SE, *p*-values) are provided in Supplementary Table S1.

Table 3. Summary of comparative performance of GPT-4o and BiomedCLIP in detecting and classifying spinal stabilization systems, aligned with research hypotheses.

Hypothesis	Task	GPT-4o Sensitivity, % (95% CI)	BiomedCLIP Sensitivity, % (95% CI)	Sensitivity Difference (z, *p*-Value)	Cohen's h	GPT-4o AC1 (95% CI)	Key Finding and Conclusion
H1: Accuracy in Detecting SSS	Presence (No Stabilization)	97.0 (94.0–100.0)	99.6 (99.6–99.6)	−2.6% (z = 2.7, p = 0.007)	−0.21	0.97 (0.94–1.00)	GPT-4o slightly less sensitive (small effect); both highly accurate, clinically negligible difference.
	Presence (PSF)	100.0 (100.0–100.0)	5.1 (3.9–6.3)	94.9% (z = 95.0, p < 0.001)	2.05	1.00 (1.00–1.00)	GPT-4o far superior (large effect), critical for clinical detection of PSF.
	Presence (MCGR)	100.0 (100.0–100.0)	6.6 (5.5–7.7)	93.4% (z = 93.0, p < 0.001)	1.95	1.00 (1.00–1.00)	GPT-4o highly reliable (large effect), BiomedCLIP inadequate for MCGR detection.
H2: Consistency of Responses	Type (No Stabilization)	97.0 (94.0–100.0)	66.9 (63.0–70.8)	30.1% (z = 13.44, p < 0.001)	0.68	0.97 (0.94–1.00)	BiomedCLIP perfectly consistent (AC1 = 1.00), GPT-4o variable but high agreement (medium effect).
	Type (PSF)	98.0 (96.0–100.0)	0.6 (0.4–0.8)	97.4% (z = 37.5, p < 0.001)	2.41	0.99 (0.97–1.00)	BiomedCLIP consistent but inaccurate, GPT-4o less consistent but accurate (large effect).
	Type (MCGR)	70.0 (51.2–88.8)	66.3 (62.8–69.8)	3.7% (z = 0.27, p = 0.790)	0.08	0.32 (0.16–0.49)	BiomedCLIP consistent, GPT-4o highly variable (low AC1, small effect).
H3: Classifying Type/Kind	Kind (PSF)	84.0 (78.8–89.2)	11.0 (7.8–14.2)	73.0% (z = 36.5, p < 0.001)	1.18	0.87 (0.80–0.94)	GPT-4o more accurate but less consistent (large effect), BiomedCLIP struggles with specificity.
	Kind (MCGR)	18.0 (4.6–31.4)	4.2 (0.9–7.5)	13.8% (z = 1.40, p = 0.160)	0.43	0.50 (0.36–0.64)	Both models suboptimal, GPT-4o slightly better but inconsistent (small to medium effect).

Notes: Sensitivity and 95% CIs are derived from Table 2. Sensitivity differences and z-tests are from the Statistical Analysis section. Cohen's h is calculated as h = 2 × (arcsin(√(p_1))-arcsin(√(p_2)), where p1 and p2are GPT-4o and BiomedCLIP sensitivities, respectively. Interpretation: small (h = 0.2), medium (h = 0.5), large (h = 0.8). GPT-4o AC1 values are from Table 2; BiomedCLIP AC1 = 1.00 for all tasks (noted in text). Conclusions summarize clinical implications, e.g., GPT-4o's superior detection sensitivity (large effect sizes for PSF/MCGR) supports its use for initial screening, while BiomedCLIP's consistency reveals the potential for structured classification with further optimization.

Detection of stabilization systems (H1: Accuracy)

GPT-4o demonstrated near-perfect sensitivity (97–100%) in detecting the presence or absence of SSS across all types (No Stabilization: 97.0%, 95% *CI* 94.0–100.0; PSF: 100.0%, 95% *CI* 100.0–100.0; MCGR: 100.0%, 95% *CI* 100.0–100.0), significantly outperforming BiomedCLIP (No Stabilization: 99.6%, 95% CI 99.6–99.6, $z = 2.7$, $p = 0.007$, $h = -0.21$; PSF: 5.1%, 95% *CI* 3.9–6.3, $z = 95.0$, $p < 0.001$, $h = 2.05$; MCGR: 6.6%, 95% *CI* 5.5–7.7, $z = 93.0$, $p < 0.001$, $h = 1.95$). The small difference in No Stabilization detection (2.6%, small effect) was clinically negligible, as both models excelled in this task. However, GPT-4o's superior sensitivity for PSF and MCGR detection (large effect sizes) highlights its reliability for initial screening in clinical settings (Table 3).

Consistency of responses (H2)

BiomedCLIP exhibited perfect consistency (AC1 = 1.00) across all tasks, reflecting its deterministic classification approach. In contrast, GPT-4o showed a high but variable agreement, particularly in complex tasks. For No Stabilization and PSF, GPT-4o maintained strong agreement (AC1 = 0.97–1.00), but consistency dropped for MCGR Type (AC1 = 0.32, 95% *CI* 0.16–0.49) and Kind (AC1 = 0.50, 95% *CI* 0.36–0.64) classifications. Sensitivity differences showed a medium effect for No Stabilization Type (30.1%, $h = 0.68$), a large effect for PSF Type (97.4%, $h = 2.41$), and a small effect for MCGR Type (3.7%, $h = 0.08$), indicating variable clinical relevance (Table 3). This supports the conclusion that BiomedCLIP is more consistent, while GPT-4o's probabilistic nature leads to response fluctuations.

Classification of SSS type and kind (H3)

For classifying SSS types (Growing vs. Non-growing), GPT-4o outperformed BiomedCLIP for PSF (98.0% vs. 0.6%, $z = 37.5$, $p < 0.001$, $h = 2.41$) but showed a comparable performance for MCGR (70.0% vs. 66.3%, z = 0.27, $p = 0.790$, h = 0.077). For specific system identification (Kind), GPT-4o was more accurate for PSF (84.0% vs. 11.0%, $z = 36.5$, $p < 0.001$, $h = 1.18$), but struggled with MCGR (18.0% vs. 4.2%, z = 1.40, $p = 0.160$, $h = 0.433$), reflecting challenges in distinguishing morphologically similar systems. Large effect sizes for PSF tasks confirmed GPT-4o's clinical advantage, while smaller effects for MCGR tasks inferred that both models need optimization (Table 3). These findings indicate that GPT-4o is more effective for initial detection and broad classification, while BiomedCLIP's structured approach offers potential for detailed classification with improved training.

3.2. Comparison of Mean Sensitivity Levels for GPT-4o's Detection of Spinal Stabilization Systems

The proportion of proper responses in Table 1 is equivalent to sensitivity, reflecting the true positive rate of GPT-4o's detection of spinal stabilization systems (SSS) in advanced scoliosis ($\geq 40°$) using posturographic radiographic images (PRIs). Figure 3 compares the mean sensitivities across the type of PRIs of the SSS and the type of request about SSS. The results are stratified by the type of SSS (Absence, PSF, MGCR) and the type of request (Presence, Type, Kind), with error bars indicating the standard error (SE) of the mean sensitivity. This analysis demonstrates the performance and variability of GPT-4o's detection capabilities, providing a comprehensive evaluation of its accuracy and reliability in identifying SSS under varying conditions.

3.3. Analysis of the Performance and Interrater Agreement of BiomedClip AI in Identifying Spinal Stabilization Systems in Severe Scoliosis ($\geq 40°$) Using Posturographic Radiographic Imaging

In contrast to GPT-4o, BiomedCLIP AI enabled the estimation of the identification proportion for the queried options with a granularity of 0.01, with the total sum equaling 1.00. This approach allowed for greater precision in performance assessment.

A key distinction was the consistency of proportion estimates across repeated analyses of the same images, resulting in perfect agreement (AC1 = 1) in the identification of all types of stabilization systems.

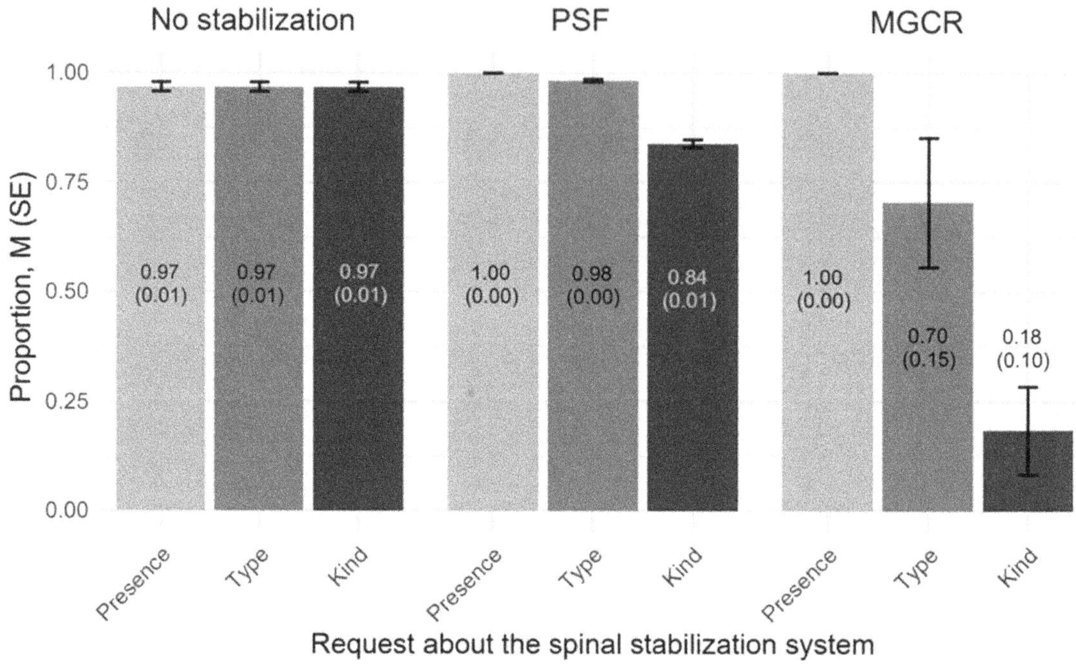

Figure 3. Comparison of detection proportions (here it is also a sensitivity level), M (SE), for GPT-4o's in advanced scoliosis (Cobb angle $\geq 40°$) using posturographic radiographic images.

3.3.1. Analysis of the Performance in Identifying Posturographic Radiographic Images with No Stabilization Systems

BiomedCLIP AI's performance differed notably depending on whether the task was simply to detect the presence or absence of stabilization hardware, to identify the 'type' of stabilization, or to specify the 'kind' of construct.

Under 'Presence of stabilization' requests, the model achieved a mean correct classification rate of 0.996 (SE = 0.00) for images containing no stabilization. In other words, the AI system successfully ruled out stabilization in nearly 99.6% of cases, with only 0.4% of images incorrectly flagged as having some form of stabilization systems (see Figure 4 for visualization).

When tasked with specifying the 'type' of stabilization (Growing rod, No growing rod, or No stabilization), BiomedCLIP AI continued to classify the majority of true No-stabilization images correctly (0.669, SE = 0.02). However, 0.106 of these images were mistakenly labeled as 'Growing rod', and 0.225 were labeled as No growing rod, indicating that the model still confused some images that should have been confidently identified as 'No stabilization'.

Performance diminishes further under 'kind' classifications (PSF, MCGR, No stabilization), where BiomedCLIP AI correctly retained the no-stabilization label in 0.302 (SE = 0.02) of cases, but mislabeled 0.673 as MCGR and 0.0252 as PSF. This observation highlights that while the BiomedCLIP AI is highly reliable for straightforward detection of absence or presence, it becomes less precise when finer distinctions are required, particularly if the request demands a specific 'kind' of hardware category.

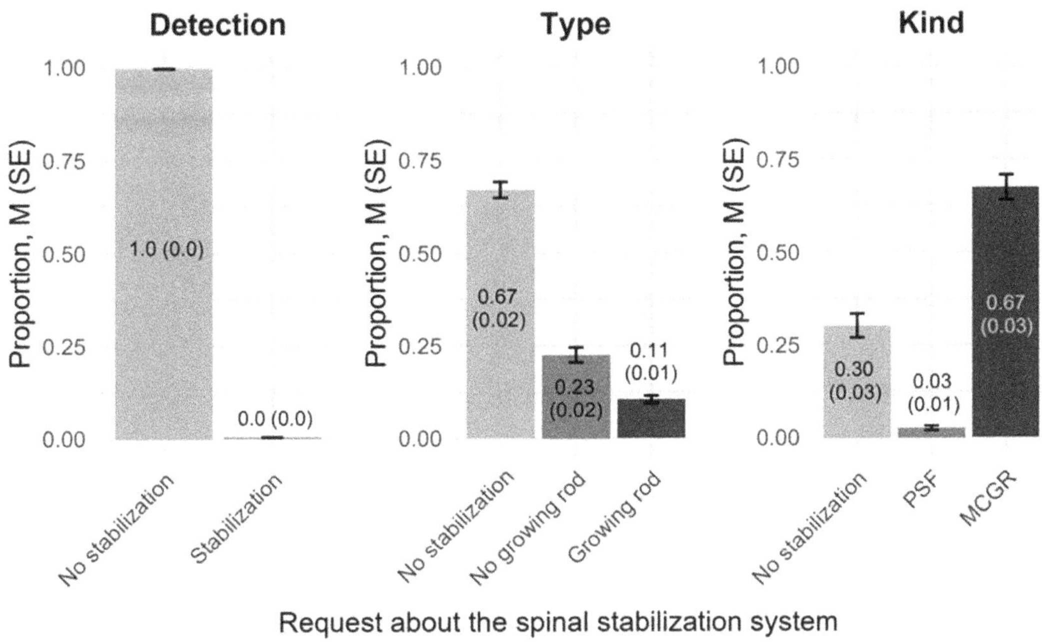

Figure 4. Comparison of detection proportions, M (SE), by BiomedClip AI in advanced scoliosis (Cobb Angle $\geq 40°$) using posturographic radiographic images without stabilization systems (N = 93).

3.3.2. Analysis of the Performance in Identifying Posturographic Radiographic Images with PSF Stabilization System

BiomedClip AI's ability to detect a posterior spinal fusion (PSF) in severe scoliosis ($\geq 40°$) posturographic imaging remained suboptimal when dissected by specific classification requests. Under the most basic 'Detection' protocol, the system correctly identified 'Stabilization' in only 5.10% (SE = 0.00568) of cases, while it incorrectly assigned 'No stabilization' 94.90% of the time (see Figure 5 for visualization results).

In the subsequent 'Type' categorization, correctness hinged on labeling these PSF images as 'No growing rod'; the model achieved a mere 0.64% success rate (SE = 0.00128), with the remaining classifications scattered among 'Growing rod' or 'No stabilization'. At the most granular 'Kind' level—where a precise PSF designation was required—the model attained a correctness rate of only 11.0% (SE = 0.0183), while disproportionately mislabeling many of these images as 'No stabilization' (86.2%) or 'MCGR' (2.77%).

These findings underscore BiomedClip AI's marked tendency to overlook PSF constructs and misinterpret them, especially in more specialized requests that demand accurate differentiation between various fixation categories. Although the system excelled in other contexts (e.g., ruling out hardware for individuals genuinely lacking instrumentation), it struggled here to recognize key radiographic hallmarks of a posterior spinal fusion.

From a clinical perspective, the low detection and classification rates for a procedure as prevalent and standardized as PSF may prompt the need for further refinement of BiomedClip's training data, specifically incorporating robust examples of routine posterior fusion hardware in advanced scoliosis.

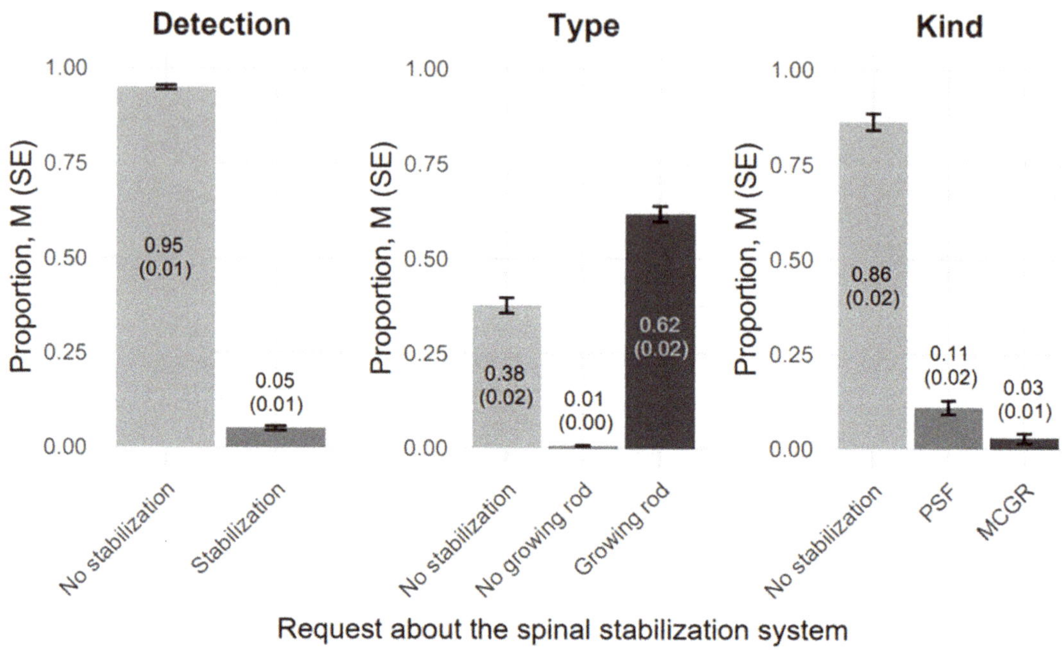

Figure 5. Comparison of the detection proportions, M (SE), by BiomedClip AI in advanced scoliosis (Cobb angle $\geq 40°$) using posturographic radiographic images with PSF No-growing-rod stabilization systems (N = 97).

3.3.3. Analysis of the Performance in Identifying Posturographic Radiographic Images with MCGR Stabilization Systems

BiomedClip AI displayed a pronounced discrepancy in classifying MCGR-based stabilization. When merely tasked with detecting whether spinal hardware was present, the model labelled only 6.62% (SE = 0.00564) of MCGR images correctly as 'Stabilization' and misclassified the remaining 93.38% as 'No stabilization' (see Figure 6 for visualization results).

Once directed to identify the 'type' of hardware, it correctly assigned 'Growing rod' status to 66.3% (SE = 0.0177) of these same images, suggesting that once it (occasionally) recognized the presence of an implant, the system was comparatively adept at recognizing it as a 'growing' construct.

However, under the most granular 'kind' classification, only 4.16% (SE = 0.0150) were labeled accurately as 'MCGR', while 86.8% remained misclassified as 'No stabilization', with another 9.05% classified as 'PSF'. The net effect ws that although BiomedClip AI could sometimes characterize the hardware as 'growing' once it surmised stabilization waas present, its overall performance for consistently detecting MCGR constructs remained suboptimal.

Clinically, these results indicate that, in the context of advanced scoliosis ($\geq 40°$), the model's failure to recognize the initial presence of hardware compromised the reliability of subsequent designations. Such gaps highlight the need for further refinement of the system's training data—especially involving subtle morphological traits of MCGR rods—to ensure both accurate detection and correct categorization of complex dynamic instrumentation.

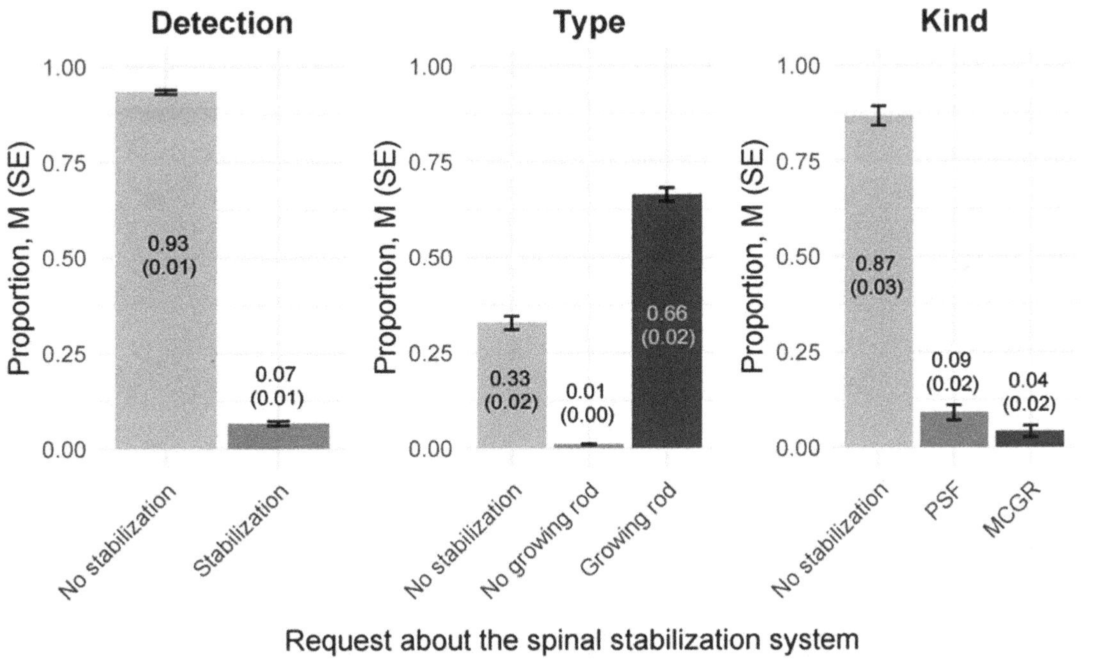

Figure 6. Comparison of detection proportions, M (SE), by BiomedClip AI in advanced scoliosis (Cobb angle $\geq 40°$) using posturographic radiographic images with MCGR growing rod stabilization systems (N = 80).

3.4. *Comparative Sensitivity Analysis of BiomedClip AI and GPT-4o in Spinal Instrumentation Classification*

3.4.1. Posturographic Radiographic Images with No Stabilization Systems

BiomedClip AI demonstrated significantly higher sensitivity in the presence-versus-absence detection of spinal instrumentation (M = 99.7%, SE = 0) compared to GPT-4o (M = 97%, SE = 1%), with a statistically significant difference (z = 2.7, $p = 0.007$).

However, as classification complexity increased, GPT-4o maintained a consistently high sensitivity (97%), whereas BiomedClip AI's performance declined substantially. For the 'type' classification task, BiomedClip AI achieved M = 66.9%, SE = 2%, significantly lower than GPT-4o (M = 97%, SE = 1%, z = −13.44, $p < 0.001$).

This performance disparity was even more pronounced in the 'kind' classification task, where BiomedClip AI's sensitivity dropped to M = 30.2%, SE = 3.2%, while GPT-4o remained stable at M = 97%, SE = 1% (z = −19.94, $p < 0.001$).

These findings indicate that while BiomedClip AI excelled in binary classification tasks, GPT-4o provided superior reliability and stability in more complex hierarchical classifications. This suggests that for clinical applications requiring detailed differentiation of spinal hardware, GPT-4o may offer a more robust and consistent solution.

3.4.2. Posturographic Radiographic Images with PSF Stabilization Systems

GPT-4o demonstrated a significantly superior performance compared to BiomedClip AI in detecting spinal stabilization systems across multiple classifications. In identifying the presence of stabilization systems, GPT-4o achieved perfect sensitivity (M = 1.00, SE = 0.00), markedly outperforming BiomedClip (M = 0.05, SE = 0.01), with a highly statistically significant difference (z = 95.00, $p < 0.001$).

Similarly, for the detection of non-growing rod systems, GPT-4o exhibited near-perfect sensitivity (M = 0.98, SE = 0.00), significantly surpassing BiomedClip (M = 0.23, SE = 0.02), as reflected in a highly significant statistical difference (z = 37.5, $p < 0.001$). A comparable trend was observed in the classification of PSF systems, where GPT-4o (M = 0.84, SE = 0.01) outperformed BiomedClip (M = 0.11, SE = 0.02), with a highly significant difference (z = 36.5, $p < 0.001$).

The above findings stress the substantial advantage of GPT-4o in accurately detecting and classifying spinal stabilization systems, highlighting its potential as a more effective tool for clinical decision-making, particularly in the management of complex scoliosis cases compared to BiomedClip.

3.4.3. Posturographic Radiographic Images with MCGR Stabilization Systems

GPT-4o demonstrated significantly superior accuracy in detecting stabilization systems, achieving perfect sensitivity (M = 1.00, SE = 0.00) compared to BiomedClip (M = 0.07, SE = 0.01), with a highly statistically significant difference (z = 93, $p < 0.001$). However, in the detection of growing-rod systems, GPT-4o (M = 0.70, SE = 0.15) and BiomedClip (M = 0.66, SE = 0.02) exhibited a comparable performance, with no statistically significant difference (z = 0.27, $p = 0.790$). For MCGR systems, GPT-4o (M = 0.18, SE = 0.10) outperformed BiomedClip (M = 0.04, SE = 0.02), although the difference did not reach statistical significance (z = 1.40, $p = 0.160$), suggesting a trend toward an improved performance.

These findings highlight GPT-4o's superior capability in detecting stabilization systems, reinforcing its potential as a more reliable tool for identifying such hardware in clinical practice. In contrast, for rowing rod systems, both models performed similarly, indicating that either may be effectively utilized in this context. However, the overall performance for MCGR classification remained suboptimal, suggesting that both models struggled with accurately identifying these systems.

4. Discussion

The findings of this study provide partial confirmation of our initial hypotheses, revealing both strengths and limitations in the performance of ChatGPT-4o and BiomedCLIP in detecting and classifying spinal stabilization systems in posturographic X-ray images.

Regarding H1 (accuracy in detecting stabilization systems), the results contradict our initial assumption, as ChatGPT-4o consistently outperformed BiomedCLIP in detecting the presence of spinal hardware, achieving near-perfect sensitivity (97–100%), while BiomedCLIP misclassified stabilization in a substantial number of cases (e.g., PSF detection: 5.10%, MCGR detection: 6.62). These results indicate that ChatGPT-4o, although not specifically trained for medical imaging, performs more reliably when identifying the presence or absence of spinal hardware.

Conversely, H2 (consistency of model responses) was confirmed, as BiomedCLIP exhibited perfect agreement (AC1 = 1.00) across repeated classifications, while ChatGPT-4o displayed variability in its responses, particularly in more complex classification tasks, such as distinguishing between stabilization types (Growing vs. Non-Growing) and specific systems (MCGR vs. PSF). This variability suggests that while ChatGPT-4o is highly effective in initial detection, its decision-making process lacks stability across repeated analyses.

The results for H3 (effectiveness in classifying the type and nature of the stabilization system) were mixed. ChatGPT-4o effectively identified the presence of stabilization systems but struggled with the precise classification of type and system (e.g., MCGR classification accuracy of only 18%). BiomedCLIP, despite its limitations in basic detection, performed slightly better in distinguishing specific types of stabilization systems once hardware was recognized, albeit with suboptimal accuracy. This indicates that while ChatGPT-4o is more effective at recognizing the presence of stabilization, BiomedCLIP provides more structured classification but requires further optimization to improve accuracy.

4.1. Generalist vs. Specialist AI: Understanding the Superior Detection Performance of ChatGPT-4o in Spinal Stabilization System Identification

The results of our study indicate that ChatGPT-4o outperformed BiomedCLIP in detecting the presence of spinal stabilization systems, contradicting H1, which hypothesized that BiomedCLIP would demonstrate superior accuracy due to its specialization in medical image analysis. Several factors may explain this unexpected finding, aligning with recent insights from AI research.

The finding that ChatGPT-4o outperformed BiomedCLIP in detecting spinal stabilization systems—despite contradicting Hypothesis 1—invites further interpretation. One possible explanation is the trade-off between generalization and specialization—ChatGPT-4o, as a generalist model, was trained on a vast and diverse dataset encompassing both text and images, which may have endowed it with the ability to detect features beyond the medical context. Its ability to detect broad patterns and high-contrast features, like stabilization systems, may explain its strong performance in binary classification tasks. In contrast, BiomedCLIP was fine-tuned for specific tasks related to matching medical images to text, suggesting a greater reliance on textual descriptions in the classification process. This study tested the model solely on image data, which could limit its ability to precisely recognize stabilization systems. A similar phenomenon has been described in the literature, indicating that generalist models like ChatGPT-4o can achieve competitive results in X-ray image analysis, particularly in tasks involving the detection of distinct contrast structures, without the need for deep semantic interpretation of the image. In summary, BiomedCLIP utilized stringent decision thresholds, while ChatGPT-4o likely had exposure to more diverse radiographic images, including variable contrast, noise levels, and different anatomical conditions, which may have enhanced its adaptation to unknown clinical cases [32]. Conversely, despite being tuned to the PMC-15 dataset (15 million image-text pairs), BiomedCLIP may not have been sufficiently trained on posturographic X-ray images of the spine with stabilization implants. This was confirmed by analyses indicating that the diversity of training datasets is crucial for models' generalization capabilities. Significant roles may also be played by differences in feature extraction mechanisms—ChatGPT-4o likely utilizes a vision model based on the transformer architecture, similar to CLIP or GPT-Vision, known for efficiently detecting objects even in complex scenes [32]. It is possible that its classification relies more heavily on detecting features of shape, contrast, and texture, facilitating the identification of metallic structures such as MCGR or PSF systems, regardless of their orientation or intensity levels. In contrast, BiomedCLIP, despite using a ViT-based vision encoder, may be optimized primarily for multimodal search, which limits its effectiveness in purely visual tasks. The results indicate that ViT models tuned to text–image retrieval may not achieve a maximum performance in tasks requiring independent image analysis [33]. Finally, key aspects may include differences in models' confidence thresholds and decision boundaries. ChatGPT-4o might have employed more lenient classification thresholds, resulting in high sensitivity in detecting stabilization systems, even with some level of uncertainty. This approach could increase the number of correctly identified cases, although, in other contexts, it might lead to a higher number of false positive results. In contrast, BiomedCLIP may have used more rigorous decision boundaries, which increased its precision, but might also have led to a higher number of missed detections (false negatives). The work *Generative Artificial Intelligence in Anatomic Pathology* suggests that more conservative models, operating at high decision thresholds, may more effectively avoid false positive errors, but might also be more susceptible to missing significant detections [34]. Jegham et al. suggested that ChatGPT-4o employs a well-calibrated mechanism for recognizing uncertainty, which could explain its high efficacy in detection tasks. Overall, the results of this study indicate that generalist models like ChatGPT-4o can achieve high effectiveness in medical image classification due to their broad exposure to diverse data and more flexible feature extraction mechanisms [35]. However, specialist models, although often characterized by greater precision in their niche applications, might be more limited in tasks requiring independent visual analysis without textual support.

4.2. Possible Explanations for the Confirmation of H2 (Model Response Consistency)

The confirmation of H2, which predicted that BiomedCLIP would demonstrate greater consistency in classifying spinal stabilization systems than ChatGPT-4o, can be attributed to several key differences in their architectures, training methodologies, and response mechanisms. Below are potential explanations for why BiomedCLIP exhibited perfect agreement (AC1 = 1.00) across repeated classifications, while ChatGPT-4o showed response variability, particularly in complex classification tasks.

4.3. Deterministic vs. Probabilistic Decision-Making

Research on multimodal AI models like BiomedCLIP and ChatGPT-4o has highlighted fundamental differences in their approach to image classification, stemming from distinct decision-making mechanisms. BiomedCLIP, optimized for medical imaging analysis, exhibits deterministic behavior—its classifications are repeatable and consistent, regardless of the number of iterations with the same image. This predictive structure is characteristic of specialist models trained on structured datasets, where precise and consistent image interpretation is critical [36]. In contrast, language–visual models like ChatGPT-4o introduce a probabilistic component to image analysis. As a transformer-based LLM, GPT-4o does not operate like a traditional deterministic classifier—its predictions can vary depending on temperature settings, token sampling methods, and subtle differences in data preprocessing [37]. This mechanism means that while ChatGPT-4o may show a high sensitivity in initial structural detection, its specific classifications may fluctuate between subsequent analyses of the same photo. Probabilistic models are commonly used in radiology and diagnostic description generation, as their ability to interpret data stems from estimating probability distributions between possible outcomes and actual labels [38]. Moreover, vision–language analysis indicates that the classification mechanisms in models like GPT-4o are based on comparing probability distributions, reinforcing the thesis about their probabilistic nature [39]. In the context of medical applications, studies on transformer-based models suggest that although they may exhibit some level of determinism in task planning, their final responses to diagnostic questions remain variable depending on the input data and result generation methods [40]. These findings highlight key differences between deterministic and probabilistic models: BiomedCLIP delivers consistent results, while ChatGPT-4o offers flexibility, but may vary depending on input conditions.

4.4. Differences in Model Training Objectives and Architecture

Studies on multimodal AI models like BiomedCLIP and GPT-4o reveal fundamental differences in their training objectives, architectures, and image processing methods. BiomedCLIP, designed for precise image–text alignment, relies on contrastive learning and uses fixed embeddings and a highly structured visual feature extraction pipeline, making its classifications consistent and repeatable upon multiple analyses of the same image [41]. Its deterministic nature has been confirmed in studies on the stability of specialist models in image analysis, which indicate that BiomedCLIP maintains a high precision by tightly matching image features to its prior representations [42]. In contrast, ChatGPT-4o, as a general-purpose model, does not rely on static embeddings in the same way. Its visual system interprets images dynamically, in the context of prior experiences and a broad range of training data, which can lead to slight variations in the classification of the same image across different iterations [43]. The literature emphasizes that such models may struggle with the fine classification of hierarchical structures, like distinguishing MCGR and PSF systems in X-ray images, due to their more abstract feature extraction strategy [44]. Unlike BiomedCLIP, tuned for medical image analysis, it exhibits higher stability in text–visual image classification, but its effectiveness may be limited in tasks not requiring direct linkage to textual data [45]. In summary, these studies confirm that BiomedCLIP, as a specialist model, achieves high precision by tightly matching visual features, while GPT-4o, with its generative nature, applies a dynamic approach to image analysis, which may result in some fluctuations in the classification of the same image between iterations.

4.5. Handling of Complex Morphological Features in X-Ray Images

Research on multimodal AI models indicates that BiomedCLIP offers greater consistency in radiographic classification than LLM-based models like ChatGPT-4o, due to its structured approach to feature extraction. As a model optimized for medical image analysis, BiomedCLIP uses precise feature mapping and is fine-tuned to specialized datasets such as PMC-15 (15 million image–text pairs), which minimizes classification ambiguity and allows for more accurate assignment of images to specific diagnostic categories [46]. Although this approach permits a degree of flexibility, it means that medical image classification may be more prone to errors, especially in cases of structures with high density and morphological similarity [47]. Furthermore, the literature suggests that in LLM models, image classification often relies on image–text matching strategies, which can lead to ambiguous results in strictly visual tasks where textual context is not available [48]. This phenomenon is particularly noticeable in the analysis of X-ray images with high-density anatomical structures, where LLM-based models exhibit greater variability in results compared to BiomedCLIP, which uses dedicated medical encoders, such as BiomedCLIP-CXR, to reduce classification discrepancies [49]. Additionally, the heuristics used by LLM models, including GPT-4o, are not precise enough to achieve effectiveness comparable to deep learning systems designed specifically for medical image analysis [50]. In the context of clinical applications, this suggests that models like BiomedCLIP may be more suitable for precise diagnostic tasks, while generative models, although potentially useful in exploratory tasks, may require additional mechanisms to stabilize results in order to obtain repeatable and reliable predictions.

4.6. Influence of Decision Thresholds and Ambiguity Tolerance

The analysis of decision thresholds used by BiomedCLIP and ChatGPT-4o points to significant differences in their approach to medical image classification, particularly regarding sensitivity in detection and prediction stability. BiomedCLIP appears to employ a stringent certainty threshold for classification, meaning it assigns labels only when the forecast meets a high criterion of reliability. This approach increases result stability and reduces the number of incorrect classifications, but it may also lead to reduced sensitivity in detecting less distinct radiographic structures [51]. Since BiomedCLIP has been fine-tuned to specialized medical datasets, its classification decisions are strongly dependent on previously learned patterns, which may limit its ability to adapt to new clinical cases and rare anomalies [52]. Conversely, ChatGPT-4o features a more flexible certainty threshold, which allows it to more effectively detect the presence of spinal stabilization systems, but also means its classifications may be less stable. As a generative model based on a probabilistic approach to image processing, GPT-4o tends to exhibit greater sensitivity in classification tasks, increasing the number of correct detections, but also making it more susceptible to erroneous identifications in cases of structurally similar objects [53]. This is because LLM models like GPT-4o apply a dynamic approach to classification decisions, where prediction is based on probability estimation and gradual alignment with the most likely category, which can lead to greater variability in results compared to deterministic models like BiomedCLIP [43]. Research on multimodal AI systems indicates that generalist language−visual models can achieve high effectiveness in detecting broad object categories, but lose precision when classification requires distinguishing fine differences between structures [38]. These findings underscore the critical role of selecting a certainty threshold in designing AI models for medical applications, and suggest that the effectiveness of image analysis systems can be optimized by combining the advantages of both specialist and generalist models.

4.7. Explaining the Results for H3: Effectiveness in Classifying the Type and Nature of Stabilization Systems

The findings for H3 suggest that ChatGPT-4o was highly effective at detecting the presence of stabilization systems, but struggled with detailed classification, whereas BiomedCLIP, despite lower overall detection rates, performed slightly better in differentiating between stabilization system types (Growing vs. Non-Growing) and specific systems (MCGR vs. PSF), albeit with suboptimal accuracy. Several factors likely contributed to these results.

4.8. BiomedCLIP's Dependence on Structured Feature Representations

BiomedCLIP features a structured approach to classification, enabling it to more accurately determine the type and structure of a spinal stabilization system once detected. Unlike general-purpose models such as ChatGPT-4o, BiomedCLIP employs a more logical and hierarchical classification scheme, which allows it to achieve a higher accuracy when differentiating between MCGR and PSF systems [42]. BiomedCLIP's lower implant detection accuracy likely results from its primary design focus on image-to-text matching, rather than direct object recognition. Research on multimodal AI systems shows that models integrating textual analysis perform better in structural classification and contextually demanding tasks, but struggle with object classification when the textual input component is absent [54]. In the context of medical classification, this may mean that BiomedCLIP is better suited for tasks where image analysis is supported by descriptive metadata, allowing it to more finely distinguish similar anatomical structures. In contrast, ChatGPT-4o relies mainly on visual patterns and more flexible heuristic classification, which enables it to effectively detect high-contrast objects, but may lead to greater variability in their subsequent classification. These differences highlight that while BiomedCLIP achieves greater accuracy in fine-grained classification after initial object detection, generative models like ChatGPT-4o may perform better in tasks requiring high-sensitivity detection, but with a greater risk of incorrect detailed classifications. This suggests that an optimal approach to medical image analysis might involve a hybrid application of both types of models—using a general model for structure detection and a specialized model like BiomedCLIP for precise hierarchical classification.

4.9. Difficulty in Differentiating Morphologically Similar Hardware

Spinal stabilization systems such as MCGR and PSF often exhibit significant visual convergence in posturographic X-ray images, especially when viewed from different angles or under varying contrast conditions. This structural similarity can pose a challenge for AI models like ChatGPT-4o, which largely base their classification decisions on shape heuristics rather than detailed morphological analysis. Research on radiological image interpretation shows that ChatGPT-4o often uses global visual features for decision-making, which can lead to erroneous classifications, especially when the analyzed objects exhibit significant visual similarity [55]. Similar limitations have been observed in other areas of medical diagnostics—for example, in zero-shot classification of lung diseases, where AI models struggled to identify unknown patterns without access to highly specialized datasets [56]. In contrast, multimodal models like BiomedCLIP may partially compensate for this issue by utilizing textual associations, which allows them to more precisely differentiate structures with a high degree of visual similarity. BiomedCLIP, fine-tuned based on large image–text pair datasets, likely uses contextual language connections to improve the hierarchical classification of stabilization systems, although its effectiveness remains limited due to inadequate coverage of these specific cases in training sets [57]. The literature has indicated that for diagnosing diseases with similar morphological progression, such as oral lichen planus, AI models, including ChatGPT-4o, struggled to differentiate subtle features of the disease without specialized training [58]. This points to a broader problem of generalist models, which despite high effectiveness in classifying structures with distinct contrast, may not perform equally well in tasks requiring detailed differentiation of similar objects.

4.10. ChatGPT-4o's Variability in Classification of Specific Systems

The inconsistency in classification observed with ChatGPT-4o stems from its probabilistic nature, which causes its results to vary between iterations, even if the initial detection of the stabilization system was correct. This issue is particularly evident in hierarchical classification tasks, where the model must first determine the general category of an object and then precisely assign it to a specific subtype. In the classification of spinal stabilization systems MCGR and PSF, it was noted that although ChatGPT-4o could effectively detect the presence of an implant, its decisions regarding the specific type of system were less consistent and showed significant variability across iterations [59]. This phenomenon has been widely documented in studies on transformer-based models, which often exhibit classification instability in tasks requiring the recognition of subtle structural differences [34].

In anatomical classification, where distinguishing minor morphological differences is necessary, AI based on probabilistic mechanisms often changes its predictions depending on subtle changes in input data, which makes their effectiveness in classifying detailed subtypes lower than in general categories. A similar problem was observed in studies on taxonomic classification, where generative models, such as TaxonGPT, struggled with transitioning from broad categories to more detailed subdivisions, leading to reduced accuracy in subtype classification [60].

In the context of medical image analysis, this means that while ChatGPT-4o achieves high effectiveness in recognizing high-contrast structures, its classification at a more detailed level is less predictable. An additional factor affecting result variability is how transformer-based models interpret visual features depending on input conditions and sampling strategies. Research shows that such AI may be prone to inaccuracies, especially if a given image lacks clear features enabling precise assignment to a specific subcategory [61].

In the classification of spinal stabilization systems, this means that while ChatGPT-4o may correctly detect an implant, its classification of the specific system type is more susceptible to fluctuations arising from contextual differences in image processing. This phenomenon suggests that models with a probabilistic architecture may require additional mechanisms to stabilize outcomes in tasks requiring consistent hierarchical classification, particularly in the context of medical diagnostics, where precision and repeatability of results are critical.

4.11. Clinical Implications of GPT-4o's Diagnostic Stability

The high stability of GPT-4o in detecting the presence of spinal stabilization systems across repeated analyses suggests important clinical implications. In particular, its consistent performance in binary classification tasks may support real-time decision-making in radiological triage, especially in resource-limited settings. Its ability to reliably identify the presence of metallic hardware could enhance workflows by pre-screening images for further specialist evaluation. While GPT-4o shows limitations in precise classification of hardware type, its robustness in identifying hardware presence highlights its potential as an effective support tool in early diagnostic pipelines or as a cross-verification step in clinical practice.

4.12. Analysis of BiomedCLIP Performance on Stabilization Classification

Initial evaluation of the BiomedCLIP model's performance indicates a moderate capability in differentiating between the presence and absence of spinal stabilization interventions. The model demonstrates reasonable accuracy when classifying images as either exhibiting evidence of stabilization or showing no such intervention. However, a significant performance degradation is observed when the task requires finer-grained classification, specifically distinguishing between different types of stabilization systems.

In scenarios requiring differentiation among specific stabilization methods, the model exhibits a pronounced bias towards selecting labels containing the term 'stabilization', irrespective of other relevant label components. This behavior suggests a potential issue related to the semantic weighting of the term 'stabilization' within the model's learned representations. The frequent occurrence of 'stabilization' in the training data, particularly in the context of the MCGR system (where the term is often used even when referring to alternative approaches), may have led to an overemphasis on this specific term. This creates an 'archetype effect', where the strong semantic association of 'stabilization' overshadows other, more nuanced, aspects of the image and label.

Furthermore, the use of negative labels, such as 'no stabilization', presents an additional challenge. Negation, while readily understood by humans, remains a significant difficulty for many machine learning models, particularly in natural language processing. One of the primary challenges arises from the complexity of negation scope detection, which affects tasks like sentiment analysis and text classification. Despite advancements in deep learning, accurately replicating human-like interpretations of negation remains an open problem [62]. The model may struggle to correctly interpret the negation of a concept ('stabilization') that has a strong, positive association in its training data. The inherent illogical nature—from the model's perspective—of negating a strongly established concept likely contributes to the observed misclassifications.

It is important to emphasize that BiomedCLIP was not specifically trained on radiographic datasets featuring spinal stabilization hardware. As an open-source model developed for broad biomedical image–text alignment, its training corpus did not explicitly include posturographic X-ray images with metallic implants such as MCGR or PSF systems. Therefore, this study aimed not to critique a misapplication of the model, but rather to explore its potential when applied to a complex diagnostic task outside its original design scope. The observed limitations in implant detection may stem from the model's lack of exposure to high-density artifacts commonly associated with surgical instrumentation, highlighting a broader challenge in transferring specialist AI models to new clinical domains without targeted fine-tuning. These findings underscore the necessity of dedicated retraining on implant-specific datasets if BiomedCLIP is to be effectively adapted for orthopedic diagnostics.

4.13. Study Limitations

This study has several limitations that should be considered when interpreting the results. First, although the dataset consisted of 270 posturographic X-ray images selected according to strict inclusion and exclusion criteria, the sample size remained relatively small compared to large-scale AI evaluation studies. The limited dataset may affect the generalizability of the findings, particularly regarding the AI models' ability to handle a broader range of anatomical variations, image quality discrepancies, and cases with atypical spinal deformities.

Second, while the study included a rigorous three-stage evaluation process for AI-based image interpretation, the methodology inherently relies on textual responses generated by ChatGPT-4o, which are subject to variability due to the model's probabilistic nature. This variability may not have been fully accounted for, even with repeated testing in this study. Future research should explore methods to quantify and mitigate variability in AI-generated responses to improve reproducibility.

Third, BiomedCLIP, although fine-tuned on the PMC-15 dataset, was not explicitly trained on pediatric posturographic spinal images, which could have influenced its performance in this domain. The model's reliance on text–image alignment suggests that its effectiveness may be enhanced with additional fine-tuning on a dataset specifically curated for pediatric scoliosis imaging. Additionally, the model's classification accuracy may have been impacted by the resolution and format of the X-ray images (JPEG, 2663 × 1277 px), as medical imaging AI models often benefit from higher-resolution DICOM formats that preserve more radiographic details.

Finally, the computational environment used for BiomedCLIP's training and evaluation, while standardized, may differ from real-world clinical deployment conditions. Factors such as processing power, inference time, and real-time interpretability were not extensively analyzed in this study. Future work should assess how these AI models perform in clinical workflows, considering integration challenges, latency, and model interpretability for radiologists and orthopedic specialists.

Another important consideration is the broader limitation of using open-source AI models in clinical settings. Although models like GPT-4o and BiomedCLIP are accessible and promote innovation, they lack regulatory approval, clinical validation, and task-specific fine-tuning. These factors may limit their reliability and trustworthiness in high-stakes diagnostic contexts. Moreover, open-source models often rely on general datasets that do not adequately represent specialized medical scenarios, such as pediatric spinal stabilization. This study contributes to addressing these gaps by highlighting specific strengths and weaknesses of such models in a controlled evaluation, offering a foundation for future refinement and clinical adaptation.

Despite these limitations, the study provides valuable insights into the comparative performance of ChatGPT-4o and BiomedCLIP in spinal stabilization system detection and classification. Future research should expand dataset diversity, explore additional AI fine-tuning strategies, and investigate clinical feasibility to enhance the practical application of AI-driven scoliosis assessment.

4.14. Future Directions for Model Validation and Improvement

To ensure clinical relevance and broader applicability, further validation of AI models for spinal stabilization system detection is essential. Future research should focus on fine-tuning models like BiomedCLIP using larger, multicenter datasets specifically curated for pediatric spinal imaging with surgical implants. Additionally, combining generalist and specialist models may enhance diagnostic accuracy. Prospective clinical testing and integration into radiology workflows will be key to evaluating the real-world utility and safety of such systems.

5. Conclusions

This study provides a comparative evaluation of ChatGPT-4o and BiomedCLIP in the detection and classification of spinal stabilization systems on pediatric posturographic X-ray images. The findings highlight key differences between these AI models in terms of detection accuracy, classification consistency, and interpretability in a clinical context.

ChatGPT-4o demonstrated a higher sensitivity in detecting the presence of a spinal stabilization system compared to BiomedCLIP. However, its probabilistic nature resulted in classification inconsistencies, particularly in distinguishing between MCGR and PSF stabilization systems. The model's reliance on general shape-based heuristics likely contributed to its misclassification of visually similar structures, reinforcing prior findings that generalist AI models may struggle with fine-grained medical classification tasks without extensive domain-specific training. Despite its high detection rate, ChatGPT-4o's variable responses across repeated trials indicate a need for stability-enhancing mechanisms in clinical applications.

In contrast, BiomedCLIP exhibited greater classification consistency, particularly in hierarchical differentiation between stabilization system types. Its structured classification approach, combined with its image–text alignment capability, allowed for more precise subtype identification once a system was detected. However, its lower sensitivity in initial detection suggests that its performance was limited by dataset constraints and its primary optimization for image–text retrieval rather than pure visual analysis. While BiomedCLIP demonstrated advantages in structured classification, its dependency on specialized training data underscores the importance of domain-specific fine-tuning for optimal medical AI performance.

The study also underscores broader challenges associated with AI-based radiological interpretation, including model variability, dataset limitations, and the need for standardized evaluation protocols. The differences observed between ChatGPT-4o and BiomedCLIP suggest that neither model, in its current state, offers a fully reliable standalone solution for automated scoliosis assessment. Instead, a hybrid approach—leveraging the detection sensitivity of generalist models like ChatGPT-4o and the classification consistency of specialized models like BiomedCLIP—may offer a more robust framework for AI-assisted spinal imaging analysis.

Future research should focus on expanding dataset diversity, refining AI training methodologies, and integrating multimodal AI models into clinical workflows to improve both detection accuracy and classification reliability. Additionally, exploring methods to enhance model interpretability and reduce response variability will be crucial for increasing the clinical trustworthiness of AI-assisted radiological assessments. Despite its limitations, this study provides valuable insights into the capabilities and challenges of AI models in pediatric spinal imaging, paving the way for further advancements in automated scoliosis evaluation.

Supplementary Materials: The following supporting information can be downloaded at: https://www.mdpi.com/article/10.3390/jcm14103282/s1, Table S1: Detailed detection levels and inter-rater agreement for GPT-4o in detecting spinal stabilization systems (SSS) in advanced scoliosis ($\geq 40°$) using posturographic radiographic images.

Author Contributions: Conceptualization, A.F., R.F. and A.Z.-F.; methodology, A.F., R.F., A.Z.-F. and B.P.; investigation, A.F., B.P., A.Z.-F. and R.F.; data curation, A.F., R.K. and B.P.; writing—original draft preparation, A.F., A.Z.-F., B.P., R.K. and R.F.; writing—review and editing, A.F., A.Z.-F., R.F.,

B.P., R.K. and E.N.; supervision, B.P. and E.N.; funding acquisition, A.F., E.N. and B.P. All authors have read and agreed to the published version of the manuscript.

Funding: This research received no external funding.

Institutional Review Board Statement: Ethical review and approval were waived for this study, due to the fact that the Bioethics Committee determined that the study does not meet the criteria of a medical experiment and therefore does not require ethical approval. This conclusion was provided in Opinion No. 58/2021 issued on 21 September 2021, by the Bioethics Committee, which explicitly stated that the study does not constitute a medical experiment under applicable regulations.

Informed Consent Statement: Not applicable.

Data Availability Statement: The data are contained within the article.

Acknowledgments: Many thanks are extended to Agnieszka Strzała for linguistic proofreading and to Robert Fabijan for the substantive support in the field of AI and for assistance in designing the presented study.

Conflicts of Interest: The authors declare no conflicts of interest.

References

1. Daeschler, S.C.; Bourget, M.H.; Derakhshan, D.; Sharma, V.; Asenov, S.I.; Gordon, T.; Cohen-Adad, J.; Borschel, G.H. Rapid, automated nerve histomorphometry through open-source artificial intelligence. *Sci. Rep.* **2022**, *12*, 5975. [CrossRef]
2. Hentschel, S.; Kobs, K.; Hotho, A. CLIP knows image aesthetics. *Front. Artif. Intell.* **2022**, *5*, 976235. [CrossRef] [PubMed]
3. Quazi, S. Artificial intelligence and machine learning in precision and genomic medicine. *Med. Oncol.* **2022**, *39*, 120. [CrossRef]
4. Takada, K. Artificial intelligence expert systems with neural network machine learning may assist decision-making for extractions in orthodontic treatment planning. *J. Evid. Based Dent. Pract.* **2016**, *16*, 190–192. [CrossRef] [PubMed]
5. Ahmed, Z.; Mohamed, K.; Zeeshan, S.; Dong, X. Artificial intelligence with multi-functional machine learning platform development for better healthcare and precision medicine. *Database* **2020**, *2020*, baaa010. [CrossRef] [PubMed]
6. Meier, J.-M.; Tschoellitsch, T. Artificial Intelligence and Machine Learning in Patient Blood Management: A Scoping Review. *Anesth. Analg.* **2022**, *135*, 524–531. [CrossRef]
7. Polis, B.; Zawadzka-Fabijan, A.; Fabijan, R.; Kosińska, R.; Nowosławska, E.; Fabijan, A. Exploring BiomedCLIP's Capabilities in Medical Image Analysis: A Focus on Scoliosis Detection and Severity Assessment. *Appl. Sci.* **2025**, *15*, 398. [CrossRef]
8. OpenAI. CLIP: Connecting Text and Images. Available online: https://openai.com/research/clip (accessed on 29 July 2024).
9. Li, Y.; Jia, S.; Song, G.; Wang, P.; Jia, F. SDA-CLIP: Surgical visual domain adaptation using video and text labels. *Quant. Imaging Med. Surg.* **2023**, *13*, 6989–7001. [CrossRef]
10. Yang, W.; Wang, Y.; Hu, J.; Yuan, T. Sleep CLIP: A Multimodal Sleep Staging Model Based on Sleep Signals and Sleep Staging Labels. *Sensors* **2023**, *23*, 7341. [CrossRef]
11. BiomedCLIP-PubMedBERT_256-vit_base_patch16_224. Available online: https://huggingface.co/microsoft/BiomedCLIP-PubMedBERT_256-vit_base_patch16_224 (accessed on 2 September 2024).
12. Suthar, P.-P.; Kounsal, A.; Chhetri, L.; Saini, D.; Dua, S.-G. Artificial Intelligence (AI) in Radiology: A Deep Dive Into ChatGPT 4.0's Accuracy with the American Journal of Neuroradiology's (AJNR) "Case of the Month". *Cureus* **2023**, *15*, e43958. [CrossRef]
13. Lee, K.-H.; Lee, R.-W.; Kwon, Y.-E. Validation of a Deep Learning Chest X-ray Interpretation Model: Integrating Large-Scale AI and Large Language Models for Comparative Analysis with ChatGPT. *Diagnostics* **2024**, *14*, 90. [CrossRef] [PubMed]
14. Sohail, S.-S. A Promising Start and Not a Panacea: ChatGPT's Early Impact and Potential in Medical Science and Biomedical Engineering Research. *Ann. Biomed. Eng.* **2023**, *52*, 1131–1135. [CrossRef]
15. Fabijan, A.; Zawadzka-Fabijan, A.; Fabijan, R.; Zakrzewski, K.; Nowosławska, E.; Polis, B. Artificial Intelligence in Medical Imaging: Analyzing the Performance of ChatGPT and Microsoft Bing in Scoliosis Detection and Cobb Angle Assessment. *Diagnostics* **2024**, *14*, 773. [CrossRef] [PubMed]
16. Maharathi, S.; Iyengar, R.; Chandrasekhar, P. Biomechanically designed Curve Specific Corrective Exercise for Adolescent Idiopathic Scoliosis gives significant outcomes in an Adult: A case report. *Front. Rehabil. Sci.* **2023**, *4*, 1127222. [CrossRef]
17. Yang, F.; He, Y.; Deng, Z.-S.; Yan, A. Improvement of automated image stitching system for DR X-ray images. *Comput. Biol. Med.* **2016**, *71*, 108–114. [CrossRef] [PubMed]
18. Hwang, Y.-S.; Lai, P.-L.; Tsai, H.-Y.; Kung, Y.C.; Lin, Y.Y.; He, R.J.; Wu, C.T. Radiation dose for pediatric scoliosis patients undergoing whole spine radiography: Effect of the radiographic length in an auto-stitching digital radiography system. *Eur. J. Radiol.* **2018**, *108*, 99–106. [CrossRef]

19. Patient examination AO Surgery Reference. Available online: https://surgeryreference.aofoundation.org/spine/deformities/adolescent-idiopathic-scoliosis/further-reading/patient-examination (accessed on 10 April 2024).
20. Pishnamaz, M.; Migliorini, F.; Blume, C.; Kobbe, P.; Trobisch, P.; Delbrück, H.; Hildebrand, F.; Herren, C. Long-term outcomes of spinal fusion in adolescent idiopathic scoliosis: A literature review. *Eur. J. Med. Res.* **2024**, *29*, 534. [CrossRef]
21. Maccaferri, B.; Vommaro, F.; Cini, C.; Filardo, G.; Boriani, L.; Gasbarrini, A. Surgical Treatment of Early-Onset Scoliosis: Traditional Growing Rod vs. Magnetically Controlled Growing Rod vs. Vertical Expandable Prosthesis Titanium Ribs. *J. Clin. Med.* **2024**, *14*, 177. [CrossRef]
22. Gwet, K.L. Computing inter-rater reliability and its variance in the presence of high agreement. *Br. J. Math. Stat. Psychol.* **2008**, *61*, 29–48. [CrossRef]
23. Gwet, K.L. *Handbook of Inter-Rater Reliability: The Definitive Guide to Measuring the Extent of Agreement Among Raters*; Advanced Analytics, LLC: Louisville, KY, USA, 2008.
24. Gwet, K.L. *Agreement Coefficients for Nominal and Ordinal Data*; Advanced Analytics, LLC: Louisville, KY, USA, 2014.
25. Wongpakaran, N.; Wongpakaran, T.; Wedding, D.; Gwet, K.L. A comparison of Cohen's Kappa and Gwet's AC1 when calculating inter-rater reliability coefficients: A study conducted with personality disorder samples. *BMC Med. Res. Methodol.* **2013**, *13*, 61. [CrossRef]
26. Gwet, K.L. irrCAC: Computing Chance-Corrected Agreement Coefficients (CAC). R Package Version 1.0, CRAN 2019. Available online: https://CRAN.R-project.org/package=irrCAC (accessed on 1 March 2025).
27. Makowski, D.; Lüdecke, D.; Patil, I.; Thériault, R.; Ben-Shachar, M.; Wiernik, B. Automated Results Reporting as a Practical Tool to Improve Reproducibility and Methodological Best Practices Adoption. CRAN 2023. Available online: https://easystats.github.io/report/ (accessed on 1 March 2025).
28. Pedersen, T. Patchwork: The Composer of Plots. R Package Version 1.2.0. 2024. Available online: https://CRAN.R-project.org/package=patchwork (accessed on 1 March 2025).
29. R Core Team. *R: A Language and Environment for Statistical Computing*; R Foundation for Statistical Computing: Vienna, Austria, 2021; Available online: https://www.R-project.org/ (accessed on 1 March 2025).
30. Sjoberg, D.; Whiting, K.; Curry, M.; Lavery, J.; Larmarange, J. Reproducible Summary Tables with the gtsummary Package. *R. J.* **2021**, *13*, 570–580. [CrossRef]
31. Wickham, H. *Ggplot2: Elegant Graphics for Data Analysis*; Springer: New York, NY, USA, 2016; ISBN 978-3-319-24277-4.
32. Hoopes, A.; Butoi, V.I.; Guttag, J.V.; Dalca, A.V. Voxelprompt: A Vision-Language Agent for Grounded Medical Image Analysis. *arXiv* **2024**, arXiv:2410.08397. Available online: https://arxiv.org/abs/2410.08397 (accessed on 6 March 2025). [CrossRef]
33. Awais, M.; Alharthi, A.H.S.A.; Kumar, A.; Cholakkal, H. AgroGPT: Efficient Agricultural Vision-Language Model with Expert Tuning. *arXiv* **2024**, arXiv:2410.08405. Available online: https://arxiv.org/abs/2410.08405 (accessed on 6 March 2025). [CrossRef]
34. Brodsky, V.; Ullah, E.; Bychkov, A. Generative Artificial Intelligence in Anatomic Pathology. *Arch. Pathol. Lab. Med.* **2025**, *149*, 298–318. Available online: https://meridian.allenpress.com/aplm/article/doi/10.5858/arpa.2024-0215-RA/505319 (accessed on 6 March 2025). [CrossRef]
35. Jegham, N.; Abdelatti, M.; Hendawi, A. Visual Reasoning Evaluation of Grok, Deepseek Janus, Gemini, Qwen, Mistral, and ChatGPT. *arXiv* **2025**, arXiv:2502.16428. Available online: https://arxiv.org/abs/2502.16428 (accessed on 6 March 2025). [CrossRef]
36. Koleilat, T.; Asgariandehkordi, H.; Rivaz, H. Medclip-samv2: Towards universal text-driven medical image segmentation. *arXiv* **2024**, arXiv:2409.19483. [CrossRef]
37. Neveditsin, N.; Lingras, P.; Mago, V. Clinical insights: A comprehensive review of language models in medicine. *arXiv* **2024**, arXiv:2408.11735. [CrossRef]
38. Soni, N.; Ora, M.; Agarwal, A.; Yang, T.; Bathla, G. A Review of The Opportunities and Challenges with Large Language Models in Radiology: The Road Ahead. *Am. J. Neuroradiol.* **2024**. [CrossRef]
39. Hartsock, I.; Rasool, G. Vision-language models for medical report generation and visual question answering: A review. *Front. Artif. Intell.* **2024**, *7*, 1430984. [CrossRef]
40. Liu, Y.; Cao, X.; Chen, T.; Jiang, Y.; You, J.; Wu, M. A Survey of Embodied AI in Healthcare: Techniques, Applications, and Opportunities. *arXiv* **2025**, arXiv:2501.07468. [CrossRef]
41. Buess, L.; Keicher, M.; Navab, N.; Maier, A. From large language models to multimodal AI: A scoping review on the potential of generative AI in medicine. *arXiv* **2025**, arXiv:2502.09242. [CrossRef]
42. Zhang, S.; Xu, Y.; Usuyama, N.; Xu, H.; Bagga, J.; Tinn, R. A multimodal biomedical foundation model trained from fifteen million image–text pairs. *NEJM AI* **2025**, *2*, AIoa2400640. [CrossRef]
43. Wang, C.; Li, M.; He, J.; Wang, Z.; Darzi, E.; Chen, Z. A survey for large language models in biomedicine. *arXiv* **2024**, arXiv:2409.00133. [CrossRef]
44. Li, Q.; Li, L.; Li, Y. Developing ChatGPT for biology and medicine: A complete review of biomedical question answering. *PMC* **2024**, *10*, 152. [CrossRef]

45. Chen, Z.; Pekis, A.; Brown, K. Advancing high resolution vision-language models in biomedicine. *arXiv* **2024**, arXiv:2406.09454. [CrossRef]
46. Chaves, J.M.Z.; Huang, S.C.; Xu, Y.; Xu, H. Towards a clinically accessible radiology foundation model: Open-access and lightweight, with automated evaluation. *arXiv* **2024**, arXiv:2403.08002. [CrossRef]
47. Bansal, H.; Israel, D.; Zhao, S.; Li, S.; Nguyen, T. MedMax: Mixed-Modal Instruction Tuning for Training Biomedical Assistants. *arXiv* **2024**, arXiv:2412.12661. [CrossRef]
48. Liang, X.; Wang, D.; Zhong, H.; Wang, Q.; Li, R.; Jia, R. Candidate-Heuristic In-Context Learning: A new framework for enhancing medical visual question answering with LLMs. *ScienceDirect* **2024**, *61*, 103805. [CrossRef]
49. Khan, W.; Leem, S.; See, K.B.; Wong, J.K.; Zhang, S.; Fang, R. A comprehensive survey of foundation models in medicine. *IEEE Rev Biomed Eng.* **2025**. [CrossRef]
50. Ikezogwo, W.O.; Zhang, K.; Seyfioglu, M.S. MedicalNarratives: Connecting Medical Vision and Language with Localized Narratives. *arXiv* **2025**, arXiv:2501.04184. [CrossRef]
51. Nie, Y.; He, S.; Bie, Y.; Wang, Y.; Chen, Z.; Yang, S. ConceptCLIP: Towards Trustworthy Medical AI via Concept-Enhanced Contrastive Language-Image Pre-training. *arXiv* **2025**, arXiv:2501.15579. [CrossRef]
52. Zheng, Q.; Zhao, W.; Wu, C.; Zhang, X.; Dai, L. Large-scale long-tailed disease diagnosis on radiology images. *Nat. Commun.* **2024**, *15*, 10147. [CrossRef] [PubMed]
53. Han, Y.; Liu, X.; Zhang, X.; Ding, C. Foundation Models in Electrocardiogram: A Review. *arXiv* **2024**, arXiv:2410.19877. [CrossRef]
54. Zhao, Z.; Liu, Y.; Wu, H.; Wang, M.; Li, Y.; Wang, S. CLIP in Medical Imaging: A Comprehensive Survey. *arXiv* **2023**, arXiv:2312.07353. Available online: https://arxiv.org/abs/2312.07353 (accessed on 6 March 2025). [CrossRef]
55. Lee, R.W.; Lee, K.H.; Yun, J.S.; Kim, M.S.; Choi, H.S. Comparative Analysis of M4CXR, an LLM-Based Chest X-Ray Report Generation Model, and ChatGPT in Radiological Interpretation. *J. Clin. Med.* **2024**, *13*, 7057. [CrossRef]
56. Wang, J.; Wang, T.; Xu, J.; Zhang, Z. Zero-Shot Diagnosis of Unseen Pulmonary Diseases via Spatial Domain Adaptive Correction and Guidance by ChatGPT-4o. In Proceedings of the2024 IEEE International Conference on Bioinformatics and Biomedicine (BIBM), Lisbon, Portugal, 3–6 December 2024; IEEE: Piscataway, NJ, USA, 2024. Available online: https://ieeexplore.ieee.org/abstract/document/10822114/ (accessed on 6 March 2025).
57. Gu, D.; Gao, Y.; Zhou, Y.; Zhou, M.; Metaxas, D. RadAlign: Advancing Radiology Report Generation with Vision-Language Concept Alignment. *arXiv* **2025**, arXiv:2501.07525. Available online: https://arxiv.org/abs/2501.07525 (accessed on 6 March 2025). [CrossRef]
58. Yu, S.; Sun, W.; Mi, D.; Jin, S.; Wu, X.; Xin, B.; Zhang, H. Artificial Intelligence Diagnosing of Oral Lichen Planus: A Comparative Study. *Bioengineering* **2024**, *11*, 1159. [CrossRef]
59. Ghanta, S.N.; Al"Aref, S.J.; Lala-Trinidade, A.; Nadkarni, G.N. Applications of ChatGPT in Heart Failure Prevention, Diagnosis, Management, and Research: A Narrative Review. *Diagnostics* **2024**, *14*, 2393. [CrossRef]
60. Huang, H.; Li, T.; Wang, Z.; Seldon, D.; Rodrigo, A. TaxonGPT: Taxonomic Classification Using Generative Artificial Intelligence. *bioRxiv*. 2024. Available online: https://www.biorxiv.org/content/10.1101/2024.10.28.618575 (accessed on 6 March 2025). [CrossRef]
61. Peng, B.; Chen, K.; Li, M.; Feng, P.; Bi, Z.; Liu, J. Securing Large Language Models: Addressing Bias, Misinformation, and Prompt Attacks. *arXiv* **2024**, arXiv:2409.08087. Available online: https://arxiv.org/abs/2409.08087 (accessed on 6 March 2025). [CrossRef]
62. Pröllochs, N.; Feuerriegel, S.; Lutz, B.; Neumann, D. Negation scope detection for sentiment analysis: A reinforcement learning framework for replicating human interpretations. *Inf. Sci.* **2020**, *512*, 1662–1676.

Journal of
Clinical Medicine

MDPI

Article

Public Perception of Robot-Assisted Spine Surgery

Luca Fumagalli [1,*], Alexandros Moniakis [1], Alberto Pagnamenta [2,3,4], Andrea Cardia [1] and Ivan Cabrilo [1]

1 Neurosurgery Department, Neurocenter of Southern Switzerland, Ente Ospedaliero Cantonale, 6900 Lugano, Switzerland; alexandros.moniakis@eoc.ch (A.M.); andrea.cardia@eoc.ch (A.C.); ivan.cabrilo@eoc.ch (I.C.)
2 Department of Intensive Care Medicine, Ospedale Regionale di Lugano, Ente Ospedaliero Cantonale, 6900 Lugano, Switzerland; alberto.pagnamenta@eoc.ch
3 Clinical Trial Unit, Ente Ospedaliero Cantonale, 6900 Lugano, Switzerland
4 Division of Pneumology, University Hospital of Geneva, 1205 Geneva, Switzerland
* Correspondence: luca.fumaga@gmail.com

Abstract

Background/Objectives: The potential advantages of robotic assistance in spinal procedures are a growing area of interest, and patient perception plays a key role in its broader acceptance. However, public perception of robotic surgery in spinal operations remains unexplored. This study aims to assess the general public's perceptions, expectations, and concerns regarding robot-assisted spine surgery. **Methods**: In the fall of 2024, a questionnaire was distributed to attendees at a public open day at the Neurocenter of Southern Switzerland, where the Globus ExcelsiusGPS™ spine surgery robot was demonstrated live on a mannequin. The 15-item questionnaire assessed demographic data, prior knowledge of medical robots, mental representations of surgical robots, expectations, and emotions after witnessing the demonstration. Data were analyzed using descriptive statistics, chi-square, Wilcoxon, McNemar tests, and logistic regression analysis. **Results**: A total of 109 questionnaires were collected. Most participants were female (64.4%) and had no direct experience with spinal pathology (79.8%). While 87.2% were aware of robotic surgery in general, only 65.1% specifically knew about its use in spine surgery. After witnessing the live demonstration, 81.9% felt reassured by the robot's presence in surgery, compared to 61.3% before the demonstration ($p = 0.007$). Preference for robot-assisted surgery increased from 50.5% to 64.5% ($p < 0.001$). Notably, individuals with back-related issues showed greater confidence in the robot's capabilities ($p = 0.032$). **Conclusions**: The general public perceives robotic spine surgery positively, viewing it as faster, more precise, and capable of performing tasks not readily performed by humans. The study highlights the importance of live demonstrations in enhancing trust and acceptance of robotic systems. Its findings have economic implications, as patients may be more likely to choose hospitals offering robot-assisted spine surgery. However, it is essential to also acknowledge alternative methods, such as computer-assisted navigation, which has demonstrated efficacy in spine surgery.

Keywords: spine surgery; robotic surgery; spinal instrumentation; navigation; enabling technology

1. Introduction

Advances in medical technology have reshaped modern healthcare, with robotics emerging as a novel innovation in various surgical disciplines, including spine surgery. Robot-assisted surgery aims to improve precision, reduce surgical invasiveness and recovery times, and thereby enhance surgical outcomes. Yet, the integration of robotic systems in the operating room has elicited mixed reactions from the general public, ranging from enthusiasm [1] to skepticism [2].

Media has been shown to influence people's perceptions of robots [3]. Science fiction books, movies, and television series often depict autonomous robots in dystopian contexts, triggering anxieties about machines replacing human control and decision-making. It can be assumed that these cultural representations contribute to public reluctance, as people project these fictional scenarios onto real-world technologies.

The transition from conventional freehand technique to robot-assisted spine surgery has unfolded over an extended period of time, progressively incorporating technological breakthroughs as they emerged. While freehand technique solely relies on surgeons' anatomical knowledge and experience to guide screw placement, the use of intraoperative radiography and subsequently fluoroscopy provided an initial form of image guidance for screw insertion from the 1970s to the present day [4]. The advent of computer-assisted 3-dimensional navigation marked a significant advancement by enabling real-time visualization without direct sight and enhancing the precision of screw placement [5]. Robotic systems became commercially available from the 2000s, offering pre-planned trajectories and automating key steps previously dependent on manual execution in an attempt to further reduce screw placement inaccuracy [6,7]. A recent web-based survey conducted in 2023 among AO Spine members found that less than half regularly used spinal navigation and that one-third had never used a spinal navigation system, while only 19% identified themselves as robotic users [8], highlighting that although there is an evolution in the development of these technologies and methods, they remain widely in contemporaneous use.

The adoption of robotic systems in spine surgery therefore remains relatively recent [9,10] when compared to other better known medical robots such as the da Vinci Surgical System (Intuitive Surgical, Sunnyvale, CA, USA), used in abdominal, urological, and gynecological surgery. Consequently, there is still only limited comprehensive data on the long-term outcomes of robotic spine surgery. While early clinical studies suggest positive results [7,11], the novelty of the technology and the lack of extensive application may contribute to uncertainty over its potential advantages. The perspective of spine surgeons has been surveyed in this regard and viewed as positively impacting surgical training and practice [12,13], but the expectations and concerns of the general public regarding robot-assisted spine surgery have not yet been explored. Although the adoption and use of novel technology is ultimately driven by its clinical utility, other factors may influence its integration, such as its costs, surgeons' willingness to adapt to new workflows, and patients' views, as their involvement in care and management decisions increases.

Given the rapid pace of technological advancement and its potential benefits in spine surgery [7], understanding public perceptions of robotic surgery systems is essential—and particularly how these perceptions are shaped by demographics and personal background and experience—to ensure the successful integration of these technologies into clinical practice [14]. The aim of this study, therefore, is to investigate public perception of robot-assisted spine surgery for the first time.

2. Materials and Methods

This article follows the "Strengthening the Reporting of Observational Studies in Epidemiology (STROBE) Statement" checklist [15].

ChatGPT (version 3.5) was solely used to assist in English language editing, after the manuscript had been completed. All content, including the interpretations of results and conclusions, was generated and reviewed by the Authors alone. No AI tool was used to generate scientific content, analyze data, or draw conclusions.

2.1. Questionnaire and Survey

In the fall of 2024, the Neurocenter of Southern Switzerland held an open day for the general public. During this event, the neurosurgery department conducted a demonstration of the Globus ExcelsiusGPS™ spine surgery robot. Participants had the opportunity to observe the robot in action, interact with spine surgeons and company representatives, and operate the robot firsthand on an anatomical training model. A model-based explanation was also provided to clarify how the procedure is typically performed without robotic assistance.

A questionnaire was distributed to explore the general public's knowledge, expectations, and concerns regarding the use of robots in spine surgery.

This 15-item questionnaire was divided into six sections: (1) demographic data; (2) prior knowledge of surgical robots; (3) mental representation of a surgical robot; (4) expectations of intraoperative robotic assistance; (5) emotions associated with its use prior to witnessing the robot demonstration; and (6) feedback after witnessing the robot demonstration. Questions 1–13 of the survey were filled out by participants before witnessing the robot demonstration, while questions 14–15 were filled out after, to capture participants' perceptions before and after exposure to the robotic system.

The initial draft was developed by the authors (L.F., A.M., and I.C.) based on expert input and iterative review. It was then evaluated by individuals from 5 different professional categories (1 neurosurgeon not involved in the study, 5 scrub nurses, 5 ward nurses, 5 medical secretaries, and 2 non-medical professionals) to assess its completeness, clarity, and ease of use. The final version of the questionnaire was revised based on the feedback received (Figure 1).

The data were collected anonymously and recorded in an Excel sheet for statistical analysis.

2.2. Statistical Analysis

Qualitative data were presented as absolute numbers with the corresponding percentages. The association between robot-specific random variables and subject-relevant variables was assessed using the chi-squared test. The impact of the robot's public presentation on concerns about its use in surgery and the choice of undergoing surgery in a robot-equipped hospital was estimated using the Wilcoxon test and the McNemar test, respectively. To identify potential predictors of the choice to undergo surgery in a robot-equipped hospital, univariable logistic regression analyses were performed.

All statistical tests were two-sided, and a p-value of <0.05 was considered statistically significant. Statistical analysis was performed using Stata version 17.0 software (StataCorp LP, College Station, TX, USA).

PERCEPTION OF ROBOTS IN SPINAL SURGERY

Participant Information

1	**Gender**			☐M		☐F	
2	**Age Range (years)**	☐18–25	☐26–35	☐36–50	☐51–65	☐66–80	☐>80
3	**Do you experience any back problems (regardless of whether they have been formally diagnosed by a doctor)?**			☐YES		☐NO	
4	**Have you ever undergone surgery to the spine?**			☐ YES		☐NO	
5	**Has anyone in your close circle (family, friends) had spinal surgery?**			☐ YES		☐NO	
6	**What is your profession?**			______________________			

Knowledge of Robots

7	**Are you aware of the existence of robots used in...**		
a	Surgery (in general)?	☐ YES	☐NO
b	Spinal surgery?	☐ YES	☐NO
8	If yes, how did you learn about it?	______________________	

Representation

9 **What shape do you think a surgical robot has?**______________________

10 **How big do you think it is?**

☐ Very small ☐ Human-sized ☐ Larger than a human

Expectations

11	**Do you think a robot... (1 = strongly disagree; 3 = strongly agree)**			
a	Is safer than a human?	1	2	3
b	Is faster than a human?	1	2	3
c	Is more precise than a human?	1	2	3
d	Is cleaner (fewer infections) than a human?	1	2	3
e	Can perform actions that a human cannot do?	1	2	3
f	Can make autonomous decisions?	1	2	3
g	Does not require the presence of a surgeon in the operating room?	1	2	3
h	Reduces the length of the hospital stay?	1	2	3
i	Increases the cost of surgery?	1	2	3

Emotions

12 **How does the idea of a robot participating in surgery make you feel?**

1	2	3
Worried	Indifferent	Reassured

13 **Would the presence of a robot in the operating theatre favour your choice of hospital?** ☐ YES ☐NO

Questions to answer after seeing the robot

14 **Now how does the idea of a robot participating in surgery make you feel?**

1	2	3
More worried	Indifferent	More reassured

15 **Now would the presence of a robot in the operating theatre favour your choice of hospital?"** ☐ YES ☐NO

Figure 1. Study questionnaire, translated into English from the original Italian. The layout and font were intentionally preserved to accurately reflect the survey as presented to participants.

3. Results

3.1. Demographics

A total of 109 questionnaires were collected. The responses are summarized in Table 1. Most participants were female (64.4%) and had no direct experience with spinal pathology: 79.8% reported no back problems, 96.3% had never undergone spine surgery, and 67.9% had no close acquaintances who had undergone spine surgery.

Table 1. Distribution of participants' responses to the questionnaire.

	n	%
Sex		
M	36	35.6
F	65	64.4
Age		
18–25	11	10.1
26–35	15	13.7
36–50	38	34.9
51–65	29	26.6
66–80	15	13.8
80+	1	0.9
Back problems		
Yes	22	20.2
No	87	79.8
Previous spine surgery		
Yes	4	3.7
No	104	96.3
Spine surgery in acquaintances		
Yes	34	32.1
No	72	67.9
Job		
Healthcare and social assistance	22	23.7
Business and finance	8	8.6
Education and academia	10	10.7
Hospitality and tourism	2	2.1
Construction and manual labor	13	14.0
Government and public administration	9	9.7
Science and research	1	1.1
Technology and engineering	3	3.2
Creative arts and media	1	1.1
Retired	24	25.8
Knowledge of robot in surgery (general)		
Yes	95	87.2
No	14	12.8
Knowledge of robot in spine surgery		
Yes	69	65.1
No	14	34.9
Source of information		
Media	41	55.4
Work-related	21	28.4
Acquaintances	12	16.2
Shape		
Robotic arm(s)	49	79.0
Computer box	1	1.6
Complex machinery	9	14.5
Other	3	4.9
Size		
Smaller than a human	28	26.7
Human-sized	48	45.7
Bigger than a human	29	27.6

Table 1. *Cont.*

	n	%
Expectations		
Safer		
1	7	6.6
2	65	61.3
3	34	32.1
Faster		
1	9	8.3
2	43	39.8
3	56	51.9
More precise		
1	5	4.6
2	27	25.0
3	76	70.4
Cleaner		
1	10	9.3
2	39	36.1
3	59	54.6
Gestures impossible for a human		
1	18	16.7
2	35	32.4
3	55	50.9
Autonomous decisions		
1	86	79.6
2	15	13.9
3	7	6.5
Independent		
1	91	84.3
2	11	10.2
3	6	5.6
Reduction in length of hospital stays		
1	20	18.5
2	43	39.8
3	45	41.7
Increased costs of surgery		
1	24	22.2
2	52	48.2
3	32	29.6
Before seeing robot		
Reassured by the presence of robot		
1	9	8.5
2	32	30.2
3	65	61.3
Choice of the hospital with robot		
Yes	54	50.5
No	53	49.5
After seeing robot		
Reassured by the presence of robot		
1	2	1.9
2	17	16.2
3	86	81.9
Choice of the hospital with robot		
Yes	69	64.5
No	38	35.5

Participants' occupations were categorized into the following fields: healthcare and social assistance, business and finance, education and academia, hospitality and tourism, construction and manual labor, government and public administration, science and research, technology and engineering, creative arts and media, and retired. The largest groups were retired individuals (25.8%) and healthcare workers (23.7%).

3.2. Knowledge, Expectations, and Concerns Regarding Robots in Spine Surgery

Most respondents were already aware of robotic technology in surgery: 87.2% knew about its general application in surgery, while 65.1% were specifically aware of its use in spine surgery. Participants' replies concerning how they learnt about robot-assisted spine surgery were categorized into the following fields: media, work-related, and acquaintances. The primary source of information was the media (55.4%).

Regarding the mental representation of the robot, most participants described it as having one or more robotic arms (79.0%) and being approximately human-sized (45.7%). However, a quarter of participants imagined it as smaller than a human (26.7%), while another quarter perceived it as larger than a human (27.6%).

In terms of expectations, compared to a surgeon, the robot was perceived as faster (51.9%), more precise (70.4%), cleaner (54.6%), and capable of performing movements impossible for a human (50.9%). However, the majority believed that the robot could not make autonomous decisions (79.6%) or perform surgery without a surgeon present in the operating room (84.3%), and 67.9% did not consider the surgical robot to be safer than a human surgeon.

Trust in the robot's capabilities was assessed before and after participants observed a live demonstration of the robotic spine system. Initially, 61.3% felt reassured by the presence of a robot during surgery, but this increased to 81.9% after the demonstration ($p = 0.007$). Similarly, before the demonstration, 50.5% stated they would prefer to be treated in a hospital using robotic systems for spinal surgery, rising to 64.5% afterward ($p < 0.001$).

Multivariable analysis found no significant association between sex, age, profession, and participants' mental image of a surgical robot (questions 7–10), expectations of robotic surgery (questions 11a–11i), or trust in robotic surgery before and after the demonstration (questions 12–15). However, individuals with back-related problems were more likely to believe that robots could perform movements impossible for a human ($p = 0.032$) and that robot-assisted surgeries were less expensive ($p = 0.036$). No significant association was found between past spinal surgeries and expectations of the robot.

4. Discussion

4.1. Key Findings

To the best of our knowledge, this study is the first to investigate public perception of robot-assisted spine surgery. Our findings indicate that while most participants were aware of robotic surgery in general, fewer knew about its specific application in spine surgery, with media being the primary source of information.

Regarding the mental representation of spine surgery robots, most participants envisioned them as having one or more robotic arms and being human-sized, though perceptions varied.

Participants generally viewed the robot as more precise, cleaner, and capable of complex—but not autonomous—movements compared to a human surgeon; however, most did not consider it necessarily safer. Trust in robot-assisted spine surgery significantly increased after witnessing a live demonstration, as did the preference for surgery in a hospital equipped with robotic systems.

Multivariable analysis found no significant associations between demographic factors or profession and expectations, but individuals with back problems were more likely to attribute unique capabilities to the robot.

4.2. Comparison with Other Studies on Public Perception of Robotic Systems in Healthcare

Although data on the general public's perception of robotic systems in spine surgery was previously lacking, a few studies—although limited in number—have explored public attitudes toward the introduction of robots in the medical field, revealing divergent views. Aymerich-Franch et al. [1] reported a generally positive attitude towards the implementation of robots in healthcare. Moreover, they found an association between female sex and religiousness with fear of robots. In contrast, our study did not observe a similar association between gender—or any other demographic factor—and expectations or concerns regarding robot-assisted spine surgery. Additionally, while our study did not assess the religiousness of our participants, it did examine their professions and found no association with expectations or emotions.

In contrast to Aymerich-Franch et al. [1], McDonnell et al. [2] found that the general public perceives robotic surgery as risky. The authors suggest that this perception may stem from the public's non-expert understanding of the modality, potentially triggering fears of increased complications. Our cohort did not significantly reflect such fears, as only 6.6% of participants strongly disagreed with the statement that the spine surgery robot is safer than a human surgeon, while 61.3% remained neutral and one-third actually considered the robot to be safer. Participants also attributed other positive characteristics to the robot: half believed it to be faster, cleaner, and capable of more complex movements than a human surgeon, while more than two-thirds felt that it was more precise. Additionally, a significant portion (41.7%) believed its use was associated with a reduction in the length of hospital stays.

The fact that the vast majority of participants did not perceive the robot as autonomous, while still recognizing the advantages stated above, suggests that it is viewed as a tool able to refine the surgeon's capabilities while remaining under human control. This is in line with findings of Aymerich-Franch et al. [1] that showed that public acceptance was higher for robots assisting a human rather than performing the role by itself.

In contrast, we found that individuals with back problems exhibited greater confidence in the robot, more often believing it could perform movements beyond human capability compared to participants without such issues—possibly due to dissatisfaction with available therapies for their chronic condition, leading to heightened expectations of emerging treatment modalities. They also assumed that robot-assisted surgery would be less expensive. This finding may again be explained by their elevated expectations of this novel technology, alongside their presumed increased awareness of healthcare costs, given that Swiss patients typically receive their medical bills directly and contribute personally up to a given threshold.

4.3. Implications

Although participants generally attributed positive baseline characteristics to the spine surgery robot, we observed that trust in the robot further increased after they viewed a live demonstration and interacted with it (61.3% before vs. 81.9% after, $p = 0.007$). Such interactions likely facilitate a better understanding of the robot's technical capabilities and advantages, while also defusing fearful misrepresentations. Furthermore, our findings suggest that opportunities to interact with the robot also positively influence participants' preference for hospitals offering robot-assisted surgery. This observation can be perceived as a marketing incentive for robot-naïve hospitals to acquire this technology, and for hospitals already equipped with a spine surgery robot to actively showcase it to the public. However, it also raises concerns about the impact of selective promotion in relation to other enabling technologies, such as non-robotic spinal navigation, which has demonstrated its clinical utility [5] and is reported to have an accuracy similar to that of robotic assistance [11]. Additionally, the overridingly critical role of surgical skill and decision-making may be overshadowed.

4.4. Study Strengths and Limitations

The questionnaire was developed through an iterative review process involving individuals with and without a healthcare background to ensure comprehensiveness and user-friendliness. To minimize hesitation in questions requiring a quantitative assessment of feelings, a three-item response scale was used instead of the five-item Likert scale, as non-experts may find it difficult to express varying degrees of opinions on such a specific topic.

Certain limitations should be considered when interpreting this study's findings. Firstly, while the decision to conduct this survey during an open day for the general public aimed to recruit a diverse and representative sample of the general population, the participant pool was relatively limited (N = 109) and may have been subject to a selection bias as attendees were likely predisposed to an interest in our Neurocenter and may not reflect broader public perspectives. Although the event was open to the general public, a significant portion of participants (23.7%) worked in healthcare, and the largest group (25.8%) was retired. This suggests that younger individuals may have been less inclined to attend, potentially limiting the generalizability of our results across broader age demographics. Additionally, participants' education level may also affect generalizability. While we had initially intended to investigate the influence of education level, we decided to collect profession data as a surrogate to avoid making participants feel uncomfortable with potentially intrusive questions. We found that profession was not significantly associated with participants' representations of the surgical robot, or with their trust in the robotic system before and after the demonstration. However, one-quarter of participants reported being "retired" without specifying their previous profession, which limits the analysis.

Furthermore, age was surveyed as a categorical rather than a continuous variable to classify participants by generation and reduce potential discomfort in disclosing their exact age.

The results of this survey provide insights into the perception of robot assistance in spine surgery. However, larger studies are needed to confirm the present findings. Notably, our study suggests that the availability of a spinal robot may positively influence patients' choice of hospital for undergoing surgery. However, this may also lead to diminished consideration of alternative methods, such as computer-assisted navigation, despite their demonstrated efficacy in pedicle screw placement.

5. Conclusions

Spine surgery is a rapidly evolving field driven by technological advancements, and the adoption of surgical robots is a key consideration for both surgeons and hospital administrators, who must weigh the benefits of this technology against its high costs, in the presence of already well-established and effective alternatives such as computer-assisted navigation. Patient perception also plays a crucial role in this process; yet, to our knowledge, this is the first such study in the context of robot-assisted spine surgery.

This study suggests that the general population holds a positive attitude toward this technology, viewing robots as faster, more precise, cleaner, and capable of performing movements beyond human ability. We found that people felt reassured by the presence of a robot in the operating theater, and this confidence was further strengthened after witnessing the robot in action. Moreover, after a live demonstration of the spinal robot, participants expressed a preference for treatment in a hospital that uses this technology over one that has not implemented it. This finding has economic implications for hospitals and also highlights the importance of exposing the general public to live demonstrations of new surgical technologies for reassurance in the face of novelty, while also prompting necessary reflection on the influence of patient perception bias on decision-making and the need to maintain a critical perspective on the benefits of new surgical techniques to mitigate that bias.

Author Contributions: Conceptualization, I.C., L.F. and A.M.; methodology, I.C., L.F., A.M. and A.P.; software, A.P.; validation, I.C. and A.C.; formal analysis, I.C., L.F., A.M. and A.P.; investigation, I.C., L.F., and A.M.; data curation, I.C., L.F. and A.M.; writing—original draft preparation, L.F., I.C. and A.M.; writing—review and editing, I.C., L.F., A.M., A.P. and A.C. All authors have read and agreed to the published version of the manuscript.

Funding: This research received no external funding.

Institutional Review Board Statement: Ethical approval was not required for this study as it involved an anonymous survey with voluntary participation and no sensitive data collection.

Informed Consent Statement: Patient consent was waived due to the nature of the study, which consisted of a survey. Attendees at the demonstration of the surgical robot were informed that the survey was intended for research purposes and could choose whether to participate.

Data Availability Statement: The raw data supporting the conclusions of this article will be made available by the authors on request.

Acknowledgments: ChatGPT (version 3.5) was solely used to assist in English language editing, after the manuscript had been completed. All content, including the interpretations of results and conclusions, was generated and reviewed by the Authors alone. No AI tool was used to generate scientific content, analyze data, or draw conclusions.

Conflicts of Interest: The authors declare no conflicts of interest.

References

1. Aymerich-Franch, L.; Gómez, E. Public Perception of Socially Assistive Robots for Healthcare in the EU: A Large-Scale Survey. *Comput. Hum. Behav. Rep.* **2024**, *15*, 100465. [CrossRef] [PubMed]
2. McDonnell, C.; Devine, M.; Kavanagh, D. The General Public's Perception of Robotic Surgery—A Scoping Review. *Surgeon* **2024**, *23*, e49–e62. [CrossRef] [PubMed]
3. Savela, N.; Turja, T.; Latikka, R.; Oksanen, A. Media Effects on the Perceptions of Robots. *Hum. Behav. Emerg. Technol.* **2021**, *3*, 989–1003. [CrossRef]
4. Wilson, J.P.; Fontenot, L.; Stewart, C.; Kumbhare, D.; Guthikonda, B.; Hoang, S. Image-Guided Navigation in Spine Surgery: From Historical Developments to Future Perspectives. *J. Clin. Med.* **2024**, *13*, 2036. [CrossRef] [PubMed]
5. Kosmopoulos, V.; Schizas, C. Pedicle Screw Placement Accuracy: A Meta-Analysis. *Spine* **2007**, *32*, E111–E120. [CrossRef] [PubMed]
6. Gajjar, A.A.; Le, A.H.D.; Lavadi, R.S.; Boddeti, U.; Barpujari, A.; Abou-Al-Shaar, H.; Agarwal, N. Evolution of Robotics in Spine Surgery: A Historical Perspective. *Interdiscip. Neurosurg.* **2023**, *33*, 101721. [CrossRef]
7. D'Souza, M.; Gendreau, J.; Feng, A.; Kim, L.H.; Ho, A.L.; Veeravagu, A. Robotic-Assisted Spine Surgery: History, Efficacy, Cost, And Future Trends. *Robot. Surg. Res. Rev.* **2019**, *6*, 9–23. [CrossRef] [PubMed]
8. Motov, S.; Butenschoen, V.M.; Krauss, P.E.; Veeravagu, A.; Yoo, K.H.; Stengel, F.C.; Hejrati, N.; Stienen, M.N. Current State and Future Perspectives of Spinal Navigation and Robotics-an AO Spine Survey. *Brain Spine* **2025**, *5*, 104165. [CrossRef] [PubMed]
9. Pham, M.H.; Brown, N.J. Evolution of Robotic Spine Surgery Technologies. *Neurosurgery* **2025**, *96*, S75–S83. [CrossRef] [PubMed]
10. Satin, A.M.; Kisinde, S.; Lieberman, I.H. Can Robotic Spine Surgery Become the Standard of Care? *Int. J. Spine Surg.* **2022**, *16*, S44–S49. [CrossRef] [PubMed]
11. Shafi, K.A.; Pompeu, Y.A.; Vaishnav, A.S.; Mai, E.; Sivaganesan, A.; Shahi, P.; Qureshi, S.A. Does Robot-Assisted Navigation Influence Pedicle Screw Selection and Accuracy in Minimally Invasive Spine Surgery? *Neurosurg. Focus* **2022**, *52*, E4. [CrossRef] [PubMed]
12. Shahi, P.; Subramanian, T.; Singh, S.; Sheha, E.; Dowdell, J.; Qureshi, S.A.; Iyer, S. Perception of Robotics and Navigation by Spine Fellows and Early Attendings: The Impact of These Technologies on Their Training and Practice. *World Neurosurg.* **2024**, *181*, e330–e338. [CrossRef] [PubMed]

13. Liounakos, J.I.; Chenin, L.; Theodore, N.; Wang, M.Y. Robotics in Spine Surgery and Spine Surgery Training. *Oper. Neurosurg.* **2021**, *21*, 35–40. [CrossRef] [PubMed]
14. AlQudah, A.A.; Al-Emran, M.; Shaalan, K. Technology Acceptance in Healthcare: A Systematic Review. *Appl. Sci.* **2021**, *11*, 10537. [CrossRef]
15. Vandenbroucke, J.P.; von Elm, E.; Altman, D.G.; Gøtzsche, P.C.; Mulrow, C.D.; Pocock, S.J.; Poole, C.; Schlesselman, J.J.; Egger, M. Strengthening the Reporting of Observational Studies in Epidemiology (STROBE): Explanation and Elaboration. *Int. J. Surg.* **2014**, *12*, 1500–1524. [CrossRef] [PubMed]

Journal of
Clinical Medicine

MDPI

Article

Vertebral Body Morphology in Neuromuscular Scoliosis with Spastic Quadriplegic Cerebral Palsy

Göker Utku Değer [1], Heon Jung Park [2], Kyeong-Hyeon Park [2], Hoon Park [3], Mohammed Salman Alhassan [2], Hyun Woo Kim [2] and Kun-Bo Park [2,*]

1 Department of Orthopedics and Traumatology, Beykoz State Hospital, Istanbul 34800, Türkiye; gokerdeger@hotmail.com
2 Division of Pediatric Orthopedic Surgery, Severance Children's Hospital, Yonsei University College of Medicine, Seoul 03722, Republic of Korea; ryan0912@naver.com (H.J.P.); ospkh@yuhs.ac (K.-H.P.); drmsalhassan@gmail.com (M.S.A.); pedhkim@yuhs.ac (H.W.K.)
3 Department of Orthopedic Surgery, Gangnam Severance Hospital, Yonsei University College of Medicine, Seoul 06273, Republic of Korea; hoondeng@yuhs.ac
* Correspondence: pedoskbp@yuhs.ac; Tel.: +82-2-2228-2180

Abstract: Background/Objectives: The distorted vertebral body has been studied in scoliosis; however, there is little knowledge about the difference between neuromuscular and idiopathic scoliosis. This study aimed to investigate the vertebral body morphology in patients with spastic quadriplegic cerebral palsy and scoliosis (CP scoliosis) and compare them with those of apex- and Cobb angle-matched patients with adolescent idiopathic scoliosis (AIS). **Methods**: Thirty-four patients with CP scoliosis and thirty-two patients with AIS were included. The pedicle diameter, chord length, and vertebral body rotation were evaluated at one level above the apex, one level below the apex, and at the apex using a reconstructed computed tomography scan. The apex of the curve and Cobb angle were too diverse between patients with CP scoliosis or AIS. Eighteen patients were matched in each group according to the apex and Cobb angle (within 5-degree differences) of the major curve, and compared between matched groups (mCPscoliosis vs. mAIS). **Results**: In the comparison of the apex and Cobb angle-matched groups, there was no statistical difference in the Cobb angle between mCPscoliosis (80.7 ± 13.8 degrees) and mAIS (78.6 ± 13.6 degrees, p = 0.426), and the vertebral body rotation (25.4 ± 15.4° in mCPscoliosis vs. 24.4 ± 6.5° in mAIS, p = 0.594). There was no difference in the pedicle diameters of either the convex (3.6 ± 1.1 mm in mCPscoliosis vs. 3.3 ± 1.2 mm in mAIS, p = 0.24) or concave side (3.1 ± 1.2 mm in mCPscoliosis vs. 2.7 ± 1.6 mm in mAIS, p = 0.127). However, the patients in the mCPscoliosis group were younger (12.7 ± 2.5 years vs. 14.6 ± 2.4 years, p = 0.001), and the chord length was shorter on the convex (38.0 ± 5.0 mm vs. 40.4 ± 4.9 mm, p = 0.025) and concave (37.7 ± 5.2 mm vs. 40.3 ± 4.7 mm, p = 0.014) sides compared with those of the mAIS group. **Conclusions**: With a similar apex and Cobb angle, the vertebral body rotation and pedicle diameter in patients with CP scoliosis were comparable to those with AIS; however, the chord length was shorter in CP scoliosis. For the selection of the pedicle screw in CP scoliosis, the length of the pedicle screw should be more considered than the diameter.

Keywords: pedicle; vertebral body; neuromuscular scoliosis; idiopathic scoliosis; cerebral palsy

1. Introduction

Scoliosis is defined as a coronal plane deformity of more than 10 degrees in the spine; however, it is a three-dimensional deformity that includes vertebral body rotation (VBR). A pedicle screw is inserted during scoliosis correction to fix all three columns and achieve sufficient correction through rod derotation, distraction, compression, and direct vertebral body rotation. Pedicle morphology must be clarified to insert the pedicle screws correctly and avoid complications. Many previous studies investigating idiopathic scoliosis involving an examination of altered pedicle morphology and the determination of the safe limits for pedicle screw applications have been performed [1–3]. In these reports, the concave-side pedicle diameter (PD) was narrower, and VBR was severe around the curved apex [4,5]. It is believed that the conditions in neuromuscular scoliosis may be similar, but the differences or similarities between neuromuscular and idiopathic scoliosis have not yet been comprehensively studied.

The Cobb angle at the time of diagnosis or operation is usually larger for neuromuscular scoliosis, and progression is more rapid than for idiopathic scoliosis. A greater-than-40-degree Cobb angle was detected in almost 40% of cerebral palsy patients (GMFCS III–V) at a mean age of 11 years, and the prevalence reached 62% in patients with non-ambulatory cerebral palsy (CP) [6]. Additionally, the highest complication rates after scoliosis surgery in patients with CP were reported, reaching up to 17% [7,8]. There are many reasons for the high complication rate, such as poor oral intake, seizure, cardiopulmonary problems, and severe curves. One of the important factors related to the complications in scoliosis with CP may be the severely distorted vertebral body at high degrees of Cobb angle. It is even more important to understand the severely distorted pedicle morphology in scoliosis with CP because scoliosis correction techniques have evolved with advances in pedicle screw instrumentation [9–12].

Several previous studies examined the vertebral morphology of neuromuscular scoliosis cases only in diverse disease groups with neurofibromatosis, spinal muscular atrophy, Chiari malformation, or a small number of mixed diagnosed groups [13–17]. No comprehensive study has yet examined pedicle morphology in only patients with spastic quadriplegic cerebral palsy and scoliosis. Furthermore, there have been few reports about the comparison of vertebral body morphology between the different disease entities. In the present study, we selected only spastic quadriplegic cerebral palsy scoliosis (CP scoliosis) and compared the altered vertebral morphology with that of adolescent idiopathic scoliosis.

Among the various forms of neuromuscular scoliosis, patients with CP scoliosis are usually non-ambulatory, the curve magnitude is severe, and the onset is very young; hence, osteoporosis may be common, and the vertebral body would be skeletally immature. We hypothesized that the vertebral body rotation and pedicle morphology in CP scoliosis may differ from adolescent idiopathic scoliosis (AIS). However, the prerequisite for comparing different etiologies is that the curve character should at least be similar between groups. In the present study, we (1) evaluated VBR and pedicle morphology in non-ambulatory patients with CP scoliosis or patients with AIS and (2) compared those parameters between patient groups of CP scoliosis and AIS with apex and Cobb angle-matches of the major curve, using reconstructed computed tomography (CT) images.

2. Materials and Methods

2.1. Patient Selection

This retrospective study was approved by the Yonsei University Health System, Severance Hospital, Institutional Review Board (approval number: 4-2022-0937), and was conducted in accordance with the Declaration of Helsinki 2013. Informed consent waiver was obtained from the Institutional Review Board. The primary outcome of this study was to compare pedicle width between CP scoliosis and AIS. While there has not been a similar study, we found some pedicle diameter data in previous research [17]. The pedicle width was 4.7 ± 1.0 mm for CP and 4.2 ± 0.9 mm for AIS between T8 and L3, the common apex of scoliosis. Based on this data, we calculated a sample size of 33 with a type I error of 0.05 and a power of 0.9 for each group.

Among all patients who underwent surgery for scoliosis in our clinic between 2019 and 2022, the data of those with available reconstructed CT images for surgery planning were extracted. Of the 129 patients who met these criteria, 76 were found to have neuromuscular scoliosis, and 35 were diagnosed with idiopathic scoliosis. Eighteen patients with congenital or syndromic scoliosis were excluded.

Forty-one patients were diagnosed with cerebral palsy and neuromuscular scoliosis. We excluded four patients who were older than 18 years, had undergone previous spine operations, or were independent ambulators. In 35 patients with idiopathic scoliosis, 3 patients were excluded because of spondylolytic spondylolisthesis, previous sternum operation, or being over 18 years old. Finally, 34 patients with spastic quadriplegic cerebral palsy and scoliosis (CP scoliosis) and 32 patients with adolescent idiopathic scoliosis (AIS) were enrolled in the study (Figure 1).

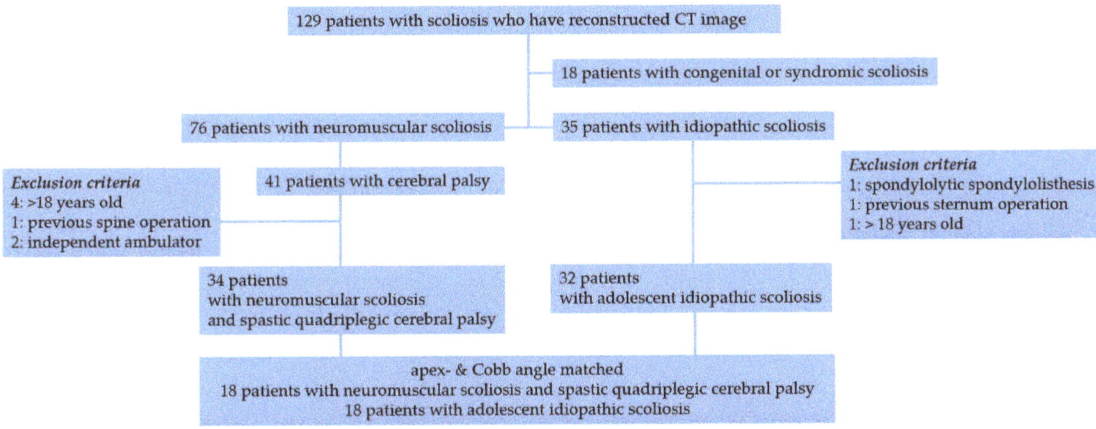

Figure 1. Flow diagram of the inclusion and exclusion process.

Many patients with AIS had smaller Cobb angles than those with CP scoliosis, and the apex in AIS was usually the middle of the thoracic spine. The apices of CP scoliosis were T8 (1), T9 (4), T10 (4), T11 (3), T12 (8), L1 (3), L2 (4), L3 (7), but those of AIS were T7 (3), T8 (4), T9 (7), T10 (5), T11 (2), T12 (4), L1 (2), L2 (4), and L3 (1). Because the vertebral body between thoracic and lumbar is different, the comparison of the vertebral body morphology should be performed at the same level. Additionally, the severity of Cobb angle may affect to the vertebral body morphology. We collected patients with same apex of the major curve and a similar major Cobb angle within 5-degree differences in both groups.

Comparison to find the difference in vertebral body morphology between CP scoliosis and AIS was performed using data for each of the 18 patients with CP scoliosis (mCPscoliosis) and AIS (mAIS) matched for apex and Cobb angle (within 5-degree differences) of the major curve. The matched apices were T8 (1), T9 (2), T10 (4), T11 (2), T12 (3), L1 (2), L2 (3), and L3 (1).

2.2. Radiographic Measurements and Reconstruction of CT Images

All patients had a whole spine posteroanterior and lateral view radiographs taken in the preoperative evaluation. Cobb angle measurements were taken from whole spine posteroanterior radiographs obtained in the sitting position for CP scoliosis and standing position for AIS using the line parallel to the upper endplate of the uppermost end vertebra and the lower endplate of the lowermost end vertebra. The curve's apex was defined as where the curvature is most pronounced or severe. If the disc was the apex in CP scoliosis, the above or below vertebra of AIS was defined as the apex for the matching.

CT scans were performed from the T1 to the S1 vertebrae with the patient in the supine position using SOMATOM (Siemens Healthineers, Erlangen, Germany). The resulting CT images were reconstructed using Syngo.via VB40 software (Siemens Healthineers, Erlangen, Germany). The image contrast levels were standardized for clear soft tissue and bone demarcation at the vertebral pedicles. The relevant vertebral body was identified by counting upward from the sacrum and confirmed by counting the rib levels superiorly and inferiorly. From the reconstructed sagittal and coronal images, a transverse image parallel to the endplate plane in both the sagittal and coronal plane was reconstructed at the center of the pedicle. When the superior and inferior endplate planes were not parallel owing to vertebral wedging, an orientation approximately halfway between (i.e., bisecting) the two endplate inclinations was selected [18,19].

In total, 102 vertebrae with CP scoliosis and 96 vertebrae with AIS were measured. Pedicle diameter (PD), chord length (CL), and vertebral body rotation (VBR) were evaluated one level above the apex, one level below the apex, and at the apex using a reconstructed CT scan [14,17–19]. PD was measured in the isthmus region, where the medial and lateral middle cortical borders were the narrowest. The CL was measured as the distance between the posterior cortical entry point of the pedicle and the anterior vertebral cortex in line with the axis of the pedicle. VBR was measured as the angle between the vertical line and the line that bisects the vertebral body (Figure 2). Additionally, the presence of neurocentral synchondroses was investigated (Figure 3) [20,21].

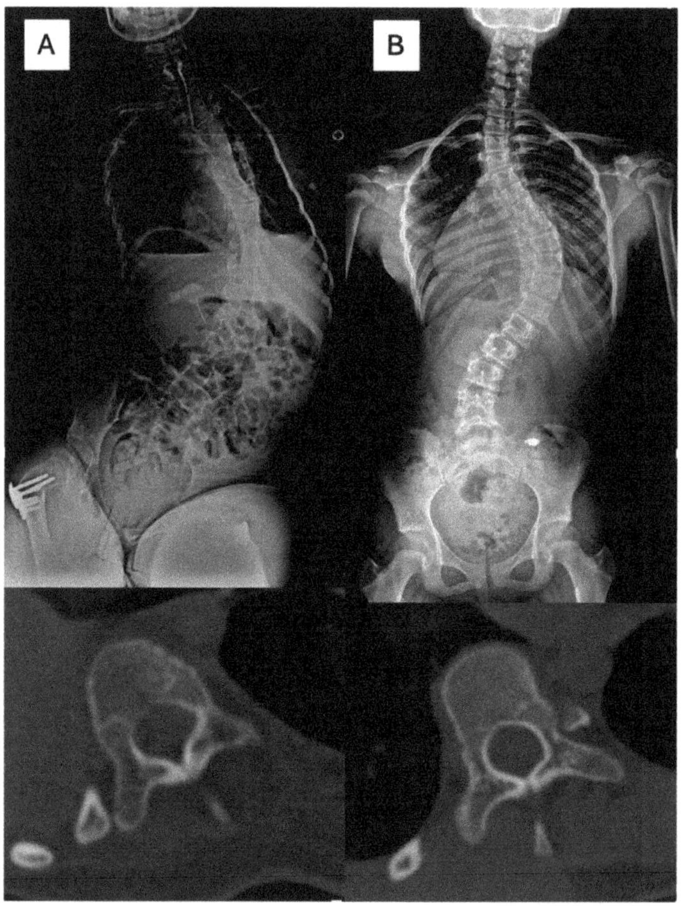

Figure 2. (**A**) A female aged 10 years and 7 months had neuromuscular scoliosis with spastic quadriplegic cerebral palsy. The Cobb angle between T6 and L4 was 79 degrees, and the apex was T10 (CT). The pedicle diameter and chord length were 3.2 and 24.9 mm at the concave side, and 4.8 and 29 mm at the convex side. (**B**) An 11 years, 6 months old female was diagnosed with adolescent idiopathic scoliosis with a Cobb angle of 74 degrees (T7-L1) and apex at T10 (CT). The pedicle diameter and chord length were 3.9 and 37.5 mm at the concave side, and 4.8 and 39 mm at the convex side.

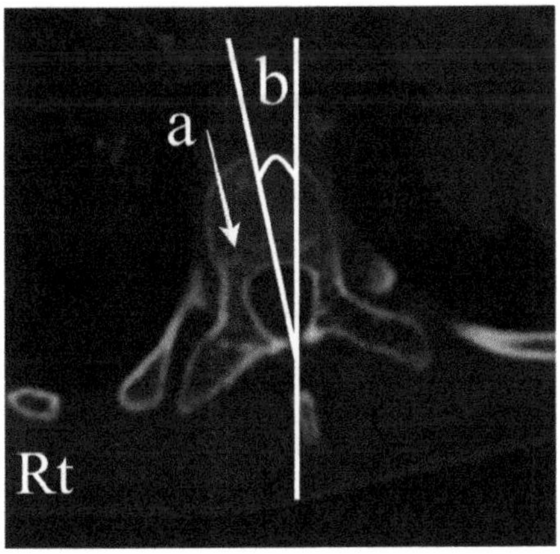

Figure 3. Exemplar vertebra with neurocentral synchondrosis (a) and a vertebral body rotation toward the right side (b).

2.3. Statistical Analyses

All statistical analyses were performed using SPSS version 25.0 (IBM Corp., Armonk, NY, USA), and $p < 0.05$ was considered statistically significant. Data were assessed for normality using the Shapiro–Wilk test. Paired t-test or independent t-tests were used to compare continuous variables between the convex and concave sides of the CP scoliosis or AIS, and between VBR, PD, and CL of the apex- and Cobb angle-matched groups (mCPscoliosis vs. mAIS). The chi-square test and Fisher's exact test were used to compare categorical variables according to expected values. Among the radiographic parameters, VBR, PD, and CL at the apex of matched groups were measured again by experienced orthopedic surgeons to estimate interobserver reliability. The intraclass correlation coefficient to define interobserver reliability was calculated as 0.982 (0.964–0.991) for VBR, 0.910 (0.857–0.944) for PD, and 0.777 (0.645–0.860) for CL.

3. Results

3.1. Patient Characteristics

The mean age at the time of surgery for CP scoliosis was 14 years and 2 months (range, 10–18 years). Fifteen patients were male, and 19 patients were female. The mean height and weight were 138.3 ± 14.5 cm (108–173 cm) and 30.1 ± 11.5 kg (15–62 kg), respectively. Thirteen patients were classified as Gross Motor Function Classification System (GMFCS) IV and 21 patients as GMFCS V. Twenty-one patients had dislocated hips and 19 patients had undergone reconstruction operations. The mean age of the AIS patients was 14 years and 7 months (range, 11–18 years). One patient was male and 31 patients were female. The mean height and weight were 154.5 ± 8.95 cm (127–170 cm) and 46.3 ± 9.8 kg (28–83 kg), respectively.

3.2. Comparison Between the Convex and Concave Side in Patients with CP Scoliosis

The average Cobb angle of the main curve was 87.7 ± 18.7°, and T12 was the most common apex of the curve. Neurocentral synchondrosis was noted in 55.8% (19/34) of the patients. Left thoracic curve was noted in 32.4% (11/34) of patients, and the average VBR was 29.9 ± 14.6°. The PD of the convex side (4.0 ± 1.5 mm) was larger than that of the concave side (3.6 ± 1.4 mm, p = 0.001). The chord length (CL) of the convex side (39.2 ± 5.0 mm) and concave side (39.0 ± 5.5 mm) showed no statistically significant differences (p = 0.550).

3.3. Comparison Between the Convex and Concave Side in Patients with AIS

The average Cobb angle of the main curve was 68.2 ± 18.8°, and T9 was the most common apex of the curve. Neurocentral synchondrosis was noted in 6.3% (2/32) of the patients. All patients had a right thoracic curve, and the average VBR was 18.7 ± 9.7°. The PD of the convex side (3.4 ± 1.2 mm) was larger than that of the concave side (2.6 ± 1.5 mm, $p < 0.001$). The chord length (CL) of the convex side (38.6 ± 5.9 mm) and concave side (39.4 ± 5.6 mm) showed no statistically significant differences ($p = 0.414$).

3.4. Comparison of Apex- and Cobb Angle-Matched Patients with CP Scoliosis and AIS

The average Cobb angles were 80.7 ± 13.8 degrees and 78.6 ± 13.6 degrees in the matched CP scoliosis (mCPscoliosis) and AIS (mAIS) groups ($p = 0.426$). The average age was younger in the mCPscoliosis (12.7 ± 2.5 years) than the mAIS (14.6 ± 2.4 years, $p = 0.001$). In mCPscoliosis, males were predominant, while the height and weight were greater in m AIS.

There was no difference between the two groups in terms of VBR (25.4 ± 15.4° in mCPscoliosis vs. 24.4 ± 6.5° in mAIS, $p = 0.594$) or PD in either the convex (3.6 ± 1.1 mm in mCPscoliosis vs. 3.3 ± 1.2 mm in mAIS, p=0.24) or concave side (3.1 ± 1.2 mm in mCPscoliosis vs. 2.7 ± 1.6 mm in mAIS, $p = 0.127$). However, the CL of the mCPscoliosis was significantly shorter than the mAIS in both the convex side (38.0 ± 5.0 mm in mCPscoliosis vs. 40.4 ± 4.9 mm in mAIS, $p = 0.025$) and concave side (37.7 ± 5.2 mm in mCPscoliosis vs. 40.3 ± 4.7 mm in mAIS, $p = 0.014$) (Table 1).

Table 1. Comparison of vertebral body morphology between Cobb angle- and apex-matched patients with spastic quadriplegic cerebral palsy and scoliosis (mCPscoliosis) and adolescent patients with idiopathic scoliosis (mAIS).

	mCPscoliosis	mAIS	*p* Value
Cobb angle (degree)	80.7 ± 13.8	78.6 ± 13.6	0.426
Age * (years)	12.7 ± 2.5	14.6 ± 2.4	0.001
Sex (M:F)	7:11	1:17	<0.001
Height * (cm)	140.3 ± 16.5	152.9 ± 8.6	<0.001
Weight * (kg)	30.7 ± 13.2	43.1 ± 7.4	<0.001
Vertebral body rotation (degree)	25.4 ± 15.4	24.4 ± 6.5	0.594
Convex pedicle diameter (mm)	3.6 ± 1.1	3.3 ± 1.2	0.24
Convex chord length * (mm)	38 ± 5	40.4 ± 4.9	0.025
Concave pedicle diameter (mm)	3.1 ± 1.2	2.7 ± 1.6	0.127
Concave chord length * (mm)	37.7 ± 5.2	40.3 ± 4.7	0.014

Values are presented as mean ± standard deviation. *: $p < 0.05$.

4. Discussion

Although it is commonly believed that scoliosis in cerebral palsy (CP) progresses with greater angular deformities and more pronounced differences in the vertebral structure compared to adolescent idiopathic scoliosis (AIS), our study revealed fewer differences than expected when we compared the CP scoliosis and AIS with matching apex and Cobb angle. While immature skeletal development is evident in both the younger average age of the CP scoliosis group and the higher prevalence of neurocentral synchondroses, it is noteworthy that, contrary to expectations, there is no significant difference in pedicle diameters and vertebral body rotation between the two matched groups. The only significant difference in vertebral structure is that cord length is smaller in the mCPscoliosis group compared with mAIS. These findings suggest that length, rather than diameter, should be prioritized when selecting implants in CP scoliosis.

Hong et al. reported 15 degrees of VBR with a Cobb angle of 60° in a diverse type of CP scoliosis [14], while Modi et al. reported 42 degrees of VBR with a Cobb angle of 74° [22]; however, only 6 of 24 patients were diagnosed with CP. In this study, the VBR of CP scoliosis was 29.9 degrees with Cobb angles of 87.7° in only patients with spastic quadriplegic cerebral palsy. In the matched groups, the VBR was 25.4 degrees with 80.7 Cobb angle. With an increase in the Cobb angle, VBR would increase, but there may be some differences according to the level of spasticity. However, the VBR increases with Cobb angle increase, regardless of the etiology. In AIS, the VBR was 18.7 degrees with Cobb angle of 68.2 degrees, and the VBR was 24.4 degrees with 78.6 Cobb angle.

Wang et al. found no statistical differences in PDs between the concave and convex sides, except at the apical area in neuromuscular scoliosis with Chiari malformation, but Chiari malformation is different from cerebral palsy [13]. Hong et al. reported that there were no significant differences between the concave and convex sides when the PD was compared in the 11 patients with CP; however, the Cobb angle was smaller than that in our study [17]. When we compared the PD in CP scoliosis, the convex side diameter was larger than that on the concave side like previous studies and it was similar in AIS groups. Although there may be differences according to the etiology of neuromuscular scoliosis or severity, the pedicle width would be larger on the convex side around the apex in patients with CP scoliosis.

In vertebral morphology studies investigating AIS, the pedicle diameter on the concave side was smaller than on the convex side, and the apical vertebra was the most rotated vertebra [4,17,18,23,24]. These findings on AIS were similar to our findings on the CP scoliosis group. Specifically, we found that patients with CP scoliosis were younger and the CL was shorter, but the PD was similar to that of the apex- and Cobb angle-matched patients with AIS. Although the etiology of AIS is uncertain, recent studies have reported the importance of neurocentral synchondrosis [20,21]. We suspected that there might be some differences in the presence of neurocentral synchondrosis and growth patterns between AIS and CP scoliosis. Neurocentral synchondrosis was commonly noted in patients with CP scoliosis compared with AIS and the patients with CP scoliosis were younger in the matched comparison. The vertebral body was immature in CP scoliosis, which may be related to the shorter CL. However, there was no difference in the PD between the groups. One of the reasons for this may be the thin cortical bone in CP scoliosis, due to the high levels of osteoporosis. Hell et al. found significantly smaller vertebral body and PDs in neuromuscular scoliosis with spinal muscular atrophy as compared to age-matched healthy controls [15], which may be related to the early onset of neuromuscular scoliosis and the long-standing adverse effects on the neurocentral synchondroses. We think that the PD in CP scoliosis may be narrower with aging than those in AIS because of earlier suppression of neurocentral synchondrosis. In CP scoliosis, CL was short due to skeletal immaturity, but the PD may not be so small because of thin cortical bone due to osteoporosis when compared with similar Cobb angle AIS. With growth, the PD would be smaller with the long-standing adverse effect on neurocentral synchondrosis, so when we operate on CP scoliosis in older patients, the PD looks very small. Future studies should be conducted to investigate the severity of osteoporosis and the effect of neurocentral synchondroses.

Several studies have reported a smaller PD in neuromuscular scoliosis, resulting in the use of hooks or wiring. Sarwahi et al. compared the pedicle morphology between different etiology like our study, although they compared neurofibromatosis type1 patients with AIS [5]. They found a higher incidence of abnormal pedicle and higher misplacement of pedicle screws compared to AIS. Abnormal pedicles were found in 69% of the scoliosis cases diagnosed with neurofibromatosis, and they include cases with cancellous pedicle diameter less than 4 mm, according to the classification developed by Sarwahi et al. [5] and revised by Li et al. [14]. However, the pedicle in neurofibromatosis is different from CP scoliosis. In this study, the PD in patients with CP scoliosis was not so small compared with those with apex- and Cobb angle-matched AIS. Instead, the results of our study suggest that a shorter pedicle screw length may be more important. The narrow PD in CP scoliosis would be related more to the larger Cobb angles with growth. For safe and correct pedicle screw placement, we recommend performing the operation in the early stages of CP scoliosis. Still, the correct pedicle screw placement in CP scoliosis is difficult. Because of the osteoporosis, the pedicle screw can easily break the inner or outer pedicle wall.

This study has several limitations which should be considered. The number of matched cases was relatively small because the Cobb angle was usually larger in patients with CP scoliosis, the apex was different (AIS has a relatively higher apex), and cases with CT images were small. Furthermore, we did not consider the curve pattern, such as a long C curve, a double curve, or a hip problem. However, we only selected spastic quadriplegic cerebral palsy of a single etiology and found a different vertebral morphology compared with apex- and Cobb angle-matched AIS using reconstructed CT images. In matching the groups, we used the standing radiography for AIS and sitting radiography for CP scoliosis because patients with CP suffered from spastic quadriplegia. There may be some differences between sitting and standing whole spine radiography. However, we do not take preoperative supine or prone radiography routinely for all patients. Later, supine or prone radiography may be used to measure the Cobb angle and matched analysis. Further studies that consider age and sex differences or supine and prone radiography should be conducted to address these limitations, and studies with larger populations should be followed to increase the power of the study.

5. Conclusions

The VBR in patients with CP scoliosis was comparable to that in patients with AIS matched for Cobb angle and apex. Although the patients were young and the vertebral body was smaller in terms of a short chord length in the patients with CP scoliosis, the pedicle diameters were similar between the two patient groups. These deformities may be related to osteoporosis caused by non-ambulation and immature vertebral body. In CP scoliosis, we should consider not only a smaller diameter but also a shorter length of pedicle screws. Pre-operative CT analyses of vertebra morphology is essential in CP scoliosis.

Author Contributions: Conceptualization, G.U.D. and K.-B.P.; methodology, H.J.P.; software, G.U.D.; validation, H.W.K.; formal analysis, H.J.P.; investigation, K.-B.P., G.U.D., H.J.P., H.P. and M.S.A.; resources, H.P. and K.-H.P.; data curation, M.S.A.; writing—original draft preparation, G.U.D. and K.-B.P.; writing—review and editing, G.U.D. and K.-B.P.; visualization, H.J.P.; supervision, H.W.K.; project administration, K.-B.P.; funding acquisition, All authors have read and agreed to the published version of the manuscript.

Funding: This study was supported by the Severance Hospital Research Fund for Clinical Excellence (SHRC) (C-2022-0014).

Institutional Review Board Statement: This retrospective study was approved by the Yonsei University Health System, Severance Hospital, Institutional Review Board (IRB No. 4-2022-0937). The Institutional Review Board waived the requirement for informed consent because of the retrospective observational nature of the study.

Informed Consent Statement: Not applicable. The Institutional Review Board waived the requirement for informed consent because of the retrospective observational nature of the study.

Data Availability Statement: The datasets used and/or analyzed in the current study are available from the corresponding author on reasonable request.

Conflicts of Interest: The authors declare no conflicts of interest. Funders had no role in the design of the study; in the collection, analyses, or interpretation of data; in the writing of the manuscript; or in the decision to publish the results.

References

1. Liljenqvist, U.R.; Allkemper, T.; Hackenberg, L.; Link, T.M.; Steinbeck, J.; Halm, H.F.H. Analysis of Vertebral Morphology in Idiopathic Scoliosis with Use of Magnetic Resonance Imaging and Multiplanar Reconstruction. *J. Bone Jt. Surg. Am.* **2002**, *84*, 359–368. [CrossRef] [PubMed]
2. Çatan, H.; Buluç, L.; Anik, Y.; Ayyildiz, E.; Şarlak, A.Y. Pedicle morphology of the thoracic spine in preadolescent idiopathic scoliosis: Magnetic resonance supported analysis. *Eur. Spine J.* **2007**, *16*, 1203–1208. [CrossRef] [PubMed]
3. Parent, S.; Labelle, H.; Skalli, W.; Latimer, B.; de Guise, J. Morphometric Analysis of Anatomic Scoliotic Specimens. *Spine* **2002**, *27*, 2305–2311. [CrossRef]

4. Brink, R.C.; Schlösser, T.P.C.; Colo, D.; Vincken, K.L.; van Stralen, M.; Hui, S.C.N.; Chu, W.C.W.; Cheng, J.C.Y.; Castelein, R.M. Asymmetry of the Vertebral Body and Pedicles in the True Transverse Plane in Adolescent Idiopathic Scoliosis: A CT-Based Study. *Spine Deform.* **2017**, *5*, 37–45. [CrossRef] [PubMed]
5. Sarwahi, V.; Sugarman, E.P.; Wollowick, A.L.; Amaral, T.D.; Lo, Y.; Thornhill, B. Prevalence, Distribution, and Surgical Relevance of Abnormal Pedicles in Spines with Adolescent Idiopathic Scoliosis vs. No Deformity: A CT-Based Study. *J. Bone Jt. Surg. Am.* **2014**, *96*, e92. [CrossRef]
6. Vinje, S.; Terjesen, T.; Kibsgård, T. Scoliosis in children with severe cerebral palsy: A population-based study of 206 children at GMFCS levels III–V. *Eur. Spine J.* **2023**, *32*, 4030–4036. [CrossRef]
7. Reames, D.L.; Smith, J.S.; Fu, K.M.G.; Polly, D.W.; Ames, C.P.; Berven, S.H.; Perra, J.H.; Glassman, S.D.; McCarthy, R.E.; Knapp, R.D.; et al. Complications in the Surgical Treatment of 19,360 Cases of Pediatric Scoliosis: A Review of the Scoliosis Re-search Society Morbidity and Mortality Database. *Spine* **2011**, *36*, 1484–1491. [CrossRef]
8. Kim, H.S.; Kwon, J.W.; Park, K.B. Clinical Issues in Indication, Correction, and Outcomes of the Surgery for Neuromuscular Scoliosis: Narrative Review in Pedicle Screw Era. *Neurospine* **2022**, *19*, 177–187. [CrossRef]
9. Tsirikos, A.I.; Mataliotakis, G.; Bounakis, N. Posterior spinal fusion for adolescent idiopathic scoliosis using a convex pedicle screw technique: A novel concept of deformity correction. *Bone Jt. J.* **2017**, 99–1080. [CrossRef]
10. Kim, H.J.; Lenke, L.G.; Pizones, J.; Castelein, R.; Trobisch, P.D.; Yagi, M.; Kelly, M.P.; Chang, D.G. Adolescent Idiopathic Scoliosis: Is the Feasible Option of Minimally Invasive Surgery Using Posterior Approach? *Asian Spine J.* **2024**, *18*, 287–300. [CrossRef]
11. Shetty, A.P.; Meena, J.; Murugan, C.; Milton, R.; Kanna, R.M.; Rajasekaran, S. Functional and Radiological Outcomes of All-Posterior Surgical Correction of Dystrophic Curves in Patients with Neurofibromatosis Type 1. *Asian Spine J.* **2024**, *18*, 174–181. [CrossRef] [PubMed]
12. Modi, H.N.; Suh, S.W.; Fernandez, H.; Yang, J.H.; Song, H.R. Accuracy and Safety of Pedicle Screw Placement in Neuro-muscular Scoliosis with Free-Hand Technique. *Eur. Spine J.* **2008**, *17*, 1686–1696. [CrossRef] [PubMed]
13. Yang, N.; Luo, M.; Zhao, S.; Wang, W.; Xia, L. Morphological Differences Between the Pedicles in Nondystrophic Scoliosis Secondary to Neurofibromatosis Type 1 and Those in Adolescent Idiopathic Scoliosis. *World Neurosurg.* **2020**, *144*, e9–e14. [CrossRef] [PubMed]
14. Li, Y.; Luo, M.; Wang, W.; Shen, M.; Xu, G.; Gao, J.; Xia, L. A Computed Tomography–Based Comparison of Abnormal Ver-tebrae Pedicles Between Dystrophic and Nondystrophic Scoliosis in Neurofibromatosis Type 1. *World Neurosurg.* **2017**, *106*, 898–904. [CrossRef] [PubMed]
15. Hell, A.K.; Grages, A.; Braunschweig, L.; Lueders, K.A.; Austein, F.; Lorenz, H.M.; Lippross, S.; Tsaknakis, K. Children with Spinal Muscular Atrophy Have Reduced Vertebral Body Height and Depth and Pedicle Size in Comparison to Age-Matched Healthy Controls. *World Neurosurg.* **2022**, *165*, e352–e356. [CrossRef] [PubMed]
16. Wang, G.; Sun, J.; Cui, X.; Jiang, Z. Pedicle Morphology of the Thoracic and Lumbar Spine in Scoliosis Associated With Chiari Malformation/Syringomyelia Comparison With Adolescent Idiopathic Scoliosis. *J. Spinal Disord. Technol.* **2012**, *25*, 168–172. [CrossRef]
17. Hong, J.Y.; Suh, S.W.; Tr, E.; Hong, S.J.; Yoon, Y.C.; Kang, H.J. Clinical Anatomy of Vertebrae in Scoliosis: Global Analysis in Four Different Diseases by Multiplanar Reconstructive Computed Tomography. *Spine J.* **2013**, *13*, 1510–1520. [CrossRef]
18. Davis, C.M.; Grant, C.A.; Pearcy, M.J.; Askin, G.N.; Labrom, R.D.; Izatt, M.T.; Adam, C.J.; Little, J.P. Is There Asymmetry Between the Concave and Convex Pedicles in Adolescent Idiopathic Scoliosis? A CT Investigation. *Clin. Orthop. Relat. Res.* **2017**, *475*, 884–893. [CrossRef] [PubMed]
19. Lee, C.S.; Cho, J.H.; Hwang, C.J.; Lee, D.H.; Park, J.W.; Park, K.B. The Importance of the Pedicle Diameters at the Proximal Thoracic Vertebrae for the Correction of Proximal Thoracic Curve in Asian Patients with Idiopathic Scoliosis. *Spine* **2019**, *44*, E671–E678. [CrossRef] [PubMed]
20. Blakemore, L.; Schwend, R.; Akbarnia, B.A.; Dumas, M.; Schmidt, J. Growth Patterns of the Neurocentral Synchondrosis (NCS) in Immature Cadaveric Vertebra. *J. Pediatr. Orthop.* **2018**, *38*, 181–184. [CrossRef]
21. Zhang, H.; Sucato, D.J. Neurocentral Synchondrosis Screws to Create and Correct Experimental Deformity: A Pilot Study. *Clin. Orthop. Relat. Res.* **2011**, *469*, 1383–1390. [CrossRef] [PubMed]
22. Modi, H.N.; Suh, S.W.; Song, H.-R.; Lee, S.-H.; Yang, J.H. Correction of Apical Axial Rotation With Pedicular Screws in Neuromuscular Scoliosis. *J. Spinal Disord. Technol.* **2008**, *21*, 606–613. [CrossRef] [PubMed]
23. Kuraishi, S.; Takahashi, J.; Hirabayashi, H.; Hashidate, H.; Ogihara, N.; Mukaiyama, K.; Kato, H. Pedicle Morphology Using Computed Tomography-Based Navigation System in Adolescent Idiopathic Scoliosis. *J. Spinal Disord. Technol.* **2013**, *26*, 22–28. [CrossRef] [PubMed]
24. Sakti, Y.M.; Lanodiyu, Z.A.; Ichsantyaridha, M.; Wijanarko, S.; Filza, M.R.; Taufan, T.; Susanto, D.B.; Tampubolon, Y.O.; Baskara, A.A.N.N.; Nurshal, A.A.; et al. Pedicle morphometry analysis of main thoracic apex adolescent idiopathic scoliosis. *BMC Surg.* **2023**, *23*, 34. [CrossRef]

Journal of
Clinical Medicine

MDPI

Article

Comparison of Revision Techniques for Rod Fracture after Adult Spinal Deformity Surgery: Rod Replacement Alone or Coupled with Lateral Lumbar Interbody Fusions or Accessory Rods

Ki Young Lee, Jung-Hee Lee *, Gil Han, Cheol-Hyun Jung and Hong Sik Park

Department of Orthopedic Surgery, Graduate School, College of Medicine, Kyung Hee University, 23 Kyungheedae-ro, Dongdaemun-gu, Seoul 02447, Republic of Korea; keyng39@hanmail.net (K.Y.L.); gilnessxiv@gmail.com (G.H.); rucky5@naver.com (C.-H.J.); maalouf@hanmail.net (H.S.P.)

* Correspondence: ljhspine@gmail.com; Tel.: +82-2-958-8346

Abstract: Background: Rod fracture (RF) is the most common cause of revision in adult spinal deformity (ASD) surgery, and various treatment strategies for preventing RF are reported in the literature. This retrospective study, involving 139 ASD patients (aged ≥65 years and a minimum 2-year follow-up) who underwent long-segment fixation from T10 to sacrum with pedicle subtraction osteotomy (PSO), analyzed long-term results, including radiographical parameters and the incidence of recurrent RF (re-RF), to determine the most effective revision method for preventing RF. **Methods:** Patients were classified into three groups according to the revision method performed for RF: simple rod replacement (RR group, $n = 17$), lateral lumbar interbody fusion around the PSO site (RR + LLIF group, $n = 8$), and accessory rod insertion (RR + AR group, $n = 22$). Baseline characteristics and radiographical and clinical parameters were analyzed. **Results:** RF occurred in 47 patients (34%) at an average of 28 months following primary deformity correction. Re-RF occurred in six patients (13%) at an average of 37 months. Re-RF occurred most commonly in the RR group ($p = 0.048$). Every re-RF in the RR group occurred at the PSO site; none occurred in the RR + LLIF group, and one in the RR + AR group occurred near the L4–5. After both primary deformity correction and revision surgery, spinopelvic parameters had shown favorable results, and clinical outcomes had improved in all three groups without significant intergroup differences. **Conclusions:** Accessory rod insertion or an additional LLIF around the PSO site seems to provide greater strength and stability to the previously fused segments than a simple rod replacement, which demonstrates the need for additional support in revision surgery for RF after a PSO.

Keywords: accessory rod; adult spinal deformity; lateral lumbar interbody fusion; pedicle subtraction osteotomy; revision surgery; rod fracture

1. Introduction

The reported complication rates following adult spinal deformity (ASD) surgery are as high as 70% [1], with pseudarthrosis being the major reason for a revision surgery [2]. In particular, rod fracture (RF), the most common form of pseudarthrosis, may occur even when radiographical findings show a solid bone union. Accordingly, various treatment strategies for reducing the incidence of RF following surgical treatment of ASD are reported in the literature [3,4].

ASD patients who receive deformity correction are not free from the risk of RF, as it can occur when patients accidently fall down or abruptly bend over. Moreover, the pedicle subtraction osteotomy (PSO) technique itself has been reported as a risk factor of RF [3]. Many studies to date have analyzed the related risk factors [4,5], compared the procedure-related complication risks between primary and revision surgeries [6], and explored the various complications after revision surgery [7] in the setting of ASD. However, long-term follow-up studies assessing the outcomes after revision surgeries due to RF are sparse.

In general, patients with RF are strongly advised to undergo revision not only to reduce associated pain but also to prevent the potential deterioration of sagittal balance that may result from the collapse of the vertebral body at the PSO site [3]. Although a revision surgery for RF is traditionally performed through rod replacement and supplementary posterior fusion, several alternative methods have been introduced in recent years to enhance fusion above and below the osteotomy site through a minimally invasive lateral approach and to increase both the stiffness and stability of the construct by inserting accessory rods into previous instrumentation [8,9].

The current study was conducted on ASD patients who underwent primary deformity correction via PSO and subsequent revision surgery due to RF with one of the three major revision techniques: (1) simple rod replacement, (2) lateral lumbar interbody fusion (LLIF) above and below the PSO site, and (3) accessory rod insertion. This study analyzed the long-term results, including the incidence of recurrent RF (re-RF) and the radiographical parameters, for each revision procedure.

2. Materials and Methods

2.1. Study Design

This retrospective study reviewed 139 consecutive ASD patients aged ≥65 years enrolled from 2002 to 2020 with a minimum 2-year follow-up after deformity correction via PSO. The inclusion criteria were as follows:

(1) Sagittal malalignment (sagittal vertical axis [SVA] > 50 mm, pelvic incidence [PI] minus lumbar lordosis [LL] mismatch > 10°, and pelvic tilt [PT] > 25°).
(2) Long-segment fixation with the uppermost and lowermost instrumented vertebrae at the T10 and S1, respectively.
(3) Atrophy of the back musculature in the cross-section area of magnetic resonance imaging and computed tomography (CT) in the diagnosis of lumbar degenerative kyphosis (LDK) and notable clinical signs, as previously described [10].
(4) Identification of RF based on rod breakage, with a recent fusion mass fracture being observed on plain radiography and CT and confirmed by uptakes in either bone scans or bone single-photon emission CT.

The patients were classified into three groups according to the received revision procedure: simple rod replacement (RR group), rod replacement with lateral lumbar interbody fusion above and below the PSO site (RR + LLIF group), and rod replacement with accessory rod insertion (RR + AR group).

2.2. Surgical Method

2.2.1. Simple Rod Replacement

With each patient in a prone position, the standard posterior midline approach was made to expose the implant and confirm the site of RF. Previously inserted rods were replaced bilaterally.

2.2.2. Accessory Rod Replacement

After previously inserted rods were replaced bilaterally with the standard posterior midline approach, accessory rods, each bent at the upper and lower ends, were connected to the newly replaced rods with connectors [3].

2.2.3. Lateral Lumbar Interbody Fusion

In the lateral decubitus position, a blunt dissection along the muscle fibers was made to reach the retroperitoneal space. Following discectomy with contralateral annular release, a polyetheretherketone cage (12°) of appropriate height and length was chosen by inserting trial cages. A mixture of demineralized bone matrix or recombinant human bone morphogenetic protein-2 (rhBMP-2) and chipped-bone allograft was used to fill in each cage, which was subsequently inserted into the disk space above and below the PSO site. Then, previously inserted rods were replaced bilaterally with the standard posterior midline approach [3].

2.3. Radiographic Measurements

Sagittal alignment was evaluated using lateral 14 × 36-inch full-spine radiographs obtained with the patients standing in a neutral unsupported position with "fists-on-clavicle" [11]. All digital radiographs were analyzed using validated software (Surgimap, version 2.3.2.1, Nemaris Inc., New York, NY, USA). We evaluated PI, sacral slope (SS), PT, thoracic kyphosis (TK), thoracolumbar junction (TL), LL, lumbosacral junction (LS), and SVA. Sagittal Cobb angles were measured for TK (T5–12), TL (T10–L2), LL (T12–S1), and LS (L4–S1) [9,10]. PI, PT, and SS were measured using a standing lateral radiograph of the pelvis according to methods described previously [12].

2.4. RF Analysis

RF occurrence, RF site (vertebral level), and RF side (unilateral vs. bilateral) were evaluated. The surgical factors (sacropelvic fixation application and the L5-S1 fusion method) were also analyzed.

2.5. Clinical Outcome Measurements

Clinical outcomes were assessed using Oswestry Disability Index (ODI) and Visual Analog Scale (VAS) preoperatively, postoperatively, and at last follow-up prior to the occurrence of RF. In addition, age, bone mineral density (BMD), and body mass index (BMI), were also analyzed.

2.6. Statistical Analysis

Statistical analyses were performed using IBM SPSS Statistics for Windows, version 20.0 (IBM Corp., Armonk, NY, USA). Continuous variables were analyzed using one-way analysis of variance (ANOVA), Welch's robust ANOVA, Bonferroni's method, the Tukey HSD method, and the Dunnett T3 method for variables with normal distributions, and a Kruskal–Wallis test and the Mann–Whitney method were used for variables without normal distributions. Categorical variables were assessed using chi-square and Fisher's exact tests, as appropriate. A p-value of <0.05 was considered statistically significant.

3. Results

3.1. Baseline Characteristics of Patients with RF

Patients were referred to the outpatient clinic after a startling crack sound with accompanying back pain. RF occurred in 47 patients (34%) at an average of 28 months after primary deformity correction with a mean age of 69.7 years. RF occurred at the PSO site in 39 patients (83%) and at the L4–5 level in eight patients (17%). Bilateral and unilateral RF were observed in 23 and 24 patients, respectively. Thirty-three patients had a sacropelvic fixation, and 31 and 16 patients had received ALIF and PLIF, respectively, for L5-S1 interbody fusion. Each patient received one of the following revision surgery procedures: (1) simple bilateral rod replacement (n = 17), (2) bilateral rod replacement with LLIF around the PSO site (n = 8), or (3) bilateral rod replacement with accessory rod insertion (n = 22).

3.2. Characteristics of Re-RF

Table 1 presents the characteristics of patients with re-RF. Re-RF occurred in six patients (13%) at an average of 37 months (one unilateral RF and five bilateral RF). Re-RF occurred most commonly in the RR group (p = 0.048), being seen in five patients (29.4%) at 15, 18, 25, 36, and 96 months, postoperatively. There was no re-RF in the RR + LLIF group. Re-RF occurred in one patient in the RR + AR group at 29 months, postoperatively. Every re-RF in the RR group occurred at the PSO site, while one bilateral re-RF in the RR + AR group occurred at L4–5 level just below each junction between the distal end of AR and the primary rod. Every patient with re-RF underwent a re-revision procedure, while one asymptomatic patient with unilateral RF underwent close observation from refusal of surgical intervention.

Table 1. Baseline characteristics of re-RF patients.

Variables	RR (n = 17)	RR + LLIF (n = 8)	RR + AR (n = 22)	p-Value
Re-RF (n = 6)	5/12 (29.4%)	0/8 (0%)	1/21 (4.5%)	0.048 *1
RF detection time (month)	38	-	29	-
RF site (level)	L2–3	-	L4–5	-
RF side	1 right 4 both	-	both	-
Sacropelvic fixation	9/8	6/2	18/4	0.182 1
ALIF/PLIF	11/6	4/4	16/6	0.508 1

RR, simple rod replacement; LLIF, lateral lumbar interbody fusion; AR, accessory rod; RF, rod fracture; ALIF, anterior lumbar interbody fusion; PLIF, posterior lumbar interbody fusion. * Statistically significant ($p < 0.05$). [1] Chi-square test.

3.3. Radiographic and Surgical Features of Re-RF Patients

Table 2 shows the radiographic parameters of the three groups. Although preoperative SVA was larger in the RR + AR group than those in the other groups ($p = 0.034$), patients in all groups showed severe sagittal malalignment before primary deformity surgery. After both deformity correction and revision surgery for RF, the spinopelvic parameters of all groups showed favorable results, and sagittal alignment was well maintained prior to the occurrence of re-RF without significant intergroup differences. Also, there were no significant differences between groups with respect to sacropelvic fixation application and the L5-S1 fusion method (ALIF or PLIF) (Table 1).

Table 2. Comparison of radiographic parameters between groups †.

Variables	RR (n = 17)	RR + LLIF (n = 8)	RR + AR (n = 22)	p-Value
Sagittal vertical axis (SVA, mm)				
Pre SVA	169.9 ± 67.1	169 ± 74.5	236.4 ± 98.1	0.034 *
Post SVA	−16.5 ± 17.3	−20.8 ± 29.6	−16.4 ± 27.7	0.901
SVA correction	−186.4 ± 72	−189.8 ± 84.7	−252.7 ± 97.8	0.047 *
Post Rev SVA	16 ± 33.8	6.3 ± 25.4	13.1 ± 37.4	0.805
Last SVA	36.5 ± 27.6	24.8 ± 9.7	22.4 ± 33	0.304
Thoracic kyphosis (TK, °)				
Pre TK	−2.8 ± 12	−1 ± 13.5	10.9 ± 37.8	0.407
Post TK	18.2 ± 15.1	22.6 ± 9.6	27.5 ± 10.1	0.069
Post Rev TK	32.1 ± 11.7	27.6 ± 13	35.6 ± 12.1	0.267
Last TK	31.9 ± 12	31.9 ± 13.3	39.7 ± 14.4	0.150
Thoracolumbar junctional angle (TL, °)				
Pre TL	7.5 ± 18.1	1.4 ± 17.2	11.2 ± 16.6	0.389
Post TL	−22.3 ± 19.1	−11.8 ± 23.1	−25.4 ± 16.1	0.345
Post Rev TL	−17.8 ± 22.2	−18.4 ± 16.9	−21.8 ± 9	0.971
Last TL	−17.4 ± 19.5	−15.4 ± 16.7	−20.4 ± 11.9	0.697
Lumbar lordosis (LL, °)				
Pre LL	7.6 ± 16.3	7.5 ± 14.5	11.2 ± 17.5	0.988
Post LL	−66.6 ± 16	−62.4 ± 7.4	−77.7 ± 24	0.093
LL correction	−74.2 ± 19.4	−70 ± 17.6	−88.9 ± 26.4	0.108
Post Rev LL	−61.6 ± 16.1	−62.6 ± 7.8	−70.4 ± 9.5	0.065
Last LL	−59 ± 23.5	−53.3 ± 25.5	−65.3 ± 18.6	0.376
Lumbosacral junctional angle (LS, °)				
Pre LS	−5.6 ± 19.1	0.4 ± 12.7	2.4 ± 15.1	0.383

Table 2. *Cont.*

Variables	RR (n = 17)	RR + LLIF (n = 8)	RR + AR (n = 22)	p-Value
Post LS	−24.8 ± 8.8	−27.4 ± 7.4	−27.7 ± 11.2	0.746
Post Rev LS	−22.1 ± 8.8	−27 ± 7.7	−29.4 ± 9.3	0.051
Last LS	−25.6 ± 8.7	−19 ± 11.9	−27.9 ± 11.7	0.214
Pelvic incidence (°)	55.5 ± 11.2	51 ± 10.2	57.5 ± 9.8	0.326
Sacral slope (SS, °)				
Preoperative SS	17.1 ± 14.5	21 ± 12.3	21.3 ± 13.1	0.604
Postoperative SS	42.3 ± 11.8	38.4 ± 6.9	45.7 ± 8.4	0.177
Post Rev SS	39.7 ± 13.3	40.1 ± 3.9	46.4 ± 7.4	0.074
Last SS	41.7 ± 13.4	39.4 ± 7.1	43.9 ± 8	0.538
Pelvic tilt (PT, °)				
Preoperative PT	38.4 ± 15.1	30 ± 11.3	36.2 ± 11.6	0.317
Postoperative PT	16.1 ± 9.5	16.3 ± 8.3	14.4 ± 15.6	0.894
Post Rev PT	15.8 ± 12.9	11.5 ± 7.2	10.8 ± 11.4	0.386
Last PT	13.8 ± 12.4	12.3 ± 8.2	13.4 ± 10.4	0.945
PI-LL (°)				
Pre PI-LL	63.1 ± 20.9	58.5 ± 17	68.7 ± 19.1	0.783
Post PI-LL	−11.1 ± 14.5	−11.5 ± 6.8	−20.2 ± 25.4	0.428
Post Rev PI-LL	−6.1 ± 16.3	−11.7 ± 8.6	−13 ± 11.7	0.263
Last PI-LL	−5.7 ± 19	−8 ± 10.7	−9.7 ± 12.5	0.714

† Data are presented as mean ± standard deviation. RR, simple rod replacement; LLIF, lateral lumbar interbody fusion; AR, accessory rod; Pre, preoperative; Post, postoperative; Rev, revision; Last, last follow-up. * Statistically significant ($p < 0.05$).

3.4. Clinical Outcomes

The VAS for back pain and radiating pain, as well as ODI, had all improved after primary deformity surgery prior to RF without significant intergroup differences (Table 3). The lack of such differences in clinical outcomes could be attributed to the fact that the patients included in this study were elderly (age ≥ 65 years) with severe baseline sagittal imbalance and both relatively high ODI and VAS scores preoperatively. Thus, along with spinopelvic harmony, the leveled horizontal gaze and normal upright posture had already been recovered through sufficient decompression and deformity correction, which enhanced their quality of life to a great extent. Additionally, patient factors, including age, BMI, and BMD, also did not significantly differ between the three groups (Table 3).

Table 3. Comparison of clinical parameters between groups †.

Variables	RR (n = 17)	RR + LLIF (n = 8)	RR + AR (n = 22)	p-Value
Age (year)	68.7 ± 6.4	69.3 ± 6.3	70.7 ± 5	0.522
BMD (gm/cm^2)	0.89 ± 0.18	1.02 ± 0.11	0.93 ± 0.16	0.184
BMD T-score (gm/cm^2)	−1.96 ± 1.56	−0.99 ± 1.08	−1.64 ± 1.45	0.301
BMI (kg/m^2)	24.8 ± 3.7	27.3 ± 2.8	24.7 ± 3.7	0.211
Pre ODI	37.5 ± 2.7	37.9 ± 3.5	38.2 ± 2.4	0.675
Post ODI	18.8 ± 6	17.3 ± 4.7	19.9 ± 4	0.419
Last ODI	10.2 ± 4.2	10 ± 4.8	9.6 ± 3.6	0.986
Pre LBP VAS	8.1 ± 1.3	8.4 ± 1.2	8.6 ± 0.9	0.654
Post LBP VAS	4.5 ± 2	4.1 ± 2.4	5 ± 1.7	0.537
Last LBP VAS	1.8 ± 1.5	2 ± 1.3	1.5 ± 1.2	0.582
Pre Leg VAS	7.8 ± 0.9	8.1 ± 1.4	8 ± 1.2	0.870
Post Leg VAS	1.9 ± 1	1.8 ± 0.7	1.6 ± 0.7	0.746
Last Leg VAS	0.9 ± 0.7	1.9 ± 2.1	1.8 ± 1.7	0.419

† Data are presented as mean ± standard deviation. RR, simple rod replacement; LLIF, lateral lumbar interbody fusion; AR, accessory rod; BMD, bone mineral density; BMI, body mass index; Pre, preoperative; Post, postoperative; Last, last follow-up; ODI, Oswestry disability index; VAS, visual analog scale; LBP, lower back pain.

4. Discussion

The restoration of sagittal balance is the main goal in the surgical treatment of ASD. Among the deformity correction methods in ASD, PSO is understandably one of the most powerful methods for achieving an ideal LL correction, which is fundamental in obtaining and maintaining optimal sagittal balance [13]. Still, there remain an array of challenges stemming from not only the complexity of the procedure itself but also from the many known complications of PSO, including RF [14,15]. Accordingly, various methods to prevent RF have been reported, such as the combination of sacropelvic fixation with long segment fusion to increase construct stability via lumbosacral fusion [16] and the insertion of multiple rod constructs for proper load distribution and posterior reinforcement at the PSO site [3].

In the setting of deformity correction of ASD, however, studies analyzing the appropriate surgical methods for revision, the long-term follow-up outcomes after revision, and the incidences of re-RF are lacking. Therefore, our study was significant in that it is the first to report on long-term outcomes, with a minimum follow-up duration of 2 years, of the three different revision methods for RF—simple bilateral rod replacement, bilateral rod replacement with LLIF around the PSO site, and bilateral rod replacement with accessory rod insertion—in ASD patients who have previously received deformity correction via long-level fusion with PSO.

4.1. Simple Bilateral Rod Replacement

Our study findings revealed the incidence of re-RF following revision surgery due to RF to be 13%. Of the three revision methods, simple bilateral rod replacement (RR group) showed the highest incidence of re-RF. We believe that the hyper-acutely contoured posterior rods paralleling a relatively large angular correction in PSO could have progressively intensified the stress concentration and lowered the fatigue strength of each rod [17–21], which consequently may have led to rod-breakage. Furthermore, the fact that every re-RF in the RR group occurred consistently at the same PSO site (Figure 1) not only suggests that simple bilateral rod replacement alone has a high risk of re-RF but also proves that additional support around the PSO site is ultimately required to prevent RF and maintain sagittal balance in PSO.

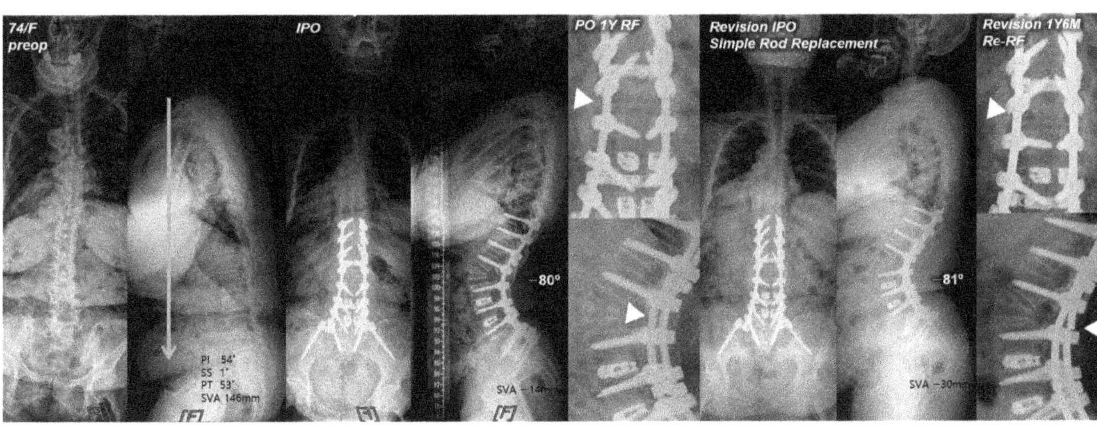

Figure 1. Pre- and postoperative standing radiographs of a 74-year-old female patient. After T10-S1 posterior instrumentation with PSO on L2, PLIF on L3–5, and ALIF on L5-S1, optimal sagittal balance was achieved (SVA, −14 mm; TK, 28°; LL, −80°; PI, 54°; PT, 4°; SS, 50°). At 1 year after primary deformity correction, RF (left rod) occurred at L2. At 1 year and 6 months following revision surgery with simple bilateral rod replacement, re-RF occurred at L2–3. White triangles indicate the site of RF.

4.2. Bilateral Rod Replacement with LLIF around the PSO Site

None of the patients in the RR + LLIF group had experienced re-RF (Figure 2). This result can be attributed to the reduced residual sagittal motion of the construct, the increased stress distribution through anterior support, and the enhanced stability via interbody fusion immediately above and below the PSO site [22]. This finding was consistent with that of a cadaveric study by Deviren et al. [23] which showed increased stability through placement of interbody cages above and below the PSO site in multiaxial bending conditions. Luca et al. [8] also reported that the management of revision surgery after PSO may require an addition of anterior column support to maintain correction and reduce complications. In the same vein, Dickson et al. [24] recommended interbody fusion above and below the PSO site to help reduce the risk of further pseudarthrosis. Therefore, providing the anterior column support through interbody work around the PSO site by either a lateral or anterior approach may be a promising method for revision due to RF. However, further comparative studies are needed to assess the effectiveness of the LLIF technique with respect to the prevention of RF and postoperative complications.

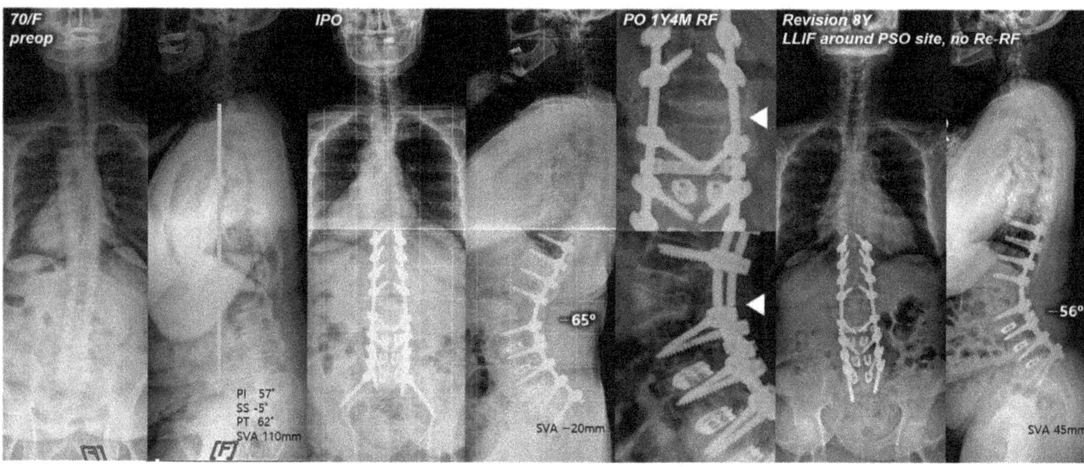

Figure 2. Pre- and postoperative standing radiographs of a 70-year-old female patient. After T10-S1 posterior instrumentation with PSO on L2, and PLIF on L3-S1, optimal sagittal balance was achieved (SVA, −20 mm; TK, 12°; LL, −65°; PI, 57°; PT, 17°; SS, 40°). At 1 year and 4 months after primary deformity correction, RF (right rod) occurred at L2–3. At 8 years following revision surgery with bilateral rod replacement and LLIF around the PSO site, sagittal alignment was well maintained without re-RF. White triangles indicate the site of RF.

4.3. Bilateral Rod Replacement with Accessory Rod Insertion

Posterior reinforcement at the PSO site with multiple-rod fixation for appropriate load distribution is a crucial preventive method for RF. Numerous finite element models have demonstrated the effectiveness of additional rods in reducing stress on the primary rods across the osteotomy site [25,26]. Several clinical studies also have reported that multiple-rod fixation reduced the occurrence of RF and increased the stability at the osteotomy site [3,9]. A biomechanical study by Scheer et al. [27] that analyzed revision strategies for RF in PSO reported that multiple-rod fixation could restore stiffness and prevent fatigue in revision constructs. Therefore, multiple-rod fixation should offer proven biomechanical stability in terms of revision for RF. However, RF can still occur even with reinforcements. In our study, re-RF occurred in one of 22 patients in the RR + AR group. Interestingly, instead of occurring at the PSO site, it occurred just below each junction between the distal end of the AR and the primary rod (Figure 3). We believe that, in the application of multiple rods, connecting the distal end of the AR to the previous instrumentation at the S1–2 area could potentially offer increased stability in conjunction with L5-S1 interbody fusion and sacropelvic fixation, and further studies to confirm this are warranted.

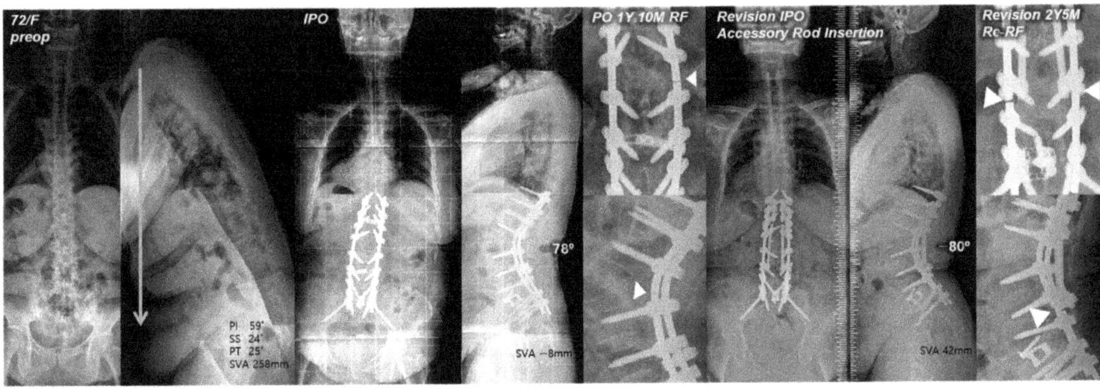

Figure 3. Pre- and postoperative standing radiographs of a 72-year-old female patient. After T10-S1 posterior instrumentation with PSO on L2, and ALIF on L5-S1, optimal sagittal balance was achieved (SVA, −8 mm; TK, 27°; LL, −78°; PI, 60°; PT, 12°; SS, 48°). At 1 year and 10 months after primary deformity correction, RF (right rod) occurred at L2–3. At 2 years and 5 months following revision surgery with bilateral rod replacement and accessory rod insertion, re-RF occurred at L4–5. White triangles indicate sites of RF.

4.4. Limitations

This study has several limitations. First, several variables may exist due to its retrospective nature. Second, this study examined only the patients who underwent deformity correction via PSO and subsequent revision procedures due to RF. Therefore, the number of patients with re-RF was relatively small, and the study findings may have limited implications. However, despite its limitations, this study is the first to compare the incidence of re-RF and analyze different revision methods for RF in the setting of ASD surgery.

5. Conclusions

For ASD patients, various revision surgery methods are available for RF following deformity correction. Our results showed that additional LLIF around the PSO site or accessory rod insertion was superior to simple rod replacement in the prevention of re-RF. Therefore, any revision surgery for RF after deformity correction with PSO should also utilize additional support to provide greater strength and stability to the previous construct. Our findings should provide an effective guideline for revisions due to RF following long posterior spinal fusion with PSO.

Author Contributions: Conceptualization, K.Y.L. and J.-H.L.; methodology, K.Y.L. and J.-H.L.; software, K.Y.L.; validation, K.Y.L., J.-H.L., G.H. and C.-H.J.; formal analysis, K.Y.L., J.-H.L., G.H., C.-H.J. and H.S.P.; investigation, K.Y.L., J.-H.L., G.H., C.-H.J. and H.S.P.; resources, J.-H.L.; data curation, J.-H.L.; writing—original draft preparation, K.Y.L., J.-H.L., G.H. and C.-H.J.; writing—review and editing, K.Y.L., J.-H.L., G.H. and C.-H.J.; visualization, K.Y.L., J.-H.L., G.H. and C.-H.J.; supervision, J.-H.L.; project administration, J.-H.L. All authors have read and agreed to the published version of the manuscript.

Funding: This research received no external funding.

Institutional Review Board Statement: This study was approved by our institutional review board (approval number: KMC IRB: 2023-03-053, approval date: 19 May 2023).

Informed Consent Statement: The need for informed consent was waived because our study was performed retrospectively.

Data Availability Statement: The data presented in this study are available on request from the corresponding author. The data are not publicly available, as participants of this study did not agree for their data to be shared publicly.

Conflicts of Interest: The authors declare no conflicts of interest.

References

1. Smith, J.S.; Klineberg, E.; Lafage, V.; Shaffrey, C.I.; Schwab, F.; Lafage, R.; Hostin, R.; Mundis, G.M., Jr.; Errico, T.J.; Kim, H.J.; et al. Prospective multicenter assessment of perioperative and minimum 2-year postoperative complication rates associated with adult spinal deformity surgery. *J. Neurosurg. Spine* **2016**, *25*, 1–14. [CrossRef] [PubMed]
2. Kim, Y.J.; Bridwell, K.H.; Lenke, L.G.; Cheh, G.; Baldus, C. Results of lumbar pedicle subtraction osteotomies for fixed sagittal imbalance: A minimum 5-year follow-up study. *Spine* **2007**, *32*, 2189–2197. [CrossRef] [PubMed]
3. Lee, K.Y.; Lee, J.H.; Kang, K.C.; Im, S.K.; Lim, H.S.; Choi, S.W. Strategies for prevention of rod fracture in adult spinal deformity: Cobalt chrome rod, accessory rod technique, and lateral lumbar interbody fusion. *J. Neurosurg. Spine* **2021**, *34*, 706–715. [CrossRef] [PubMed]
4. Smith, J.S.; Shaffrey, E.; Klineberg, E.; Shaffrey, C.I.; Lafage, V.; Schwab, F.J.; Protopsaltis, T.; Scheer, J.K.; Mundis, G.M., Jr.; Fu, K.M.; et al. Prospective multicenter assessment of risk factors for rod fracture following surgery for adult spinal deformity. *J. Neurosurg. Spine* **2014**, *21*, 994–1003. [CrossRef]
5. Smith, J.S.; Shaffrey, C.I.; Ames, C.P.; Demakakos, J.; Fu, K.M.; Keshavarzi, S.; Li, C.M.; Deviren, V.; Schwab, F.J.; Lafage, V.; et al. Assessment of symptomatic rod fracture after posterior instrumented fusion for adult spinal deformity. *Neurosurgery* **2012**, *71*, 862–867. [CrossRef]
6. Diebo, B.G.; Passias, P.G.; Marascalchi, B.J.; Jalai, C.M.; Worley, N.J.; Errico, T.J.; Lafage, V. Primary Versus Revision Surgery in the Setting of Adult Spinal Deformity: A Nationwide Study on 10,912 Patients. *Spine* **2015**, *40*, 1674–1680. [CrossRef]
7. Cho, S.K.; Bridwell, K.H.; Lenke, L.G.; Yi, J.S.; Pahys, J.M.; Zebala, L.P.; Kang, M.M.; Cho, W.; Baldus, C.R. Major complications in revision adult deformity surgery: Risk factors and clinical outcomes with 2- to 7-year follow-up. *Spine* **2012**, *37*, 489–500. [CrossRef]
8. Luca, A.; Lovi, A.; Galbusera, F.; Brayda-Bruno, M. Revision surgery after PSO failure with rod breakage: A comparison of different techniques. *Eur. Spine J.* **2014**, *23* (Suppl. 6), 610–615. [CrossRef]
9. Hyun, S.J.; Lenke, L.G.; Kim, Y.C.; Koester, L.A.; Blanke, K.M. Comparison of standard 2-rod constructs to multiple-rod constructs for fixation across 3-column spinal osteotomies. *Spine* **2014**, *39*, 1899–1904. [CrossRef]
10. Takemitsu, Y.; Harada, Y.; Iwahara, T.; Miyamoto, M.; Miyatake, Y. Lumbar degenerative kyphosis. Clinical, radiological and epidemiological studies. *Spine* **1988**, *13*, 1317–1326. [CrossRef]
11. Horton, W.C.; Brown, C.W.; Bridwell, K.H.; Glassman, S.D.; Suk, S.I.; Cha, C.W. Is there an optimal patient stance for obtaining a lateral 36" radiograph? A critical comparison of three techniques. *Spine* **2005**, *30*, 427–433. [CrossRef] [PubMed]
12. Legaye, J.; Duval-Beaupère, G.; Hecquet, J.; Marty, C. Pelvic incidence: A fundamental pelvic parameter for three-dimensional regulation of spinal sagittal curves. *Eur. Spine J.* **1998**, *7*, 99–103. [CrossRef] [PubMed]
13. Lee, J.-H.; Kim, K.-T.; Lee, S.-H.; Kang, K.-C.; Oh, H.-S.; Kim, Y.-J.; Jung, H. Overcorrection of lumbar lordosis for adult spinal deformity with sagittal imbalance: Comparison of radiographic outcomes between overcorrection and undercorrection. *Eur. Spine J.* **2016**, *25*, 2668–2675. [CrossRef] [PubMed]
14. Bridwell, K.H.; Lewis, S.J.; Edwards, C.; Lenke, L.G.; Iffrig, T.M.; Berra, A.; Baldus, C.; Blanke, K. Complications and outcomes of pedicle subtraction osteotomies for fixed sagittal imbalance. *Spine* **2003**, *28*, 2093–2101. [CrossRef] [PubMed]
15. Hyun, S.J.; Rhim, S.C. Clinical outcomes and complications after pedicle subtraction osteotomy for fixed sagittal imbalance patients: A long-term follow-up data. *J. Korean Neurosurg. Soc.* **2010**, *47*, 95–101. [CrossRef]
16. Lee, K.Y.; Lee, J.H.; Kang, K.C.; Shin, S.J.; Shin, W.J.; Im, S.K.; Park, J.H. Strategy for obtaining solid fusion at L5-S1 in adult spinal deformity: Risk factor analysis for nonunion at L5-S1. *J. Neurosurg. Spine* **2020**, *33*, 323–331. [CrossRef]
17. Tang, J.A.; Leasure, J.M.; Smith, J.S.; Buckley, J.M.; Kondrashov, D.; Ames, C.P. Effect of severity of rod contour on posterior rod failure in the setting of lumbar pedicle subtraction osteotomy (PSO): A biomechanical study. *Neurosurgery* **2013**, *72*, 276–282, discussion 283. [CrossRef]
18. Lindsey, C.; Deviren, V.; Xu, Z.; Yeh, R.F.; Puttlitz, C.M. The effects of rod contouring on spinal construct fatigue strength. *Spine* **2006**, *31*, 1680–1687. [CrossRef]
19. Kotani, Y.; Cunningham, B.W.; Parker, L.M.; Kanayama, M.; McAfee, P.C. Static and fatigue biomechanical properties of anterior thoracolumbar instrumentation systems. A synthetic testing model. *Spine* **1999**, *24*, 1406–1413. [CrossRef]
20. Cunningham, B.W.; Sefter, J.C.; Shono, Y.; McAfee, P.C. Static and cyclical biomechanical analysis of pedicle screw spinal constructs. *Spine* **1993**, *18*, 1677–1688. [CrossRef]
21. Dick, J.C.; Bourgeault, C.A. Notch sensitivity of titanium alloy, commercially pure titanium, and stainless steel spinal implants. *Spine* **2001**, *26*, 1668–1672. [CrossRef] [PubMed]
22. Godzik, J.; Haglin, J.M.; Alan, N.; Hlubek, R.J.; Walker, C.T.; Bach, K.; Mundis, G.M., Jr.; Turner, J.D.; Kanter, A.S.; Okonwko, D.O.; et al. Retrospective Multicenter Assessment of Rod Fracture after Anterior Column Realignment in Minimally Invasive Adult Spinal Deformity Correction. *World Neurosurg.* **2019**, *130*, e400–e405. [CrossRef] [PubMed]

23. Deviren, V.; Tang, J.A.; Scheer, J.K.; Buckley, J.M.; Pekmezci, M.; McClellan, R.T.; Ames, C.P. Construct Rigidity after Fatigue Loading in Pedicle Subtraction Osteotomy with or without Adjacent Interbody Structural Cages. *Glob. Spine J.* **2012**, *2*, 213–220. [CrossRef] [PubMed]
24. Dickson, D.D.; Lenke, L.G.; Bridwell, K.H.; Koester, L.A. Risk factors for and assessment of symptomatic pseudarthrosis after lumbar pedicle subtraction osteotomy in adult spinal deformity. *Spine* **2014**, *39*, 1190–1195. [CrossRef]
25. Luca, A.; Ottardi, C.; Sasso, M.; Prosdocimo, L.; La Barbera, L.; Brayda-Bruno, M.; Galbusera, F.; Villa, T. Instrumentation failure following pedicle subtraction osteotomy: The role of rod material, diameter, and multi-rod constructs. *Eur. Spine J.* **2017**, *26*, 764–770. [CrossRef]
26. Januszewski, J.; Beckman, J.M.; Harris, J.E.; Turner, A.W.; Yen, C.P.; Uribe, J.S. Biomechanical study of rod stress after pedicle subtraction osteotomy versus anterior column reconstruction: A finite element study. *Surg. Neurolo. Int.* **2017**, *8*, 207. [CrossRef]
27. Scheer, J.K.; Tang, J.A.; Deviren, V.; Buckley, J.M.; Pekmezci, M.; McClellan, R.T.; Ames, C.P. Biomechanical analysis of revision strategies for rod fracture in pedicle subtraction osteotomy. *Neurosurgery* **2011**, *69*, 164–172, discussion 172. [CrossRef]

Journal of
Clinical Medicine

MDPI

Article

Characterization of Patients with Poor Clinical Outcome after Adult Spinal Deformity Surgery: A Multivariate Analysis of Mean 8-Year Follow-Up Data

Se-Jun Park [1], Hyun-Jun Kim [2,*], Jin-Sung Park [1], Dong-Ho Kang [1], Minwook Kang [1], Kyunghun Jung [1] and Chong-Suh Lee [3]

1 Department of Orthopedic Surgery, Spine Center, Samsung Medical Center, Sungkyunkwan University School of Medicine, Seoul 06351, Republic of Korea; sejunos@gmail.com (S.-J.P.); paridot@daum.net (J.-S.P.); kang9451@gmail.com (D.-H.K.); npng4eve@gmail.com (M.K.); ilucky7ik@gmail.com (K.J.)

2 Department of Orthopedic Surgery, Hanyang University Guri Hospital, Hanyang University School of Medicine, Guri-si 11923, Republic of Korea

3 Department of Orthopedic Surgery, Haeundae Bumin Hospital, Busan 48094, Republic of Korea; csl3503@gmail.com

* Correspondence: hyunjun89.kim@gmail.com; Tel.: +82-31-1644-9118

Abstract: Background/Objective: Limited data exist regarding the long-term clinical outcomes and related factors after adult spinal deformity (ASD) surgery. This study aims to characterize patients who experienced poor clinical outcomes during long-term follow-up after ASD surgery. **Methods:** Patients who underwent ASD surgery with ≥5-vertebra fusion including the sacrum and ≥5-year follow-up were included. They were divided into two groups according to the Oswestry Disability Index (ODI) at the last follow-up: group P (poor outcome, ODI > 40) and group NP (non-poor outcome, ODI ≤ 40). Clinical variables, including patient factors, surgical factors, radiographic parameters, and mechanical complications (proximal junctional kyphosis [PJK] and rod fracture), were compared between the groups. **Results:** A total of 105 patients were evaluated, with a mean follow-up of 100.6 months. The mean age was 66.3 years, and 94 patients (89.5%) were women. There were 52 patients in group P and 53 patients in group NP. Univariate analysis showed that low T-score, postoperative correction relative to age-adjusted pelvic incidence-lumbar lordosis, T1 pelvic angle (TPA) at last follow-up, and PJK development were significant factors for poor clinical outcomes. Multivariate analysis identified PJK as the single independent risk factor (odds ratio [OR] = 3.957 for PJK development relative to no PJK, OR = 21.141 for revision surgery for PJK relative to no PJK). **Conclusions:** PJK development was the single independent factor affecting poor clinical outcomes in long-term follow-up. Therefore, PJK prevention appears crucial for achieving long-term success after ASD surgery.

Keywords: adult spinal deformity; poor clinical outcome; risk factor; proximal junctional kyphosis; long-term follow-up; health-related quality of life

1. Introduction

Adult spinal deformity (ASD) is a disabling condition that causes significant pain and disability, resulting in a marked decline in the patient's health-related quality of life (HRQOL) [1]. Since sagittal imbalance leads to poor HRQOL [2–5], proper spinopelvic malalignment correction has been prioritized as a crucial surgical goal. Previous ASD-related studies have uniformly emphasized the importance of correcting spinopelvic malalignment for the success of surgery [2–8]. However, this evidence is insufficient to determine whether the role of optimal sagittal alignment in clinical outcomes remains valid during long-term follow-up or if other factors influence clinical outcomes over time.

Along with adequate postoperative sagittal alignment, other factors that might negatively affect the clinical outcomes should be considered when assessing the long-term outcomes after ASD surgery. First, whether postoperatively restored sagittal alignment will be maintained over long-term follow-up should be considered, as many patients experience some degree of correction loss over time [9–11]. The loss of correction can occur within the fusion segments and unfused thoracic spine, both of which may deteriorate the global sagittal balance. Second, mechanical complications such as proximal junctional kyphosis (PJK) and rod fracture can arise, negatively impacting final clinical outcomes [12–14]. It is known that the development of mechanical complications is associated with postoperative sagittal alignment status [15,16]. However, the adequate correction of sagittal alignment cannot completely prevent mechanical failure [17]. Moreover, the incidence of these mechanical complications and the risk of related revision surgery continuously increase over time [18,19].

For assessing the long-term clinical outcome after ASD surgery, it is necessary to comprehensively consider various clinical parameters, including demographics, immediate postoperative and final radiographic findings, and mechanical complications, because these factors may be closely related and can affect the final clinical outcome. In the literature, data regarding the long-term clinical outcomes are limited. Furthermore, it has not been clearly established which factors are most responsible for poor clinical outcomes after ASD surgery. Therefore, this study aims to characterize patients who experience poor clinical outcomes using multivariate analysis of mean 8-year follow-up data.

2. Materials and Methods

This study received approval from Samsung Medical Center's institutional review board (IRB No. SMC 2024-07-144). Given its retrospective design, the requirement for informed consent was waived.

2.1. Study Cohort

This research involved a retrospective case series utilizing data extracted from our hospital's prospective ASD database. The study population comprised consecutive patients who underwent surgery for degenerative ASD (i.e., degenerative flatback [DFB] or degenerative lumbar scoliosis [DLS]) during 2010–2019. Patients were included based on the following criteria: ASD was defined by radiographic measurements, including a C7 sagittal vertical axis (C7SVA) of 50 mm or greater, a pelvic incidence (PI)-lumbar lordosis (LL) mismatch of 10° or more, a pelvic tilt (PT) of 25° or more, or a lumbar coronal Cobb angle of 20° or greater. In addition, the fusion involved at least five vertebral levels, all of which included the sacrum to minimize bias related to fusion length. Patients were also required to have at least five years of complete radiographic and HRQOL data. Exclusion criteria were incomplete radiographs, failure to complete the HRQOL questionnaire at the final follow-up, prior thoracic or lumbar fusion, or the presence of syndromic, neuromuscular, inflammatory, or non-degenerative pathological conditions.

2.2. Surgical Details

All surgeries were performed by one of three surgeons (clinical experience: >25 years for C.-S.L., 12 years for S.-J.P., and 7 years for J.-S.P.). The correction surgery was performed either through posterior-only surgery using posterior column osteotomy with or without pedicle subtraction osteotomy (PSO), or through a combined anterior–posterior approach using oblique or anterior lumbar interbody fusion. The choice of surgical technique was guided by the patient's preoperative deformity. While the choice of surgical technique was based on the preoperative deformity status, our institution favored the combined anterior–posterior approach in the later study period.

2.3. Clinical Outcome Measurements

At the final follow-up, patient outcomes were assessed using the Oswestry Disability Index (ODI), the Scoliosis Research Society-22r (SRS-22r) questionnaire, and the 36-item Short Form Survey (SF-36) score. In this study, ODI scores were converted to percentage values (%). Poor clinical outcomes were defined by ODI scores > 40 points, as in the previous studies [20–22]. Patients were divided into two groups according to their ODI score: group P (poor outcome group, ODI score > 40 points) and group NP (non-poor outcome group, ODI score ≤ 40 points). Although the groups were established based on ODI scores, other HRQOL measures, such as SRS-22r and SF-36 scores, were also compared between the two groups.

2.4. Study Variables

To identify the factors affecting poor clinical outcomes, various clinical variables were compared between the P and NP groups for patient factors, surgical factors, radiographic parameters, and mechanical complications.

The patient factors at the index surgery included age, sex, diagnosis (DFB or DLS), American Society of Anesthesiologists (ASA) grade, T-score on bone mineral density (BMD), body mass index (BMI), diabetes mellitus (DM), and smoking status. Surgical factors evaluated in the study included the number of fused segments, the surgical technique used, whether PSO was performed, and the use of pelvic fixation. Whole-spine radiographs in standing posteroanterior and lateral views were taken at three time points: preoperatively, immediate postoperatively (around two weeks post-surgery), and at the final follow-up. These images were assessed to determine radiographic measures such as PI, LL, SS, PT, thoracic kyphosis (TK), T1 pelvic angle (TPA), and the C7SVA. Additionally, in assessing the conventional parameters, the amount of correction was evaluated qualitatively on immediate postoperative radiographs according to the categorical criteria suggested in previous studies [21,23–25]. First, postoperative PI-LL mismatch was categorized based on Schwab's criteria into three groups: under (greater than 10°), matched (within ±10°), and over (less than −10°) [23]. Second, PI-LL was analyzed according to the age-adjusted PI-LL target [21]. The age-adjusted PI-LL target was determined using a previous formula: PI-LL = (age − 55 years)/2 + 3 [25]. Patients were then categorized into three groups based on the difference between their actual PI-LL mismatch and the age-adjusted PI-LL target: under-corrected (offset greater than 10°), matched (offset within ±10°), and over-corrected (offset less than −10°). Additionally, global alignment and proportion (GAP) scores were determined and grouped into three categories: proportioned (P) with scores from 0 to 2, moderately disproportioned (MD) with scores between 3 and 6, and severely disproportioned (SD) with scores of 7 or higher [24].

Regarding mechanical complications, PJK and rod fracture were investigated. In this study, PJK was broadly defined to encompass any kyphotic events at the proximal junction. This included cases where the postoperative proximal junctional angle (PJA) was ≥10°, vertebral fractures at the uppermost instrumented vertebra (UIV) or UIV + 1, failure of UIV fixation, and instances of myelopathy [26]. Rod fracture was defined as discontinuation of the rod at ≥1 site in the construct. The clinical impacts of PJK and rod fracture were further investigated according to the presence of these complications and whether revision surgery was performed.

2.5. Statistical Analysis

Categorical variables were presented as frequencies and percentages, while continuous variables were expressed as means with standard deviations. To compare categorical variables between the two groups, Fisher's exact test was employed, and differences in continuous variables were assessed using Student's t-test. A multivariate logistic regression analysis was then conducted, incorporating all variables that showed significance in the univariate analysis, to determine independent predictors of poor clinical outcomes. Professional statisticians performed the statistical analyses using SPSS (version 29.0.2.0; IBM Corp., Armonk, NY, USA). A p-value of less than 0.05 was regarded as statistically significant.

3. Results

Among 320 patients who underwent deformity correction during the study period, 105 patients were included in the final study cohort. The mean follow-up duration was 100.6 ± 32.8 months. The mean age was 66.3 ± 6.8 years at the time of index surgery and 74.7 ± 6.6 years at the final follow-up, and there were 94 women (89.5%). The diagnosis was DFB in 59 patients (56.2%) and DLS in 46 patients (43.8%), and the total number of fused segments was 6.2 levels. Front–back surgery was performed on 56 patients (53.3%), while PSO was carried out in 18 patients (17.1%). At the last follow-up, 52 patients were classified into group P, and 53 into group NP. The mean ODI score in group P was 60.7 points, while 25.7 points in group NP. Other HRQOL measures like both the scores of all individual items and the total sums of SRS-22r and SF-36 scores were significantly better in group NP compared with group P (Table 1).

Table 1. Comparison of the last-follow-up HRQOLs according to the two groups.

		Group P	Group NP	*p* *
ODI		60.7 ± 13.8	25.7 ± 11.4	**<0.001**
SRS-22r	Function	2.3 ± 0.6	3.4 ± 0.8	**<0.001**
	Pain	2.6 ± 0.9	4.0 ± 0.5	**<0.001**
	Appearance	2.3 ± 0.6	3.5 ± 0.7	**<0.001**
	Mental health	2.3 ± 0.7	3.7 ± 0.8	**<0.001**
	Satisfaction	2.9 ± 0.7	3.9 ± 0.7	**<0.001**
	Total	2.4 ± 0.5	3.7 ± 0.6	**<0.001**
SF-36	Physical functioning	18.2 ± 17.1	51.3 ± 25.2	**<0.001**
	Role—physical	40.0 ± 25.9	64.3 ± 29.7	**<0.001**
	Bodily pain	39.6 ± 21.5	63.2 ± 20.5	**<0.001**
	General Health	26.4 ± 15.6	50.9 ± 22.2	**<0.001**
	Vitality	34.2 ± 18.6	51.4 ± 21.5	**<0.001**
	Social functioning	36.6 ± 26.9	79.0 ± 21.3	**<0.001**
	Role—emotional	40.4 ± 20.1	66.8 ± 25.0	**0.002**
	Mental health	41.3 ± 20.1	66.8 ± 25.0	**<0.001**
	Physical component summary	31.1 ± 15.1	57.4 ± 18.3	**<0.001**
	Mental component summary	37.8 ± 18.4	67.9 ± 20.4	**<0.001**

Data are presented as the mean ± SD. * Bold *p* values mean statistical significance. HRQOL indicates health-related quality of life; Group P, poor clinical outcome group; Group NP, non-poor clinical outcome group; ODI, Oswestry disability index; SRS-22r, Scoliosis Research Society-22r; SF-36, 36-item short-form health survey.

In terms of the factors that could affect the clinical outcomes, there were no differences in patient factors between the P and NP groups except for the T-score on BMD, which was significantly lower in group P (−1.6 g/cm^2) than in group NP (−0.8 g/cm^2) (Table 2).

Table 2. Comparison of patient's and surgical factors according to the two groups.

	Group P	Group NP	*p* *
Patient factors			
Age at the index surgery (yr)	66.8 ± 7.3	65.9 ± 6.3	0.473
Age at the last follow-up (yr)	75.5 ± 6.6	73.9 ± 6.6	0.212
Female:male, *n* (%)	48:4 (92.3%:7.7%)	46:7 (86.8%:13.2%)	0.526
DFB:DLS, *n* (%)	31:21 (59.6%:40.4%)	28:25 (52.8%:47.2%)	0.557
ASA grade	2.0 ± 0.4	1.9 ± 0.5	0.552
T-score on BMD (g/cm^2)	−1.6 ± 1.7	−0.8 ± 1.7	**0.024**
BMI (kg/m^2)	26.2 ± 3.7	25.4 ± 3.6	0.244
DM, *n* (%)	13 (25.0%)	6 (11.3%)	0.081
Smoking status, *n* (%)	6 (11.5%)	3 (5.7%)	0.067

Table 2. *Cont.*

	Group P	Group NP	p *
Surgical factors			
No. of total segments fused	6.3 ± 2.2	6.1 ± 2.7	0.689
Front–back surgery, n (%)	23 (44.2%)	26 (49.1%)	0.697
Application of PSO, n (%)	12 (23.1%)	6 (11.3%)	0.127
Pelvic fixation, n (%)	29 (55.8%)	30 (56.6%)	1.000

Data are presented as the mean ± SD or as the number of patients (percentage). * Bold p values mean statistical significance. Group P indicates poor clinical outcome group; Group NP, non-poor clinical outcome group; DFB, degenerative flatback; DLKS, degenerative lumbar scoliosis; ASA, American Society of Anesthesiologists; BMD, bone mineral density; BMI, body mass index; DM, diabetes mellitus; PSO, pedicle subtraction osteotomy.

No notable differences were found in surgical factors, such as the total number of fused segments, use of anterior-posterior surgery, execution of PSO, or pelvic fixation. Similarly, no differences were observed between the two groups in preoperative radiographic factors (Table 3).

Table 3. Comparison of radiographic factors and mechanical failure according to the two groups.

	Group P	Group NP	p *
Preoperatively			
PI (°)	55.1 ± 10.6	53.8 ± 10.5	0.516
LL (°)	16.1 ± 21.0	21.1 ± 19.7	0.209
PI-LL (°)	39.1 ± 21.7	32.7 ± 16.9	0.096
SS (°)	22.7 ± 11.2	23.8 ± 11.0	0.616
PT (°)	32.4 ± 12.2	30.0 ± 8.5	0.239
TK (°)	11.7 ± 14.4	16.2 ± 15.4	0.127
TPA (°)	32.3 ± 11.9	28.8 ± 9.9	0.113
C7SVA (mm)	81.1 ± 53.3	66.7 ± 49.4	0.153
Immediate postoperatively			
LL (°)	41.9 ± 11.2	41.8 ± 10.1	0.953
PI-LL (°)	13.0 ± 12.9	12.1 ± 9.6	0.684
SS (°)	31.4 ± 7.9	32.1 ± 8.9	0.668
PT (°)	23.2 ± 8.9	21.9 ± 8.4	0.428
TK (°)	21.1 ± 10.1	22.7 ± 10.5	0.438
TPA (°)	20.7 ± 8.8	18.1 ± 27.9	0.091
C7SVA (mm)	28.2 ± 31.3	18.4 ± 27.8	0.092
Grouping by Schwab's criteria			0.559
Under (PI-LL mismatch > 10°), n (%)	30 (57.7%)	27 (50.9%)	
Matched (PI-LL mismatch ≤ ±10°), n (%)	22 (42.3%)	26 (49.1%)	
Over (PI-LL mismatch < −10°), n (%)	0	0	
Grouping by age-adjusted PI-LL target †			**0.026**
Under (PI-LL offset > 10°), n (%)	17 (32.7%)	12 (22.6%)	
Matched (PI-LL offset ≤ ±10°), n (%)	25 (48.1%)	38 (71.7%)	
Over (PI-LL offset < −10°), n (%)	10 (19.2%)	3 (5.7%)	
Grouping by GAP score ‡			0.632
Proportioned, n (%)	11 (21.2%)	9 (17.0%)	
Moderately disproportioned, n (%)	17 (32.7%)	22 (41.5%)	
Severely disproportioned, n (%)	24 (46.2%)	22 (41.5%)	
At the last follow-up			
LL (°)	33.9 ± 12.9	33.3 ± 11.7	0.799
PI-LL (°)	23.2 ± 17.9	20.6 ± 11.9	0.378
SS (°)	27.9 ± 8.2	27.9 ± 8.7	0.983
PT (°)	29.2 ± 10.4	25.9 ± 8.7	0.087
TK (°)	29.3 ± 14.8	27.3 ± 13.7	0.491
TPA (°)	30.0 ± 11.9	24.6 ± 7.6	**0.007**
C7SVA (mm)	77.0 ± 53.0	60.0 ± 42.2	0.077

Table 3. *Cont.*

	Group P	Group NP	p *
Mechanical complications (PJK)			**<0.001**
No PJK, n (%)	12 (23.1%)	35 (66.0%)	
PJK, but no revision surgery, n (%)	28 (53.8%)	16 (30.2%)	
Revision surgery for PJK, n (%)	12 (23.1%)	2 (3.8%)	
Mechanical complications (Rod fracture)			0.792
No rod fracture, n (%)	41 (78.8%)	43 (81.1%)	
Rod fracture, but no revision surgery, n (%)	8 (15.4%)	6 (11.3%)	
Revision surgery for rod fracture, n (%)	3 (5.8%)	4 (7.5%)	

Data are presented as the mean ± SD or as the number of patients (percentage). * Bold p values mean statistical significance. † Age-adjusted PI-LL target was calculated as follows: Age-adjusted PI-LL target = (Age − 55)/2 + 3. Offset was calculated as the following formula: (actual PI-LL) − (age-adjusted PI-LL target). According to offset, Under means offset > 10°, Matched means offset within ±10°, and Over means offset < −10°. ‡ "Proportioned" in GAP score means a total score of 0–2, "moderately disproportioned" 3–6, and "severely disproportioned" ≥ 7. Group P indicates a poor clinical outcome group; Group NP, a non-poor clinical outcome group; PI, pelvic incidence; LL, lumbar lordosis; SS, sacral slope; PT, pelvic tilt; TPA, T1 pelvic angle; C7SVA, C7 sagittal vertical axis; GAP, global alignment and proportion; PJK, proximal junctional kyphosis.

Among immediate postoperative radiographic parameters, only the correction amounts relative to the age-adjusted PI-LL target significantly differed between the two groups (Table 3). A relatively higher percentage of patients with overcorrection in group P (19.2%) compared with group NP (5.7%). In contrast, the percentage of patients who achieved matched correction was significantly greater in group NP (71.7%) than in group P (48.1%). There were no differences in terms of Schwab's PI-LL mismatch criteria or GAP score (Table 3).

At the last follow-up, TPA was the only parameter that showed a significant difference between the two groups (30.0° in group P vs. 24.6° in group NP, P = 0.007). Both PT and C7SVA tended to be higher in group P than in group NP, but these differences did not reach statistical significance. Regarding mechanical complications, PJK development significantly affected the clinical outcomes, while the development of rod fracture did not regardless of revision surgery. There were significantly more patients with PJK development in group P than in group NP (53.8% vs. 30.2%). Revision surgery for PJK was performed in significantly more patients in group P than in group NP (23.1% vs. 3.8%) (Table 3). From immediately postoperative to the last follow-up, there were significant decreases in LL and SS, along with significant increases in PT, TK, TPA, and SVA. A similar pattern of correction loss was observed in both patient groups, regardless of whether mechanical failures occurred (Figure 1A,B).

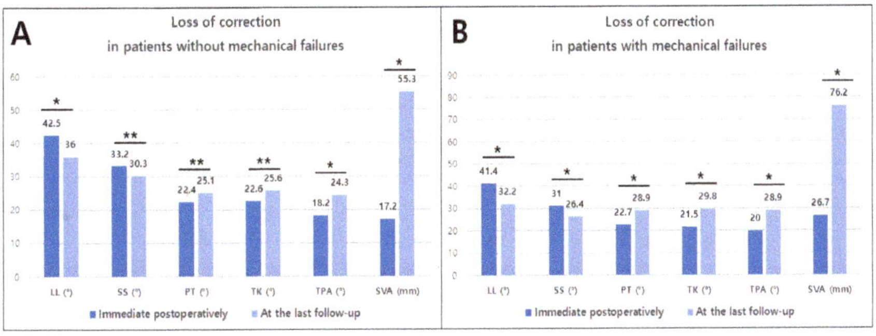

Figure 1. Changes in sagittal parameters between immediate postoperative and at the last follow-up among patients with (**A**) and without (**B**) mechanical failures. * Means $p < 0.001$ and ** means $p < 0.05$. LL indicates lumbar lordosis; SS, sacral slope; PT, pelvic tilt; TK, thoracic kyphosis; TPA, T1 pelvic angle; SVA, sagittal vertical axis.

Multivariate analysis identified PJK development as the sole independent risk factor associated with poor clinical outcomes, with an odds ratio (OR) of 3.957 for PJK development and 21.141 for revision surgery related to PJK (Table 4).

Table 4. Multivariate logistic regression analysis of risk factors to cause poor clinical outcome.

Variables	B	S.E	Wald	p *	Exp (B) (95% CI)
T-score on BMD (g/cm^2)	−0.141	0.156	0.817	0.366	0.868 (0.639–1.180)
Categories by age-adjusted PI-LL target †			3.304	0.192	
Matched (vs. Under)	−0.372	0.641	0.336	0.562	0.690 (0.196–2.423)
Over (vs. Under)	1.053	1.024	1.056	0.304	2.865 (0.385–21.325)
Last TPA	0.058	0.032	3.189	0.074	1.060 (0.994–1.129)
Presence of PJK			14.918	**0.001**	
PJK (vs. no PJK)	1.375	0.500	7.570	**0.006**	3.957 (1.485–10.540)
Revision surgery for PJK (vs. no PJK)	3.051	0.897	11.559	**0.001**	21.141 (3.641–122–754)

Stepwise multivariate analysis was performed using variables that had a significance of <0.05 in the univariate analyses. B means regression coefficient; S.E, standard error. * Bold p-values indicate statistical significance. † Age-adjusted PI-LL target was calculated as follows: Age-adjusted PI-LL target = (Age − 55)/2 + 3. Offset was calculated as the following formula: (actual PI-LL) − (age-adjusted PI-LL target). According to offset, Under means offset > 10°, Matched means offset within ±10°, and Over means offset < −10°. BMD indicates bone mineral density; PI, pelvic incidence; LL, lumbar lordosis; TPA, T1 pelvic angle; PJK, proximal junctional kyphosis.

Other factors such as T-score, correction amount according to age-adjusted PI-LL, and TPA at the final follow-up, were not significant in multivariate analysis. However, both TPA and SVA values at the last follow-up were significantly greater in patients who developed PJK compared with those who did not. There was no significant difference in these values between patients without PJK and those who underwent revision surgery for PJK (Figure 2).

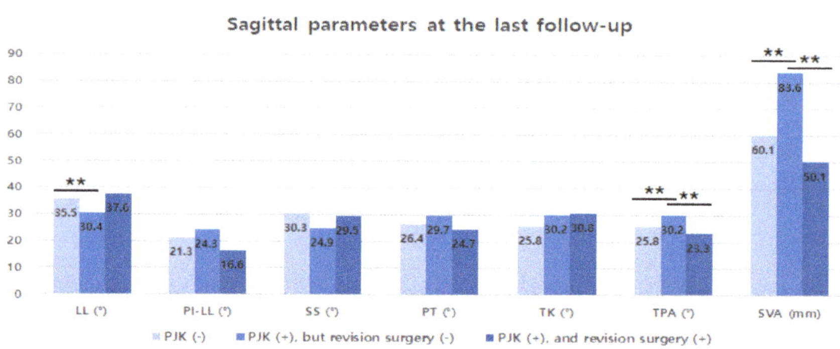

Figure 2. Sagittal parameters at the last follow-up according to PJK development and related revision surgery. Note that TPA and SVA values at the last follow-up were significantly greater in patients with PJK development but were not different between patients without PJK and those who underwent revision surgery for PJK. ** means $p < 0.05$.

At the last follow-up, HRQOL measures, such as ODI, several items of SRS-22r, and SF-36 scores, showed a trend of worse outcomes in patients with PJK development and revision surgery followed by patients with PJK but did not undergo revision surgery, and finally, patients without PJK development (Table 5).

Table 5. The last-follow-up HRQOLs according to PJK development.

		PJK (−) (N = 47)	PJK (+), Revision (−) (N = 44)	PJK (+), Revision (+) (N = 14)	p * (ANOVA)
	ODI	34.9 ± 21.0	47.6 ± 18.5	56.4 ± 23.5	**0.001**
SRS-22r	Function	3.4 ± 0.8	2.6 ± 0.7	2.6 ± 0.7	**<0.001**
	Pain	3.9 ± 0.8	3.2 ± 0.9	2.7 ± 0.9	**0.004**
	Appearance	3.5 ± 0.8	2.6 ± 0.8	2.8 ± 0.8	**0.001**
	Mental health	3.7 ± 0.9	2.7 ± 1.0	2.7 ± 0.5	**<0.001**
	Satisfaction	3.7 ± 0.8	3.5 ± 0.8	2.9 ± 0.9	0.054
	Total	3.6 ± 0.7	2.9 ± 0.7	2.7 ± 0.6	**0.001**
SF-36	Physical functioning	46.3 ± 28.6	29.4 ± 24.7	25.0 ± 24.0	**0.049**
	Role—physical	62.8 ± 32.6	47.7 ± 29.1	41.7 ± 22.7	0.124
	Bodily pain	59.0 ± 23.4	44.0 ± 23.8	56.5 ± 20.9	0.081
	General Health	49.3 ± 20.5	32.9 ± 23.7	32.2 ± 16.6	**0.030**
	Vitality	47.8 ± 22.6	38.9 ± 22.2	43.1 ± 18.1	0.392
	Social functioning	72.5 ± 29.9	51.4 ± 32.8	44.4 ± 25.1	**0.031**
	Role—emotional	65.8 ± 36.7	56.4 ± 34.5	38.9 ± 17.7	0.142
	Mental health	60.3 ± 27.3	50.2 ± 27.6	51.7 ± 14.6	0.410
	Physical component summary	54.3 ± 21.7	38.5 ± 21.2	38.8 ± 11.4	**0.027**
	Mental component summary	61.1 ± 25.3	49.5 ± 26.1	52.8 ± 24.6	0.151

Data are presented as the mean ± SD. (+) indicates that the event has occurred; (−) indicates that the event has not occurred. * Bold *p* values mean statistical significance. HRQOL indicates health-related quality of life; PJK, proximal junctional kyphosis; ODI, Oswestry disability index; SRS-22r, Scoliosis Research Society-22r; SF-36, 36-item short-form health survey.

4. Discussion

In assessing ASD surgery success, pertinent restoration of the optimal spinopelvic alignment has received the most attention. Numerous studies have shown a strong correlation between radiographic alignment and pain or disability in patients with ASD [3,23,27]. However, most of these previous studies were based on 2-year follow-up data. Few studies have reported the predictive factors affecting clinical outcomes over the long-term follow-up period. It is important to ensure good clinical outcomes even during long-term follow-up following any surgical treatment for spinal diseases because as the follow-up period increases, various adverse events can happen, such as loss of correction or mechanical complications, after ASD surgery. Therefore, we believe it is necessary to include such probable adverse events as well as postoperative spinopelvic alignment when evaluating the long-term clinical outcome.

To the best of our knowledge, no previous research has examined long-term clinical outcomes following ASD surgery by combining demographic and radiographic data, and mechanical complications. In this study, we used ODI scores to define the poor outcome group because ODI is a widely recognized tool for assessing disability levels [20,21,28]. However, we also found that other HRQOL measures such as SRS-22r, and SF-36, were significantly worse in group P compared with group NP. Therefore, we believe that the two groups based on ODI scores well represent the poor and non-poor outcome groups.

In the current study, multivariate analysis revealed that the most important factor that led to poor clinical outcomes was PJK development. It is quite understandable that patients with PJK would have inferior clinical outcomes to those of patients without PJK because numerous studies have documented clinical deterioration following PJK development. Kim et al. have reported that pain was prevalent in 0.9% of patients without PJK development compared with 29.4% of patients with PJK, resulting in a lower composite SRS-22r pain score (mean change +12 vs. +0.8) [29]. Bridwell et al. proposed the threshold of PJA of 20° to define the symptomatic PJK. They observed that changes in SRS-22r score were lower in PJK patients, although not significantly different from those in the non-PJK group [30].

At this point, it is notable that PJK development outweighs other factors such as T-score, correction amount relative to the age-adjusted PI-LL, and last TPA, which were only significant in univariate analyses. Although these values were not significant in our multivariate analysis, they are linked to PJK development. Low bone density is a strong risk factor for PJK development, especially bony-failure type PJK [31]. The concept of age-adjusted PI-LL, first introduced by Lafage et al. in 2016 [21], has been regarded as important in PJK prevention. Several studies have demonstrated that aligning with the age-adjusted PI-LL target significantly lowers the risk of developing PJK [32,33]. Recently, Park et al. demonstrated that overcorrection relative to the age-adjusted PI-LL target is associated with a higher risk of PJK and poor clinical outcomes [34]. In this study, we observed a significantly higher number of patients in group P who had overcorrection compared with the age-adjusted PI-LL target, in contrast to those in group NP (Table 3). We infer from this result that overcorrection relative to the age-adjusted PI-LL target correlates with poor clinical outcomes by increasing the risk of PJK.

Finally, TPA at the last follow-up was significantly greater in group P than in group NP. It is well-known that a higher TPA is associated with poorer clinical outcomes [22,28]. The increased TPA at the last follow-up compared with immediate postoperatively might result from correction loss during the follow-up period, as we documented a significant loss of correction over time (Figure 1A,B). However, a high TPA could also be the result of PJK development. Once the PJK occurs, C7SVA tends to increase, and the pelvis rotates backward to compensate for the forward posture. Due to these coupled mechanisms, TPA would increase after PJK development, as shown in Figure 2. Although a low T-score on BMD, overcorrection relative to the age-adjusted PI-LL at immediate postoperative and the final high TPA were not significant in the multivariate analysis, and we believe that all these factors are related to PJK development (Figure 3).

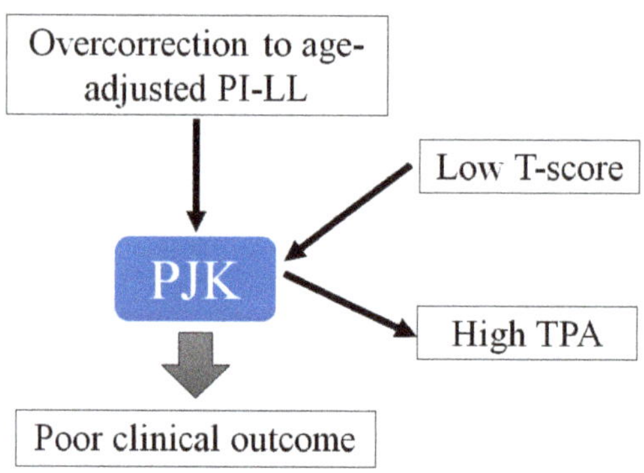

Figure 3. Diagram showing the factors affecting the PJK and clinical outcomes. PI indicates pelvic incidence; LL, lumbar lordosis; PJK, proximal junctional kyphosis; TPA, T1 pelvic angle.

Therefore, we suggest that the active management of poor bone quality before and after surgery, combined with proper alignment restoration according to the age-adjusted PI-LL target during surgery, is crucial for preventing PJK and achieving favorable long-term clinical outcomes.

Lastly, we found that patients who underwent revision surgery for PJK had worse clinical outcomes compared with patients with PJK but without revision surgery, despite significant improvement in critical radiographic parameters like TPA and SVA after the revision surgery (Figure 2). This might be because a few patients in this study underwent revision surgery due to spinal cord compression. In a recent study, Ha et al. reported that the prognosis of neurologic deficit after revision surgery for PJK with neurologic involvement is not favorable, with over 50% of patients experiencing no improvement in their neurologic status [35].

A few limitations should be acknowledged in this study. First, the number of enrolled patients was relatively small compared with recent ASD studies. However, this might be attributed to our strict inclusion and exclusion criteria regarding radiographic and clinical data, as well as the long follow-up duration. Second, although we demonstrated that PJK development is most responsible for poor clinical outcomes during long-term follow-up, there might be a few patients who did not experience clinical deterioration despite PJK development. Lastly, our study is limited by its single-center design and the lack of diversity in patient populations. Future multicenter studies are necessary to enhance the generalizability and cohort size.

5. Conclusions

This study identified PJK development as the sole independent factor contributing to poor clinical outcomes during long-term follow-up. In contrast, rod fractures were not significantly associated with poor outcomes, even in cases requiring revision surgery. While low T-scores, overcorrection relative to the age-adjusted PI-LL, and high TPAs at the last follow-up were linked to poor outcomes in univariate analysis, these factors are closely related to PJK development. Thus, preventing PJK is crucial for ensuring long-term success following ASD surgery.

Author Contributions: Conceptualization, S.-J.P. and C.-S.L.; Methodology, S.-J.P., H.-J.K. and J.-S.P.; Data acquisition, H.-J.K., D.-H.K., M.K., K.J. and C.-S.L.; Data interpretation, S.-J.P., H.-J.K., J.-S.P., D.-H.K. and C.-S.L.; Formal analysis, S.-J.P., H.-J.K. and M.K.; Writing—original draft preparation, S.-J.P., H.-J.K., M.K. and K.J.; Writing—review and editing, J.-S.P., H.-J.K., D.-H.K. and K.J. All authors have read and agreed to the published version of the manuscript.

Funding: No external funding was provided for this research.

Institutional Review Board Statement: The study protocol was approved by the Institutional Review Board (IRB) of Samsung Medical Center (Seoul, Republic of Korea; approval no. SMC 2024-07-144; Approval date: 1 July 2024) and the IRB of NHIS approved this study protocol. This study was performed in accordance with the relevant guidelines and regulations and the principles of the Declaration of Helsinki.

Informed Consent Statement: An informed consent exemption was granted by the board owing to the retrospective nature of the study.

Data Availability Statement: Data used in this study can be shared upon reasonable request from the journal. However, it can be limited due to patient privacy and ethical restrictions.

Conflicts of Interest: The authors declare no conflicts of interest.

References

1. Kim, H.J.; Yang, J.H.; Chang, D.G.; Lenke, L.G.; Suh, S.W.; Nam, Y.; Park, S.C.; Suk, S.I. Adult Spinal Deformity: A Comprehensive Review of Current Advances and Future Directions. *Asian Spine J.* **2022**, *16*, 776–788. [CrossRef] [PubMed]
2. Scheer, J.K.; Lafage, R.; Schwab, F.J.; Liabaud, B.; Smith, J.S.; Mundis, G.M.; Hostin, R.; Shaffrey, C.I.; Burton, D.C.; Hart, R.A.; et al. Under Correction of Sagittal Deformities Based on Age-adjusted Alignment Thresholds Leads to Worse Health-related Quality of Life Whereas over Correction Provides No Additional Benefit. *Spine* **2018**, *43*, 388–393. [CrossRef] [PubMed]
3. Smith, J.S.; Klineberg, E.; Schwab, F.; Shaffrey, C.I.; Moal, B.; Ames, C.P.; Hostin, R.; Fu, K.-M.G.; Burton, D.; Akbarnia, B.; et al. Change in classification grade by the SRS-Schwab Adult Spinal Deformity Classification predicts impact on health-related quality of life measures: Prospective analysis of operative and nonoperative treatment. *Spine* **2013**, *38*, 1663–1671. [CrossRef] [PubMed]
4. Takemoto, M.; Boissiere, L.; Vital, J.M.; Pellise, F.; Perez-Grueso, F.J.S.; Kleinstuck, F.; Acaroglu, E.R.; Alanay, A.; Obeid, I. Are sagittal spinopelvic radiographic parameters significantly associated with quality of life of adult spinal deformity patients? Multivariate linear regression analyses for pre-operative and short-term post-operative health-related quality of life. *Eur. Spine J.* **2017**, *26*, 2176–2186. [CrossRef]
5. Hayashi, K.; Boissière, L.; Guevara-Villazón, F.; Larrieu, D.; Núñez-Pereira, S.; Bourghli, A.; Gille, O.; Vital, J.-M.; Pellisé, F.; Sánchez Pérez-Grueso, F.J.; et al. Factors influencing patient satisfaction after adult scoliosis and spinal deformity surgery. *J. Neurosurg. Spine* **2019**, *31*, 408–417. [CrossRef]
6. Alshabab, S.; Gupta, M.C.; Lafage, R.; Bess, S.; Shaffrey, C.; Kim, H.J.; Ames, C.P.; Burton, D.C.; Smith, J.S.; Eastlack, R.K.; et al. Does Achieving Global Spinal Alignment Lead to Higher Patient Satisfaction and Lower Disability in Adult Spinal Deformity? *Spine* **2021**, *46*, 1105–1110. [CrossRef]

7. Hasegawa, T.; Ushirozako, H.; Yamato, Y.; Yoshida, G.; Yasuda, T.; Banno, T.; Arima, H.; Oe, S.; Yamada, T.; Ide, K.; et al. Impact of Spinal Correction Surgeries with Osteotomy and Pelvic Fixation in Patients with Kyphosis Due to Osteoporotic Vertebral Fractures. *Asian Spine J.* **2021**, *15*, 523–532. [CrossRef]
8. Kim, H.J.; Yang, J.H.; Chang, D.G.; Suk, S.I.; Suh, S.W.; Kim, S.I.; Song, K.S.; Park, J.B.; Cho, W. Proximal Junctional Kyphosis in Adult Spinal Deformity: Definition, Classification, Risk Factors, and Prevention Strategies. *Asian Spine J.* **2022**, *16*, 440–450. [CrossRef]
9. Lee, S.H.; Kim, K.T.; Suk, K.S.; Lee, J.H.; Seo, E.M.; Huh, D.S. Sagittal decompensation after corrective osteotomy for lumbar degenerative kyphosis: Classification and risk factors. *Spine* **2011**, *36*, E538–E544. [CrossRef]
10. Cho, K.J.; Suk, S.I.; Park, S.R.; Kim, J.H.; Kang, S.B.; Kim, H.S.; Oh, S.J. Risk factors of sagittal decompensation after long posterior instrumentation and fusion for degenerative lumbar scoliosis. *Spine* **2010**, *35*, 1595–1601. [CrossRef]
11. Kim, Y.J.; Bridwell, K.H.; Lenke, L.G.; Rhim, S.; Cheh, G. Sagittal thoracic decompensation following long adult lumbar spinal instrumentation and fusion to L5 or S1: Causes, prevalence, and risk factor analysis. *Spine* **2006**, *31*, 2359–2366. [CrossRef] [PubMed]
12. Kim, Y.J.; Bridwell, K.H.; Lenke, L.G.; Glattes, C.R.; Rhim, S.; Cheh, G. Proximal junctional kyphosis in adult spinal deformity after segmental posterior spinal instrumentation and fusion: Minimum five-year follow-up. *Spine* **2008**, *33*, 2179–2184. [CrossRef] [PubMed]
13. Lertudomphonwanit, T.; Kelly, M.P.; Bridwell, K.H.; Lenke, L.G.; McAnany, S.J.; Punyarat, P.; Bryan, T.P.; Buchowski, J.M.; Zebala, L.P.; Sides, B.A.; et al. Rod fracture in adult spinal deformity surgery fused to the sacrum: Prevalence, risk factors, and impact on health-related quality of life in 526 patients. *Spine J.* **2018**, *18*, 1612–1624. [CrossRef] [PubMed]
14. How, N.E.; Street, J.T.; Dvorak, M.F.; Fisher, C.G.; Kwon, B.K.; Paquette, S.; Smith, J.S.; Shaffrey, C.I.; Ailon, T. Pseudarthrosis in adult and pediatric spinal deformity surgery: A systematic review of the literature and meta-analysis of incidence, characteristics, and risk factors. *Neurosurg. Rev.* **2019**, *42*, 319–336. [CrossRef]
15. Park, S.J.; Park, J.S.; Lee, C.S.; Shin, T.S.; Lee, K.H. Proximal Junctional Failure after Corrective Surgery: Focusing on Elderly Patients with Severe Sagittal Imbalance. *Clin. Orthop. Surg.* **2023**, *15*, 975–982. [CrossRef]
16. Park, S.J.; Park, J.S.; Lee, C.S.; Shin, T.S.; Kim, I.S.; Lee, K.H. Radiographic Factors of Proximal Junctional Failure According to Age Groups in Adult Spinal Deformity. *Clin. Orthop. Surg.* **2023**, *15*, 606–615. [CrossRef]
17. Teles, A.R.; Aldebeyan, S.; Aoude, A.; Swamy, G.; Nicholls, F.H.; Thomas, K.C.; Jacobs, W.B. Mechanical Complications in Adult Spinal Deformity Surgery: Can Spinal Alignment Explain Everything? *Spine* **2022**, *47*, E1–E9. [CrossRef]
18. Lafage, R.; Bass, R.D.; Klineberg, E.; Smith, J.S.; Bess, S.; Shaffrey, C.; Burton, D.C.; Kim, H.J.; Eastlack, R.; Mundis, G., Jr.; et al. Complication Rates Following Adult Spinal Deformity Surgery: Evaluation of the Category of Complication and Chronology. *Spine* **2024**, *49*, 829–839. [CrossRef]
19. Kim, Y.-H.; Ha, K.-Y.; Chang, D.-G.; Park, H.-Y.; Jeon, W.-K.; Park, H.-C.; Kim, S.-I. Relationship between iliac screw loosening and proximal junctional kyphosis after long thoracolumbar instrumented fusion for adult spinal deformity. *Eur. Spine J.* **2020**, *29*, 1371–1378. [CrossRef]
20. Schwab, F.; Patel, A.; Ungar, B.; Farcy, J.P.; Lafage, V. Adult spinal deformity-postoperative standing imbalance: How much can you tolerate? An overview of key parameters in assessing alignment and planning corrective surgery. *Spine* **2010**, *35*, 2224–2231. [CrossRef]
21. Lafage, R.; Schwab, F.; Challier, V.; Henry, J.K.; Gum, J.; Smith, J.; Hostin, R.; Shaffrey, C.; Kim, H.J.; Ames, C.; et al. Defining Spino-Pelvic Alignment Thresholds: Should Operative Goals in Adult Spinal Deformity Surgery Account for Age? *Spine* **2016**, *41*, 62–68. [CrossRef] [PubMed]
22. Ryan, D.J.; Protopsaltis, T.S.; Ames, C.P.; Hostin, R.; Klineberg, E.; Mundis, G.M.; Obeid, I.; Kebaish, K.; Smith, J.S.; Boachie-Adjei, O.; et al. T1 pelvic angle (TPA) effectively evaluates sagittal deformity and assesses radiographical surgical outcomes longitudinally. *Spine* **2014**, *39*, 1203–1210. [CrossRef] [PubMed]
23. Schwab, F.; Ungar, B.; Blondel, B.; Buchowski, J.; Coe, J.; Deinlein, D.; DeWald, C.; Mehdian, H.; Shaffrey, C.; Tribus, C.; et al. Scoliosis Research Society-Schwab adult spinal deformity classification: A validation study. *Spine* **2012**, *37*, 1077–1082. [CrossRef] [PubMed]
24. Yilgor, C.; Sogunmez, N.; Boissiere, L.; Yavuz, Y.; Obeid, I.; Kleinstück, F.; Sánchez Pérez-Grueso, F.J.; Acaroglu, E.; Haddad, S.; Mannion, A.F.; et al. Global Alignment and Proportion (GAP) Score: Development and Validation of a New Method of Analyzing Spinopelvic Alignment to Predict Mechanical Complications After Adult Spinal Deformity Surgery. *J. Bone Joint Surg. Am.* **2017**, *99*, 1661–1672. [CrossRef]
25. Passias, P.G.; Jalai, C.M.; Diebo, B.G.; Cruz, D.L.; Poorman, G.W.; Buckland, A.J.; Day, L.M.; Horn, S.R.; Liabaud, B.; Lafage, R.; et al. Full-Body Radiographic Analysis of Postoperative Deviations From Age-Adjusted Alignment Goals in Adult Spinal Deformity Correction and Related Compensatory Recruitment. *Int. J. Spine Surg.* **2019**, *13*, 205–214. [CrossRef]
26. Maruo, K.; Ha, Y.; Inoue, S.; Samuel, S.; Okada, E.; Hu, S.S.; Deviren, V.; Burch, S.; Schairer, W.; Ames, C.P.; et al. Predictive factors for proximal junctional kyphosis in long fusions to the sacrum in adult spinal deformity. *Spine* **2013**, *38*, E1469–E1476. [CrossRef]
27. Hallager, D.W.; Hansen, L.V.; Dragsted, C.R.; Peytz, N.; Gehrchen, M.; Dahl, B. A Comprehensive Analysis of the SRS-Schwab Adult Spinal Deformity Classification and Confounding Variables: A Prospective, Non-US Cross-sectional Study in 292 Patients. *Spine* **2016**, *41*, E589–E597. [CrossRef]

28. Protopsaltis, T.; Schwab, F.; Bronsard, N.; Smith, J.S.; Klineberg, E.; Mundis, G.; Ryan, D.J.; Hostin, R.; Hart, R.; Burton, D.; et al. The T1 pelvic angle, a novel radiographic measure of global sagittal deformity, accounts for both spinal inclination and pelvic tilt and correlates with health-related quality of life. *J. Bone Joint Surg. Am.* **2014**, *96*, 1631–1640. [CrossRef]
29. Kim, H.J.; Bridwell, K.H.; Lenke, L.G.; Park, M.S.; Ahmad, A.; Song, K.S.; Piyaskulkaew, C.; Hershman, S.; Fogelson, J.; Mesfin, A. Proximal junctional kyphosis results in inferior SRS pain subscores in adult deformity patients. *Spine* **2013**, *38*, 896–901. [CrossRef]
30. Bridwell, K.H.; Lenke, L.G.; Cho, S.K.; Pahys, J.M.; Zebala, L.P.; Dorward, I.G.; Cho, W.; Baldus, C.; Hill, B.W.; Kang, M.M. Proximal junctional kyphosis in primary adult deformity surgery: Evaluation of 20 degrees as a critical angle. *Neurosurgery* **2013**, *72*, 899–906. [CrossRef]
31. Koike, Y.; Kotani, Y.; Terao, H.; Iwasaki, N. Risk Factor Analysis of Proximal Junctional Kyphosis after Surgical Treatment of Adult Spinal Deformity with Oblique Lateral Interbody Fusion. *Asian Spine J.* **2021**, *15*, 107–116. [CrossRef] [PubMed]
32. Lafage, R.; Schwab, F.; Glassman, S.; Bess, S.; Harris, B.; Sheer, J.; Hart, R.; Line, B.; Henry, J.; Burton, D.; et al. Age-Adjusted Alignment Goals Have the Potential to Reduce PJK. *Spine* **2017**, *42*, 1275–1282. [CrossRef] [PubMed]
33. Byun, C.W.; Cho, J.H.; Lee, C.S.; Lee, D.H.; Hwang, C.J. Effect of overcorrection on proximal junctional kyphosis in adult spinal deformity: Analysis by age-adjusted ideal sagittal alignment. *Spine J.* **2022**, *22*, 635–645. [CrossRef] [PubMed]
34. Park, S.J.; Lee, C.S.; Kang, B.J.; Shin, T.S.; Kim, I.S.; Park, J.S.; Lee, K.H.; Shin, D.H. Validation of Age-adjusted Ideal Sagittal Alignment in Terms of Proximal Junctional Failure and Clinical Outcomes in Adult Spinal Deformity. *Spine* **2022**, *47*, 1737–1745. [CrossRef] [PubMed]
35. Ha, K.Y.; Kim, E.H.; Kim, Y.H.; Jang, H.D.; Park, H.Y.; Cho, C.H.; Cho, R.K.; Kim, S.I. Surgical outcomes for late neurological deficits after long segment instrumentation for degenerative adult spinal deformity. *J. Neurosurg. Spine* **2021**, *35*, 340–346. [CrossRef]

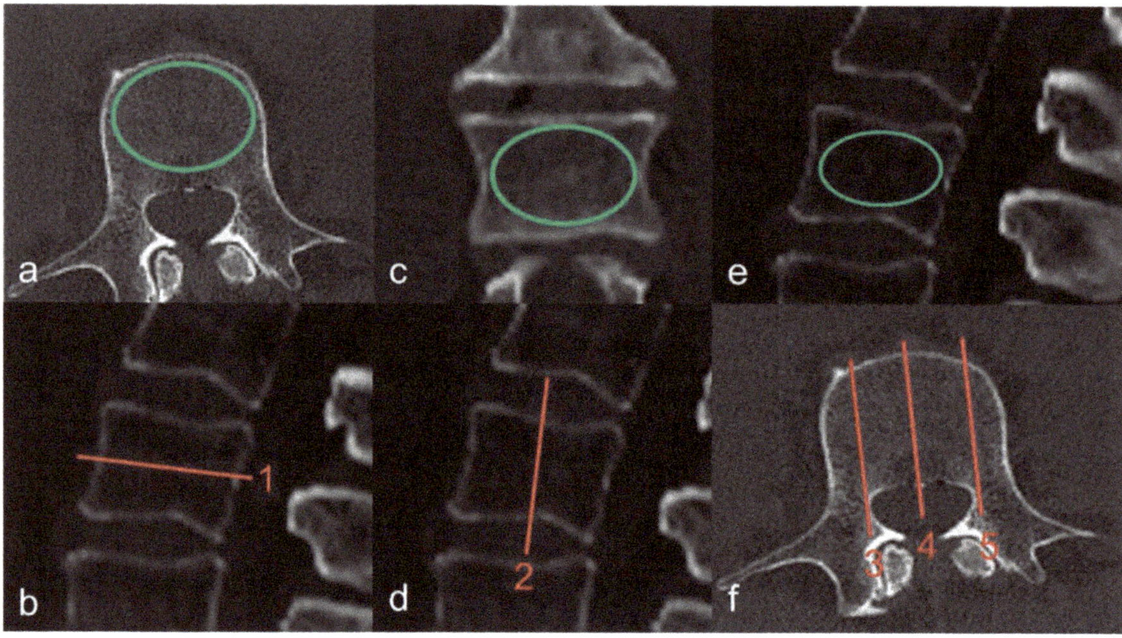

Figure 1. Determining Hounsfield units based on a mid-vertebral region of interest in the axial (**a**,**b**), coronary (**c**,**d**), and sagittal (**e**,**f**) plane. (**b**) shows the mid-vertebral height of the axial section (1). (**d**) displays the mid-vertebral height of the coronal section (2). (**f**) illustrates the mid-vertebral height of the sagittal section centrally (4), as well as laterally on the **right** (3) and **left** (5) sides.

2.6. Statistics

All descriptive statistics of quantitative characteristics (age, BMI, BMD) are shown as means ± standard deviation (SD). The study design with multiple measurements for the outcome of cancellous bone density was reflected by a General Linear Model Repeated Measures. The procedure provides an analysis of variance for several subgroups and factor levels. The model was fitted to the bone density values obtained from micro-CT (BVF%) and CT (HU) in the 3 sectional planes and measured quadrants QI, QII, QIII for 22 vertebrae using the binary predictors gender [female, male] and fracture status [$\leq$1 fracture, >1 fracture], adjusted for covariates age [years] and BMI [kg/m^2]. The assumption of normality was tested with the Shapiro–Wilk test. The resulting bone density values of investigated subgroups and factor levels are given as estimated marginal means ± SD, obtained from the model. Null hypotheses about the effects of factors, covariates, and interactions were tested; *p*-values of post hoc multiple comparison tests were Sidak-adjusted; the level of significance was set to $p < 0.05$. All data were analyzed using the statistical software package IBM® SPSS® 29.0.

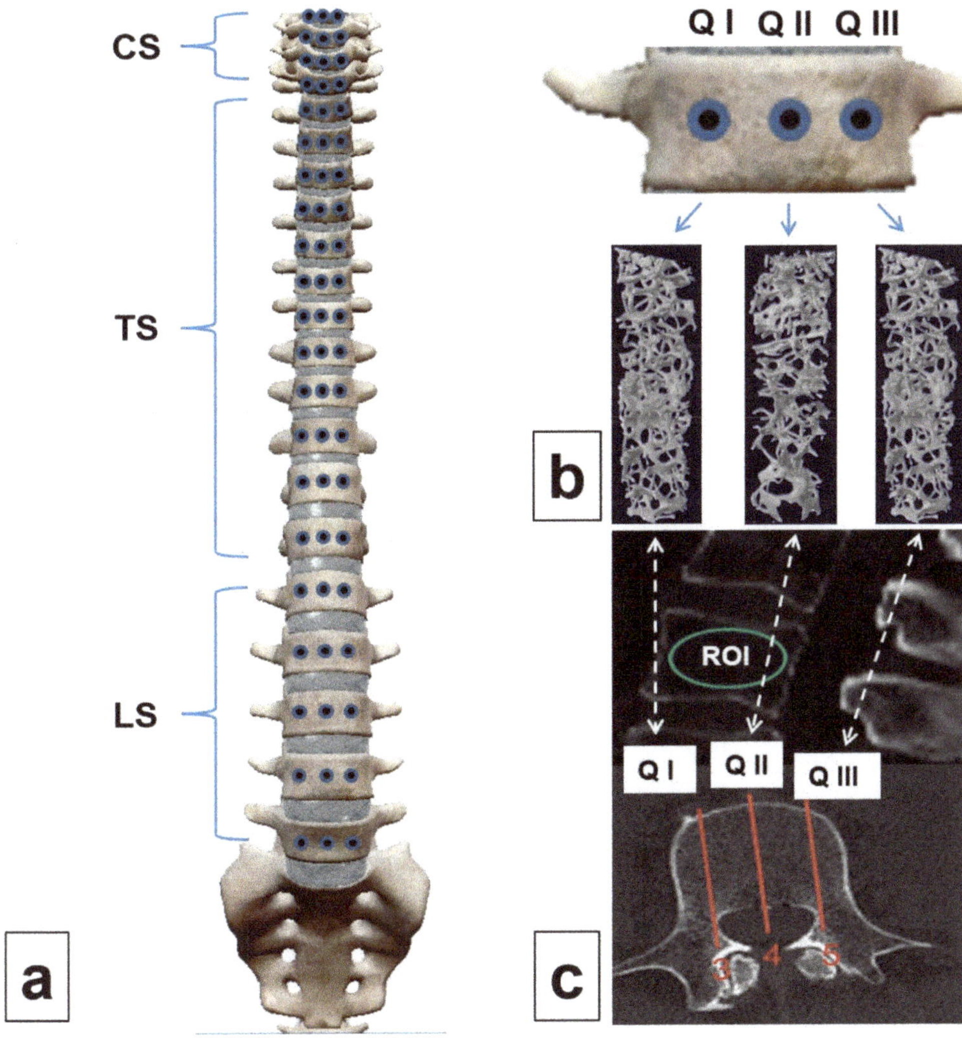

Figure 2. Schematic illustration of the extraction of cancellous bone cylinders (**a**) from the cervical (CS), thoracic (TS), and lumbar spine (LS); quadrant biopsies (**b**) from the marginal areas (QI and QIII) and the central quadrant (QII) for the determination of bone volume fraction (BVF) on micro-CT; determination of Hounsfield units using a region of interest in the sagittal (**c**) sectional plane in a central region (4) and in 2 marginal areas (3 and 5), which were deemed comparable to the biopsy quadrants on micro-CT. This was followed by a comparison of cancellous bone density determined on CT and micro-CT (QI or right-sided edge equals area 3, QII or the central region equals area 4, and Q III or the left-sided edge equals area 5).

3. Results

A total of 11 spines, each with 22 vertebrae, were extracted from human body donors. Per vertebra, we obtained three cancellous bone cylinders. Finally, 726 micro-CT samples were compared with 726 sagittal sections on CT with regard to cancellous bone density. The 11 spines were derived from five male and six female donors, 66 to 91 years old (79.1 ± 7.5). The available information about medical histories is limited to the cause of death. A summary is provided in Table 1.

Table 1. Medical history data of the entire group.

	Body Donors (n = 11)
Age (years)	79.1 ± 7.5
Gender (male/female)	5/6
Body mass index (kg/m^2)	21.9 ± 5.5
Number of sustained fractures (≤1 fracture/>1 fracture)	3/8
Extracted segments	C3-L5
Bone density in the lumbar vertebrae 1 to 3 (mg/cm^3) *	58.7 ± 27.3
Number of vertebral body fractures	1.8 ± 1.1
Number of vertebral fractures in relation to gender: overall/male/female (n)	
Th5	1/0/1
Th6	1/1/0
Th7	3/2/1
Th8	3/2/1
Th9	2/1/1
Th10	1/0/1
Th12	2/2/0
L1	5/1/4
L2	2/0/2
Number of investigated vertebrae (n)	242
Number of investigated cancellous bone cylinders (n)	726
Hounsfield units in the sagittal plane in QI to Q III (n)	726
Comparison of sectional planes in Hounsfield units (axial, coronary, sagittal) (n)	726

Data shown as numbers (n) or mean ± standard deviation (SD); * measurements based on quantitative computed tomography (QCT).

3.1. QCT

The mean overall bone mineral density of 11 spines, measured from lumbar vertebra L1 to L3, yielded a value of 58.7 ± 27.2 mg/cm^3, which indicates severe OP. In general, a bone mineral density below 80 mg/cm^3 is interpreted as osteoporosis [5]. At a bone mineral density below 60 mg/cm^3, we found more fusion fractures in the thoracic and thoracolumbar regions (p = 0.012). No fractures were seen in the cervical spine.

Density of Cancellous Bone in Hounsfield Units on the CT Image

Cancellous bone density (HU) fell from C3 downward (186 ± 25.9) to L5 (88.1 ± 29.1: p < 0.001) (Figure 3). Generally, the axial section (119 ± 17.2) yielded higher HU values than the sagittal (116 ± 16.8) or coronary sections (117 ± 16.4). Men (157 ± 22.3; n = 5) had higher bone densities than women (77.6 ± 18.9; n = 6; p = 0.002). All three sectional planes reflected the gender difference to the same degree (p = 0.003 each). Men had higher density values on the axial image than on the sagittal (p < 0.001) or coronary images (p = 0.007), but the latter two planes did not differ from each other (p = 0.256). In women, we found no significant density differences in the sectional planes (p ≥ 0.111).

On average, the donors had experienced 1.8 ± 1.1 fractures (Table 1). Vertebral fractures (VF) differed in numbers and showed the following differences in density: ≤1 fracture 146 ± 15.8; more than 1 fracture 89.1 ± 14.4 (p = 0.002). At a maximum number of one VF, there were differences between the axial and sagittal sections (p = 0.001), as well as the axial and coronary sections (p = 0.017). On the other hand, the comparison of HU values from the sagittal and coronary images revealed no significant difference (p = 0.236). In body donors with more than one VF, we also found significant differences in the comparison of HU values in the axial and sagittal sections (p < 0.001), as well as the axial and coronary sections (p = 0.024). Again, the comparison of sagittal and coronary sections revealed no significant difference ($p = 0.060$). Men with a maximum of one fracture had higher cancellous bone densities (206 ± 17.6) than men with more than one sustained fracture (109 ± 15.3; $p = 0.003$); the same was not observed in women (85.5 ± 19.0; 69.7 ± 13.8; $p = 0.335$). However, men with ≤1 fracture ($p = 0.005$) and more than 1 fracture ($p = 0.014$) had higher cancellous bone densities than women in the respective fracture groups.

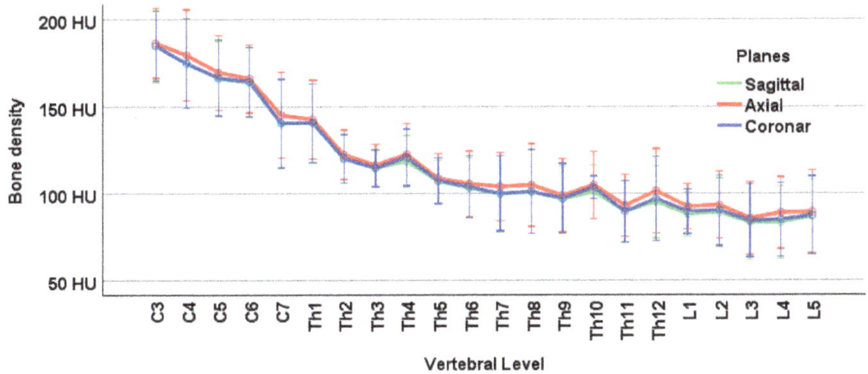

Figure 3. Cancellous bone density in Hounsfield units (HU) reduces along the spine from C3 to L5 ($p < 0.001$). Each vertebra was measured in 3 sectional planes (sagittal, axial, coronary). In all sections, we observed similar reducing values of bone density along the spine. Bone density is greater in the axial section than in the other two sectional planes. The average vertebral bone density ($n = 11$) of each sectional plane is shown as estimated marginal mean with the respective 95% confidence interval. Covariates appearing in the linear model are evaluated with age = 79.1 years and body mass index = 21.9 kg/m^2.

3.2. Micro-CT Compared with CT

3.2.1. Micro-CT and CT Scans Show Graphically Different Courses of Bone Density Values

A reduction in cancellous bone density from C3 to L5 was seen in CT investigations, as well as in the BVF values on micro-CT (C3: 25.0 ± 3.42; L5: 21.1 ± 7.56; $p = 0.018$). The values registered by the two procedures ran different courses (Figure 4). The differences were clearly seen on longitudinal sections over the 22 vertebrae in general (A vs. B), as well as divided into the 3 quadrants (C vs. D), and also in the 11 body donors (E vs. F).

3.2.2. Gender and Fracture Status Influence Bone Density Measurements

Gender ($p = 0.002$) and the number of existing VF (≤1 vs. >1; $p = 0.001$) were independent factors influencing cancellous bone density, regardless of the procedure used. However, age ($p = 0.227$) and BMI ($p = 0.091$) had no effect.

3.2.3. Micro-CT and CT Investigations Reveal Gender Differences with Varying Clarity

The two procedures (micro-CT and CT investigation) differed in their degrees of reflecting gender-related differences in cancellous bone density (Figure 5A vs. Figure 5B). Micro-CT investigation (A) revealed higher BVF values in men ($n = 5$) than in women ($n = 6$). On CT investigation (B), the gender difference was seen graphically on the fine scale in the individual vertebrae of the cervical, thoracic, and lumbar spine, and it was also statistically significant ($p = 0.002$).

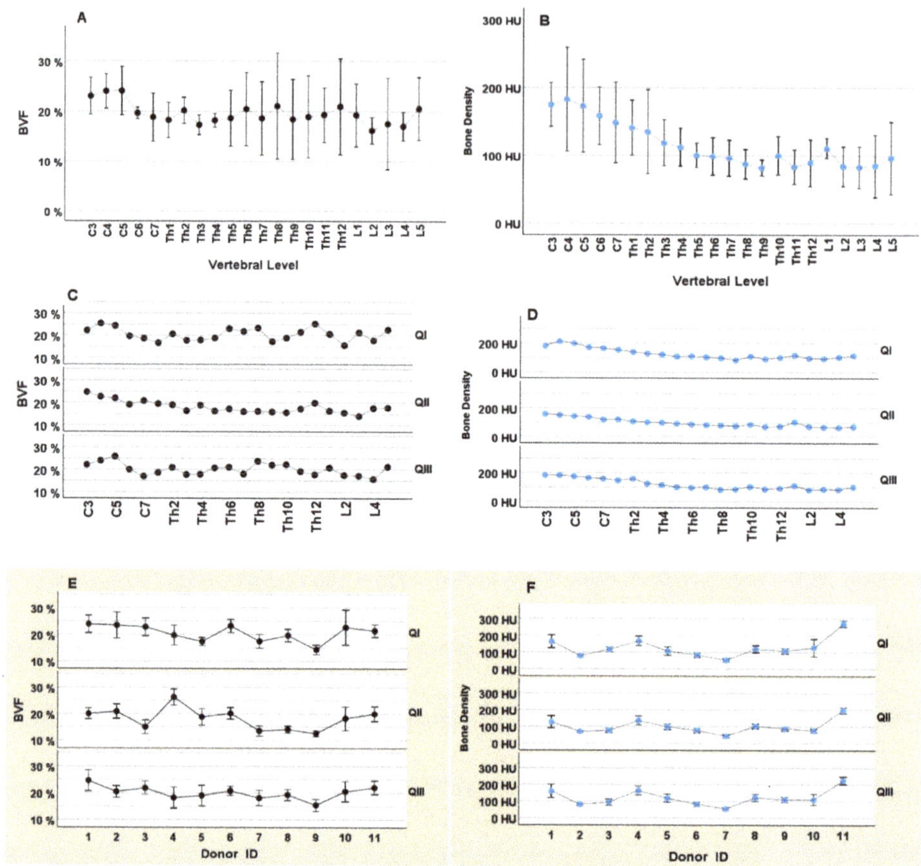

Figure 4. Graphic comparison of the two procedures for the determination of cancellous bone density with the aid of micro-CT (BVF%; left-sided panel, black dots) and CT (HU; right-sided panel, blue dots) with reference to the three quadrants QI, QII, QIII. **Above** (**A**) BVF% and (**B**) HU: Overall values for $n = 11$ body donors as profiles along the vertebrae C3-L5, averaged for 3 quadrants. A reduction in bone density along the spine is observed with both procedures but in different degrees. Data are given as means with their 95% confidence intervals. **Center** (**C**) BVF% and (**D**) HU: Individual views of the quadrants QI, QII, QIII. Each data point expresses the mean value for $n = 11$ body donors. The CT measurement yields, independent of the measured quadrant, uniformly reducing values. The micro-CT measurement shows different profiles in the quadrants, highlighting the importance of the measured quadrant. **Below** (**E**) BVF% and (**F**) HU: profiles of bone density for 11 donors in the investigated quadrants. In this regard as well, CT yields uniform profiles independent of the quadrant, but micro-CT does not. Data are given as means with their 95% confidence intervals.

3.2.4. Gender Differences Based on HU Values Were Independent of the Investigated Quadrants

The CT investigation showed higher HU values in men than in women for each of the three quadrants: Q1 ($p = 0.002$), QII ($p = 0.003$), and QIII ($p = 0.003$). In contrast, the micro-CT investigation showed no significant gender difference in QI ($p = 0.850$), QII ($p = 0.870$) or QIII ($p = 0.378$). In women, both procedures revealed no differences between the three quadrants ($p \geq 0.061$); the same was true of micro-CT measurements in men ($p \geq 0.672$). Only CT measurements in men showed differences in the quadrants ($p \leq 0.011$).

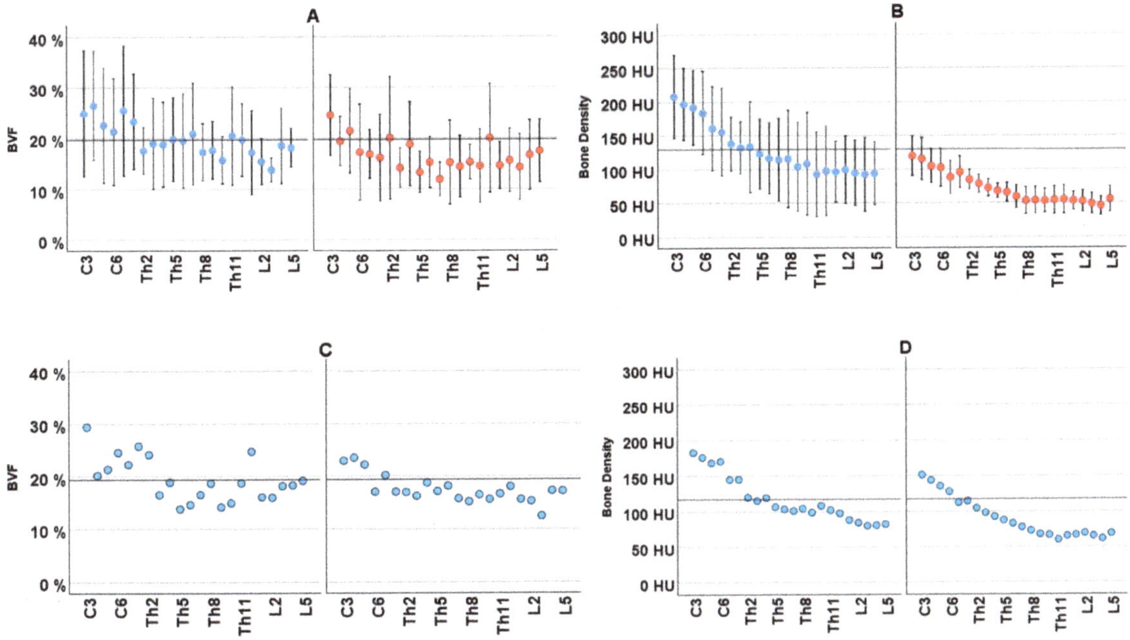

Figure 5. Bone density measurements (on the left side as bone volume fraction BVF%, on the right side in Hounsfield units HU) in relation to the two influencing factors: gender (**upper panel**) and the number of sustained vertebral fractures (VF), (**lower panel**), in relation to the location of the vertebral body. (**A**) BVF% of male (blue, $n = 5$, group mean = 19.7% as reference line) vs. female (red, $n = 6$). The mean density values in men serve as a reference line so that the below-average values in women become obvious. Data are shown as means with their 95% confidence intervals. (**B**) HU of male (blue, $n = 5$, group mean = 130 HU as reference line) vs. female (red, $n = 6$). (**C**) BVF% of the group with at most one experienced VF (**left**, $n = 3$, group mean = 19.4% as reference line) vs. the group with more than one VF (**right**, $n = 8$). Most of the shown vertebral BVF means of those with more than one fracture are smaller than the reference value of 19.4%. (**D**) HU of the group with at most one experienced VF (**left**, $n = 3$, group mean = 117 HU as reference line) vs. the group with more than one VF (**right**, $n = 8$). Data are given as means. Expected gender- and fracture-related differences in bone density are seen with both procedures. The higher bone density values on CT in HU were statistically confirmed in men as well as in the group with a maximum of one VF ($p = 0.002$ for each).

3.2.5. CT and Micro-CT Investigations Differ in Their Depiction of Fracture Status

The CT measurements showed differences between the subgroups of ≤ 1 fracture ($n = 3$) and more than 1 fracture ($n = 8$; $p = 0.002$, Figure 5D). The micro-CT measurements (C) were 21.9 ± 3.03 and 18.5 ± 2.77 ($p = 0.162$). Micro-CT revealed no differences between fracture groups for women ($p = 0.246$) or for men ($p = 0.431$). The CT investigation, on the other hand, revealed higher HU values in men at a maximum number of one versus more than one sustained vertebral fracture ($p = 0.003$).

4. Discussion

The present investigation permitted a comparison of cancellous bone densities in all segments of the spine from 11 body donors aged 66 to 91 years, measured with two different procedures. Besides, for the first time a study yielded data from aspirations of different quadrants in a micro-CT investigation, and Hounsfield units from similar quadrants of a CT investigation. The BMI in the entire group is considered normal, BMI values below 22 are related to a rising fracture rate [13]. All investigated probands had bone mineral density values below 80 mg/cm^3 on densitometry and therefore suffered from OP [14]; fusion fractures are obligatory at values below 60 mg/cm^3 [8]. The age of the body donors contributed significantly to these findings [15–17]. A rise in fracture rates was seen especially beyond the age of 70 years [18]. Fractures were typically distributed in the thoracolumbar and lumbar portions of the axial skeleton [9]. One explanation for this fracture cascade along the spine could be the pre-existing curvatures of the spine [19]. The turning point of the curvature of thoracic kyphosis is in the mid-region of the thoracic spine (Th7, Th8). Due to the greater curvature, there are higher bending moments and compression loads at this site. This notion is supported by the fact that an increase in curvature—which is equivalent to greater kyphosis which develops in the course of life and is especially significant in osteoporosis—results in greater bending loads. Likewise, the elevated fracture risk at the junction of Th12 and L1 is possibly explained by greater mobility in the lumbar spine and consequently higher compression loads. Vertebral fractures of the thoracic and lumbar spine belong to the 10 most frequent fracture entities in Germany [3].

In the present investigation, L1 was affected most frequently by a fracture, independent of gender. It was interesting to note that L1 had a model-adjusted mean value of 90.2 HU and thus a higher cancellous bone density than L4 with 86.0 HU. Thus, it may be assumed that, in addition to cancellous bone density, the above-mentioned factors play an important role in the number of sustained fractures.

No fractures of the cervical spine were observed in the present study. Montemurro et al. [20] investigated the significance of a Y-shaped trabecular bone structure (TBS) in the odontoid process of the axis (C2 vertebra) in patients with cervical spine injuries. The researchers concluded that the Y-shaped TBS plays a crucial role in the biomechanical structural dynamics of the C1-C2 joint and has significant clinical relevance for dens fractures [20]. These results suggest that the absence of this specific bone structure may be associated with an increased risk of dens fractures in cervical spine injuries.

After analyzing their data from human vertebral bodies, Shin et al. [21] conclude that the superior region of the vertebral bodies shows a higher biomechanical susceptibility, which could explain its dominant role in osteoporotic vertebral fractures. The authors recommend paying particular attention to the use of bone mineral density measurements of the superior vertebral body region using lateral DXA (Dual-energy X-ray absorptiometry) when diagnosing osteoporosis. Lateral spine DXA offers several advantages over conventional posterior–anterior measurement. It allows for a more accurate assessment of trabecular bone density in the vertebral body by excluding posterior elements and degenerative changes. Studies have shown that lateral DXA correlates better with trabecular bone density measured by quantitative computed tomography [22,23]. Additionally, lateral DXA demonstrates a stronger association with age and shows a steeper decline in bone density with increasing age compared with anterior–posterior measurement [23]. Lateral DXA can detect osteopenia and osteoporosis more frequently than anterior–posterior measurement, especially in patients with degenerative changes in the spine [23,24]. This makes it a useful tool for early detection of bone mass loss. However, there are some limitations: the precision and accuracy of lateral measurement are slightly lower than anterior–posterior measurement [23], and there is a lack of established reference values and diagnostic criteria for lateral DXA. Therefore, lateral spine DXA is currently not routinely recommended for the diagnosis of osteoporosis or monitoring of bone mass loss. However, it can provide valuable information as a complementary measurement, particularly in patients with significant degenerative changes in the spine, where anterior–posterior measurement might overestimate bone density [24].

A study by Zhao [25] and colleagues examined the differences between cranial and caudal endplates of the spine. The researchers found that the upper (cranial) endplates were significantly thinner than the lower (caudal) ones. In midsagittal sections, the difference was approximately 14%, while in pedicular sections, a difference of about 11% was observed. In addition to thickness, the optical density of the trabecular bone immediately adjacent to the endplates was also investigated. Here, it was shown that the density in the cranial region was about 6% lower than in the caudal region. Based on these findings, the scientists concluded that the thickness of the endplate alone is not sufficient to explain the more frequent failure in the upper region of the vertebral body. Rather, the biomechanical properties of the endplate seem to be closely linked to the characteristics of the underlying trabecular bone. These results highlight the complexity of vertebral body structure and indicate that multiple factors must be considered when assessing the stability and load-bearing capacity of the spine.

Measurements of HU from nearly complete spines (C3-L5), including micro-CT investigations, have rarely been performed so far. HU shows a normalized index of attenuation of the X-ray beam, based on a scale from 1000 for air and 0 for water. The HU value of bone is typically between 300 and 3000 [26]. With the aid of HU, we can make statements about bone density. Schreiber et al. [26] determined a significant correlation between T-scores on bone densitometry and HU of the same vertebra.

Our data showed a reduction in bone density in HU from cervical vertebra C3 to lumbar vertebra L5. Schröder et al. [9] investigated 624 vertebrae from cervical vertebra C3 to sacral vertebra S2, extracted from 26 body donors by using a manually positioned region of interest in cancellous bone. The authors determined the mean value from axial, sagittal, and coronary sections. Their investigation revealed a similar course of HU values over the spine as those registered in the present investigation. The highest HU was noted in the cervical spine. They conclude that a loss of bone mineral density in vertebral cancellous bone leads to a higher risk of fractures, but a value lower than the fracture-critical threshold is not achieved in the cervical spine even in the presence of evident osteoporosis.

In contrast to Schröder et. al. [9], the present investigation compared HU values from the axial, sagittal, and coronary sections of the same vertebrae in order to detect differences, if any, in the various sectional planes. The highest HU values were noted in the axial sections. Marinova et al. [27] routinely evaluated chest and abdomen CT data from 234 patients aged on average 59 years and found no significant intra-individual differences between HU values in the axial, sagittal, and coronary planes. The authors assume that HU values are similar regardless of the sectional plane. In a further investigation performed by Kim et al. [28], the CT data of the lumbar spines of 100 patients aged over 50 years were evaluated. The authors also found no difference between the axial, sagittal, and coronary planes when screening for osteoporosis on CT, and concluded that all three planes could be used equally for the measurement of bone mineral density on CT. For the sectional planes, the authors compared the areas under the ROC curve (AUC) and the intra-class correlation coefficient (ICC). Kim et al. [28] achieved cut-off values of 110 HU in the coronary plane, 112 HU in the axial, and 112 HU in the sagittal planes.

In contrast, Zhang et al. [29] investigated 1338 patients aged on average 61.9 years and showed that measurements in the axial plane were on average 9 HU higher than those on sagittal measurements. The authors used the thoracic vertebra 7 for their measurements. With regard to the differentiation between osteoporosis and no osteoporosis, the sagittal plane showed greater diagnostic efficacy. For each one-unit reduction in the sagittal CT attenuation value, the risk of osteopenia or osteoporosis rose by 3.6 percent. The authors recommend a bone densitometry investigation for all patients with a sagittal CT attenuation value of <113.7 HU in the 7th thoracic vertebra.

The observation made in the present investigation that the HU values in the axial plane are higher than those in the sagittal and coronary planes can be explained by several radiological and anatomical factors. On the one hand, the partial volume effect [30] plays a decisive role in this phenomenon. In the axial plane, the region of interest (ROI) can be defined more precisely in cancellous bone, whereas sagittal and coronary reconstructions frequently include cortical bone or surrounding soft tissue. This results in the averaging of density values and, consequently, lower HU values in these planes. On the other hand, the trabecular structure of cancellous bone in the vertebrae is not isotropic. Due to the vertical arrangement of trabeculae, more bone substance per volume is registered in the axial plane, resulting in higher density values in this plane. Technical aspects of CT imaging, such as the selected slice thickness and reconstruction are also worthy of mention. The non-contrasted axial acquisition of CT data frequently yields a higher resolution than reconstructed sagittal and coronary images. Thinner sections in the axial plane may lead to more precise measurements and consequently higher HU values. The algorithms used for sagittal and coronary reconstructions may lead to a slight smoothing of data, which may influence the determined HU values. In order to minimize this discrepancy and obtain consistent values, the ROI should be established carefully in all three planes while avoiding cortical bone and marginal structures. Furthermore, if one wishes to obtain representative values, the formation of a mean value from the measurements of all three planes [9] appears to be meaningful only when there are no significant differences between the sectional planes. These conclusions underline the importance of a careful and consistent technique of measurement when determining HU values in vertebral bodies, especially in the context of bone density measurements and for the assessment of fracture risk.

Micro-CT investigations of the cancellous bone density of vertebrae from all segments of the spine are laborious and have been scarcely described so far. More recent studies [10,11] support our data showing that the bone volume fraction (BVF) reduces from the cervical to the lumbar spine.

In the present investigation, gender and fracture numbers, in contrast to age and BMI, were independent factors influencing cancellous bone density. In their study of 299 patients aged 65 to 90 years, Zou et al. [31] showed that, independent of age and gender, patients with a fragility fracture in the vertebrae had significantly lower HU values (on average 66 HU) than patients without a vertebral fracture (101.5 HU). The authors assume that HU values may serve as useful indicators, with high specificity (60 HU) and sensitivity (100 HU) for the identification of patients with a fracture risk [31]. In contrast to Zhou et al., our study was not limited to vertebrae in the thoracolumbar junction. Rather, we studied all segments of the spine.

In our study, the gender-specific differences in bone density values were significant and were shown in different degrees of clarity by the two methods. In the HU analysis, men had, as expected, significantly higher density values than women, especially in the axial section, which is indicative of differences in bone density and possibly also differences in bone quality and loads between genders. Women, on the other hand, had no significant differences in the sectional planes, which may be a sign of a more homogeneous distribution of bone structure. The micro-CT method revealed no significant gender differences in any of the quadrants, which is indicative of its limitations in clinical use.

Our results show that HU values on CT and BVF values on micro-CT investigation have different properties in terms of sensitivity in the determination of bone density. While HU values revealed uniform profiles of bone density over the vertebrae in the various quadrants and in individual body donors, BVF values were more heterogeneous in the quadrants. Particularly the bone density profile over the vertebral body in the central quadrant II showed the expected uniform reduction in values. The "noisy" data on micro-CT investigation may be an indication of the fact that this method of measurement is more strongly influenced by the choice of the quadrant. At the same time, the direction of aspiration used for the sampling procedure appears to play a role. Schröder et al. [12] compared ventrodorsal cancellous bone puncture with the craniocaudal one in 20 body donors aged on average 79.4 years. After completion of their study, the authors concluded that ventrodorsal puncture yields more subcortical structures, especially from the marginal areas of the vertebrae. Furthermore, on the Bland–Altman diagram, the authors showed the presence of a bias related to the selected direction of puncture in that a low BVF provides similar values, but a higher BVF yields markedly deviating values.

In contrast, the HU measurements on CT appear to be independent of the quadrants, which makes them more robust for clinical diagnostic investigation in order to obtain a comprehensive view of bone density.

Knowledge of HU for individual vertebral bodies offers significant advantages in the surgical treatment of osteoporotic fractures, enabling more precise preoperative risk assessment. Studies have demonstrated that low HU values (<120–150 HU) indicate reduced bone density and an increased risk of osteoporosis, allowing for better estimation of the risks of screw loosening, implant failure, or adjacent fractures [32,33]. This information can substantially influence operative planning, with consideration given to additional stabilization measures such as cement augmentation or extended instrumentation in cases of low HU values [32,34]. Compared with conservative management, HU-based surgical planning offers the advantage of improved patient selection. Patients with very low HU values may benefit more from conservative therapy due to increased surgical risks, while those with sufficient HU values may achieve better functional outcomes through surgical intervention [35]. Furthermore, preoperative HU measurement can provide insight into long-term prognosis, as low HU values are associated with an increased risk of adjacent fractures and poorer clinical outcomes [36]. In conclusion, knowledge of HU values enables more precise and individualized treatment planning for osteoporotic vertebral fractures. It can contribute to minimizing complication risks and improving long-term outcomes [37,38]. Compared with purely conservative therapy, this approach offers a more informed basis for decision-making regarding surgical versus non-surgical management and allows for better risk stratification [6,39]. The integration of HU measurements into clinical practice could thus lead to the optimization of treatment strategies for patients with osteoporotic vertebral fractures [40,41].

Comparison of HU determined on CT and BVF measured on micro-CT shows that HU is probably more suitable for the demonstration of gender differences, especially in the cervical, thoracic, and lumbar spine, whereas these differences are not seen clearly on micro-CT. These data confirm that the HU method might be more suitable for clinical applications in which the investigator wishes to perform a more detailed assessment of bone density in various anatomical regions. On the other hand, Parsa et al. [42] performed a correlation analysis between BVF and HU in 20 mandibles of human cadavers and noted an excellent correlation. Furthermore, given the high resolution and sensitivity of the micro-CT investigation with regard to microstructural properties of bone, it permits a more detailed analysis of trabecular microarchitecture, which makes it valuable for research applications. Chen et al. [43], as well as Gong et al. [44], report that the central and anterosuperior regions of the vertebra have a lower bone volume fraction (BVF) than the posterior region. The spatial distribution of bone density within vertebrae exhibits significant variations, as demonstrated by Banse and colleagues [45] in their study. Their findings suggest that the upper and anterior half of the vertebral body tends to have a lower density. These observations regarding regional variability in microstructure are of great importance for understanding gender- and age-related changes in bone substance within the spine. Consideration of structural aspects can contribute to a deeper understanding of various fracture patterns and risks [46]. Furthermore, microdamage to trabeculae plays a non-negligible role in assessing bone strength. These micro-injuries are partly related to a reduction in bone volume fraction (BVF) [47]. Microdamage in the microarchitecture of vertebral bodies in osteoporosis refers to small structural defects in the trabecular bone that accumulate with increasing age and progressive osteoporosis. These microdamages occur in the form of linear microcracks, diffuse damage, or trabecular microfractures [48]. Understanding these microdamages and their relationship to bone architecture is crucial for assessing fracture risk and developing strategies to prevent osteoporotic VF.

Future research should be focused on establishing standardized values for bone density in various anatomical regions and demographic groups and utilize this information to improve clinical practice and personalized medicine.

The present investigation was conducted to compare two radiological procedures. It was confined to a case number limited by the existing material. The values obtained with both procedures for the demonstration of cancellous bone density differed by a power of ten. The results of subgroup ($n \leq 6$) comparisons may be considered exploratory, and graphic comparisons were used to elucidate the statements. We exclusively used body donors of advanced age; no statements can be made about the bone structure of younger body donors. We also had very little medical history data about the donors, especially about the type and duration of any drug treatment or physical treatment they may have received for osteoporosis.

5. Conclusions

The present investigation provides more extensive insights into the complex relationship between bone density, gender, fracture status, and methods of measurement than hitherto known. It underlines the significance of selecting the suitable imaging procedure and parameters such as sectional planes and quadrants in order to perform an accurate diagnosis and administer specific treatment for osteoporosis, as well as other associated bone diseases.

The presented investigation shows that CT, as well as micro-CT, may contribute to a better understanding of osteoporosis.

A major advantage of the CT investigation is its clinical applicability. HU measurements from routine CT scans can be used as a screening tool for osteoporosis, especially in patients who undergo CT investigations for other reasons. This would dispense with additional imaging procedures and radiation. In view of the limited availability of dual-energy X-ray absorptiometry, this makes CT scans an interesting tool for smaller clinics.

Author Contributions: Conceptualization, G.S., H.-C.S. and Ä.G.; investigation, E.A., J.H., J.R.A., R.A., T.M., S.S.I.F., A.G. and D.F.-B.; resources, L.H. and A.G.; data curation, Ä.G.; writing—original draft preparation, Ä.G. and G.S.; supervision, G.S., Ä.G. and H.-C.S. All authors have read and agreed to the published version of the manuscript.

Funding: This research received no external funding.

Institutional Review Board Statement: This study was conducted in accordance with the Declaration of Helsinki and approved by the Institutional Review Board of Rostock University (approval code: A 2017-0072; date of approval: 13 November 2017).

Informed Consent Statement: Written informed consent to publish this paper has been obtained from patients in their lifetimes.

Data Availability Statement: The data presented in this study are available upon request from the corresponding author.

Conflicts of Interest: The authors declare no conflicts of interest.

Abbreviations

Al	aluminum
AUC	area under the curve
BMD	bone mineral density (mg/cm^3)
BMI	body mass index
BVF	bone volume fraction
cm	centimeter
CS	cervical spine
CT	computed tomography
C1-7	cervical vertebra 1-7
DXA	dual-energy X-ray absorptiometry
EMM	estimated marginal means
Fig.	figure
g/cm^3	gram/cubic centimeter
GE	General Electric
HU	Hounsfield units
IBM	International Business Machines Corporation
ICC	intra-class correlation coefficient
kV	kilovolt
L1-5	lumbar vertebra 1-5
LS	lumbar spine
mg/cm^3	milligram/cubic centimeter
mg/mL	milligram/milliliter
Micro-CT	micro-computed tomography
Mio.	millions
Ml	milliliter
Mm	millimeter
OP	osteoporosis
PMMA	polymethylmethacrylat
Q I	Quadrant I
Q II	Quadrant II
Q III	Quadrant III
QCT	quantitative computed tomography
ROC	receiver operating characteristic
ROI	region of interest
SD	standard deviation
TBS	trabecular bone structure
Th1-12	thoracic vertebra 1-12
TS	thoracic spine
VF	vertebral fractures
µm	micrometer
µA	microampere
°C	degrees Celsius

References

1. Consensus development conference: Diagnosis, prophylaxis, and treatment of osteoporosis. *Am. J. Med.* **1993**, *94*, 646–650. [CrossRef] [PubMed]
2. Kanis, J.A.; Norton, N.; Harvey, N.C.; Jacobson, T.; Johansson, H.; Lorentzon, M.; McCloskey, E.V.; Willers, C.; Borgström, F. SCOPE 2021: A new scorecard for osteoporosis in Europe. *Arch. Osteoporos.* **2021**, *16*, 82. [CrossRef] [PubMed]
3. Rupp, M.; Walter, N.; Pfeifer, C.; Lang, S.; Kerschbaum, M.; Krutsch, W.; Baumann, F.; Alt, V. The Incidence of Fractures Among the Adult Population of Germany—An Analysis from 2009 through 2019. *Dtsch. Arztebl. Int.* **2021**, *118*, 665–669. [CrossRef] [PubMed]

4. Zanker, J.; Duque, G. Osteoporosis in Older Persons: Old and New Players. *J. Am. Geriatr. Soc.* **2019**, *67*, 831–840. [CrossRef] [PubMed]
5. Issever, A.S.; Link, T.M. Radiologische Diagnostik der Osteoporose. *Z. Rheumatol.* **2011**, *70*, 135–144, quiz 145. [CrossRef]
6. Scheyerer, M.J.; Ullrich, B.; Osterhoff, G.; Spiegl, U.A.; Schnake, K.J. "Hounsfield units" als Maß für die Knochendichte—Anwendungsmöglichkeiten in der Wirbelsäulenchirurgie. *Unfallchirurg* **2019**, *122*, 654–661. [CrossRef]
7. Burghardt, A.J.; Link, T.M.; Majumdar, S. High-resolution Computed Tomography for Clinical Imaging of Bone Microarchitecture. *Clin. Orthop. Relat. Res.* **2011**, *469*, 2179–2193. [CrossRef]
8. Andresen, R.; Radmer, S.; Banzer, D. Bone mineral density and spongiosa architecture in correlation to vertebral body insufficiency fractures. *Acta Radiol.* **1998**, *39*, 538–542. [CrossRef]
9. Schröder, G.; Flachsmeyer, D.; Kullen, C.M.; Andresen, J.R.; Schulze, M.; Hiepe, L.; Schober, H.-C.; Andresen, R. Insuffizienzfrakturen der Wirbelsäule in Abhängigkeit von der spongiösen Knochendichte: Eine in-vitro-Studie. *Orthopadie* **2022**, *51*, 547–555. [CrossRef]
10. Schröder, G.; Jabke, B.; Schulze, M.; Wree, A.; Martin, H.; Sahmel, O.; Doerell, A.; Kullen, C.M.; Andresen, R.; Schober, H.-C. A comparison, using X-ray micro-computed tomography, of the architecture of cancellous bone from the cervical, thoracic and lumbar spine using 240 vertebral bodies from 10 body donors. *Anat. Cell Biol.* **2021**, *54*, 25–34. [CrossRef]
11. Schröder, G.; Hiepe, L.; Moritz, M.; Vivell, L.-M.; Schulze, M.; Martin, H.; Götz, A.; Andresen, J.R.; Kullen, C.-M.; Andresen, R.; et al. Warum sich in der Halswirbelsäule auch bei Osteoporose nur selten Insuffizienzfrakturen finden. *Z. Orthop. Unfall.* **2022**, *160*, 657–669. [CrossRef]
12. Schröder, G.; Mittlmeier, T.; Gahr, P.; Ulusoy, S.; Hiepe, L.; Schulze, M.; Götz, A.; Andresen, R.; Schober, H.-C. Regional Variations in the Intra- and Intervertebral Trabecular Microarchitecture of the Osteoporotic Axial Skeleton with Reference to the Direction of Puncture. *Diagnostics* **2024**, *14*, 498. [CrossRef] [PubMed]
13. De Laet, C.; Kanis, J.A.; Odén, A.; Johanson, H.; Johnell, O.; Delmas, P.; Eisman, J.A.; Kroger, H.; Fujiwara, S.; Garnero, P.; et al. Body mass index as a predictor of fracture risk: A meta-analysis. *Osteoporos. Int.* **2005**, *16*, 1330–1338. [CrossRef] [PubMed]
14. Engelke, K.; Adams, J.E.; Armbrecht, G.; Augat, P.; Bogado, C.E.; Bouxsein, M.L.; Felsenberg, D.; Ito, M.; Prevrhal, S.; Hans, D.B.; et al. Clinical use of quantitative computed tomography and peripheral quantitative computed tomography in the management of osteoporosis in adults: The 2007 ISCD Official Positions. *J. Clin. Densitom.* **2008**, *11*, 123–162. [CrossRef] [PubMed]
15. Kanis, J.A.; Borgstrom, F.; de Laet, C.; Johansson, H.; Johnell, O.; Jonsson, B.; Oden, A.; Zethraeus, N.; Pfleger, B.; Khaltaev, N. Assessment of fracture risk. *Osteoporos. Int.* **2005**, *16*, 581–589. [CrossRef] [PubMed]
16. Bagger, Y.Z.; Tankó, L.B.; Alexandersen, P.; Hansen, H.B.; Qin, G.; Christiansen, C. The long-term predictive value of bone mineral density measurements for fracture risk is independent of the site of measurement and the age at diagnosis: Results from the Prospective Epidemiological Risk Factors study. *Osteoporos. Int.* **2006**, *17*, 471–477. [CrossRef]
17. Pluijm, S.M.F.; Koes, B.; de Laet, C.; van Schoor, N.M.; Kuchuk, N.O.; Rivadeneira, F.; Mackenbach, J.P.; Lips, P.; Pols, H.A.; Steyerberg, E.W. A simple risk score for the assessment of absolute fracture risk in general practice based on two longitudinal studies. *J. Bone Miner. Res.* **2009**, *24*, 768–774. [CrossRef]
18. Bässgen, K.; Westphal, T.; Haar, P.; Kundt, G.; Mittlmeier, T.; Schober, H.-C. Population-based prospective study on the incidence of osteoporosis-associated fractures in a German population of 200,413 inhabitants. *J. Public Health* **2013**, *35*, 255–261. [CrossRef]
19. Christiansen, B.A.; Bouxsein, M.L. Biomechanics of vertebral fractures and the vertebral fracture cascade. *Curr. Osteoporos. Rep.* **2010**, *8*, 198–204. [CrossRef]
20. Montemurro, N.; Cocciaro, A.; Liberti, G.; Cosottini, M.; Perrini, P. The internal trabecular bone structure of the odontoid process of the axis. A retrospective single-center comparative study in patients following cervical trauma. *J. Neurol. Surg. A Cent. Eur. Neurosurg.* **2022**. [CrossRef]
21. Shin, D.E.; Lee, Y.; An, H.-J.; Hwang, T.-S.; Cho, J.-W.; Oh, J.; Ahn, W.; Lee, J.; Hong, C.G.; Lee, Y.; et al. Trabecular structural difference between the superior and inferior regions of the vertebral body: A cadaveric and clinical study. *Front. Endocrinol.* **2023**, *14*, 1238654. [CrossRef]
22. Perilli, E.; Briggs, A.M.; Kantor, S.; Codrington, J.; Wark, J.D.; Parkinson, I.H.; Fazzalari, N.L. Failure strength of human vertebrae: Prediction using bone mineral density measured by DXA and bone volume by micro-CT. *Bone* **2012**, *50*, 1416–1425. [CrossRef] [PubMed]
23. Finkelstein, J.S.; Cleary, R.L.; Butler, J.P.; Antonelli, R.; Mitlak, B.H.; Deraska, D.J.; Zamora-Quezada, J.C.; Neer, R.M. A comparison of lateral versus anterior-posterior spine dual energy x-ray absorptiometry for the diagnosis of osteopenia. *J. Clin. Endocrinol. Metab.* **1994**, *78*, 724–730. [CrossRef] [PubMed]

24. Lunt, M.; Felsenberg, D.; Adams, J.; Benevolenskaya, L.; Cannata, J.; Dequeker, J.; Dodenhof, C.; Falch, J.A.; Johnell, O.; Khaw, K.T.; et al. Population-based geographic variations in DXA bone density in Europe: The EVOS Study. European Vertebral Osteoporosis. *Osteoporos. Int.* **1997**, *7*, 175–189. [CrossRef]
25. Zhao, F.-D.; Pollintine, P.; Hole, B.D.; Adams, M.A.; Dolan, P. Vertebral fractures usually affect the cranial endplate because it is thinner and supported by less-dense trabecular bone. *Bone* **2009**, *44*, 372–379. [CrossRef] [PubMed]
26. Schreiber, J.J.; Anderson, P.A.; Rosas, H.G.; Buchholz, A.L.; Au, A.G. Hounsfield units for assessing bone mineral density and strength: A tool for osteoporosis management. *J. Bone Jt. Surg. Am.* **2011**, *93*, 1057–1063. [CrossRef]
27. Marinova, M.; Edon, B.; Wolter, K.; Katsimbari, B.; Schild, H.H.; Strunk, H.M. Use of routine thoracic and abdominal computed tomography scans for assessing bone mineral density and detecting osteoporosis. *Curr. Med. Res. Opin.* **2015**, *31*, 1871–1881. [CrossRef]
28. Kim, Y.; Kim, C.; Lee, E.; Lee, J.W. Coronal plane in opportunistic screening of osteoporosis using computed tomography: Comparison with axial and sagittal planes. *Skelet. Radiol.* **2024**, *53*, 1103–1109. [CrossRef]
29. Zhang, J.; Luo, X.; Zhou, R.; Dai, Z.; Guo, C.; Qu, G.; Li, J.; Zhang, Z. The axial and sagittal CT values of the 7th thoracic vertebrae in screening for osteoporosis and osteopenia. *Clin. Radiol.* **2023**, *78*, 763–771. [CrossRef]
30. Kalender, W.A. *Computertomographie: Grundlagen, Gerätetechnologie, Bildqualität, Anwendungen; [mit Mehrschicht-Spiral-CT]*; Publicis-MCD-Verl.: München, Germany, 2000; ISBN 978-3-89578-082-0.
31. Zou, D.; Ye, K.; Tian, Y.; Li, W.; Zhou, F.; Zhang, Z.; Lu, Z.; Xu, Z. Characteristics of vertebral CT Hounsfield units in elderly patients with acute vertebral fragility fractures. *Eur. Spine J.* **2020**, *29*, 1092–1097. [CrossRef]
32. Yu, J.; Xiao, Z.; Yu, R.; Liu, X.; Chen, H. Diagnostic Value of Hounsfield Units for Osteoporotic Thoracolumbar Vertebral Non-Compression Fractures in Elderly Patients with Low-Energy Injuries. *Int. J. Gen. Med.* **2024**, *17*, 3221–3229. [CrossRef] [PubMed]
33. Yao, Y.-C.; Chao, H.; Kao, K.-Y.; Lin, H.-H.; Wang, S.-T.; Chang, M.-C.; Liu, C.-L.; Chou, P.-H. CT Hounsfield unit is a reliable parameter for screws loosening or cages subsidence in minimally invasive transforaminal lumbar interbody fusion. *Sci. Rep.* **2023**, *13*, 1620. [CrossRef] [PubMed]
34. Spiegl, U.J.A.; Schenk, P.; Schnake, K.J.; Ullrich, B.W.; Osterhoff, G.; Scheyerer, M.J.; Schmeiser, G.; Bäumlein, M.; Scherer, M.A.; Müller, M.; et al. Treatment and Outcome of Osteoporotic Thoracolumbar Vertebral Body Fractures With Deformation of Both Endplates With or Without Posterior Wall Involvement (OF 4): Short-Term Results from the Prospective EOFTT Multicenter Study. *Glob. Spine J.* **2023**, *13*, 36S–43S. [CrossRef]
35. Ji, C.; Rong, Y.; Wang, J.; Yu, S.; Yin, G.; Fan, J.; Tang, P.; Jiang, D.; Liu, W.; Gong, F.; et al. Risk Factors for Refracture following Primary Osteoporotic Vertebral Compression Fractures. *Pain Physician* **2021**, *24*, E335–E340. [CrossRef] [PubMed]
36. Korovessis, P. Osteoporotic Vertebral Body Fractures: New Trends in Differential Diagnosis, Bracing and Surgery. *J. Clin. Med.* **2022**, *11*, 5172. [CrossRef]
37. Jiang, L.-M.; Tong, Y.-X.; Jiang, J.-J.; Pi, Y.-W.; Gong, Y.; Tan, Z.; Zhao, D.-X. The vertebral Hounsfield units can quantitatively predict the risk of adjacent vertebral fractures after percutaneous kyphoplasty. *Quant. Imaging Med. Surg.* **2023**, *13*, 1036–1047. [CrossRef]
38. Metzner, F.; Reise, R.; Heyde, C.-E.; von der Höh, N.H.; Schleifenbaum, S. Side specific differences of Hounsfield-Units in the osteoporotic lumbar spine. *J. Spine Surg.* **2024**, *10*, 232–243. [CrossRef]
39. Chen, J.; Li, Y.; Zheng, H.; Li, H.; Wang, H.; Ma, L. Hounsfield unit for assessing bone mineral density distribution within lumbar vertebrae and its clinical values. *Front. Endocrinol.* **2024**, *15*, 1398367. [CrossRef]
40. Xu, F.; Zou, D.; Li, W.; Sun, Z.; Jiang, S.; Zhou, S.; Li, Z. Hounsfield units of the vertebral body and pedicle as predictors of pedicle screw loosening after degenerative lumbar spine surgery. *Neurosurg. Focus* **2020**, *49*, E10. [CrossRef]
41. Ye, K.; Zou, D.; Zhou, F.; Li, W.; Tian, Y. Low vertebral CT Hounsfield units: A risk factor for new osteoporotic vertebral fractures after the treatment of percutaneous kyphoplasty. *Arch. Osteoporos.* **2022**, *17*, 137. [CrossRef]
42. Parsa, A.; Ibrahim, N.; Hassan, B.; van der Stelt, P.; Wismeijer, D. Bone quality evaluation at dental implant site using multislice CT, micro-CT, and cone beam CT. *Clin. Oral Implants Res.* **2015**, *26*, e1–e7. [CrossRef] [PubMed]
43. Chen, H.; Shoumura, S.; Emura, S.; Bunai, Y. Regional variations of vertebral trabecular bone microstructure with age and gender. *Osteoporos. Int.* **2008**, *19*, 1473–1483. [CrossRef] [PubMed]
44. Gong, H.; Zhang, M.; Yeung, H.Y.; Qin, L. Regional variations in microstructural properties of vertebral trabeculae with aging. *J. Bone Miner. Metab.* **2005**, *23*, 174–180. [CrossRef] [PubMed]
45. Banse, X.; Devogelaer, J.P.; Munting, E.; Delloye, C.; Cornu, O.; Grynpas, M. Inhomogeneity of human vertebral cancellous bone: Systematic density and structure patterns inside the vertebral body. *Bone* **2001**, *28*, 563–571. [CrossRef]
46. Chen, H.; Zhou, X.; Fujita, H.; Onozuka, M.; Kubo, K.-Y. Age-related changes in trabecular and cortical bone microstructure. *Int. J. Endocrinol.* **2013**, *2013*, 213234. [CrossRef]

47. Follet, H.; Farlay, D.; Bala, Y.; Viguet-Carrin, S.; Gineyts, E.; Burt-Pichat, B.; Wegrzyn, J.; Delmas, P.; Boivin, G.; Chapurlat, R. Determinants of Microdamage in Elderly Human Vertebral Trabecular Bone. *PLoS ONE* **2013**, *8*, e55232. [CrossRef]
48. Arlot, M.E.; Burt-Pichat, B.; Roux, J.-P.; Vashishth, D.; Bouxsein, M.L.; Delmas, P.D. Microarchitecture influences microdamage accumulation in human vertebral trabecular bone. *J. Bone Miner. Res.* **2008**, *23*, 1613–1618. [CrossRef]

Journal of
Clinical Medicine

MDPI

Article

Low-Dose Vitamin D3 Supplementation: Associations with Vertebral Fragility and Pedicle Screw Loosening

Jun Li [1,*], André Strahl [2], Beate Kunze [1], Stefan Krebs [1], Martin Stangenberg [3], Lennart Viezens [4], Patrick Strube [5] and Marc Dreimann [1]

[1] Spine Center for Neuroorthopaedics, Spinal Cord Injuries, and Scoliosis, RKH Orthopedic Clinic Markgröningen, 71706 Markgröningen, Germany
[2] Department of Psychosomatic Medicine and Psychotherapy, Centre for Internal Medicine, University Medical Center Hamburg-Eppendorf, 20246 Hamburg, Germany
[3] Department of Spinal Surgery and Neurosurgery, Tabea Hospital Hamburg, 22587 Hamburg, Germany
[4] Department of Trauma and Orthopaedic Surgery, Division of Spine Surgery, University Medical Center Hamburg-Eppendorf, 20246 Hamburg, Germany
[5] Department of Orthopaedics, Jena University Hospital, Campus Waldkliniken Eisenberg, 07607 Eisenberg, Germany
* Correspondence: jun.li@rkh-gesundheit.de

Abstract

Background/Objectives: Vitamin D deficiency contributes to pathological vertebral fragility (path-VF), including fragility fractures and early pedicle screw loosening after posterior instrumented spinal fusion (PISF). Supplementation practices remain inconsistent. This retrospective study evaluated whether patients with path-VF receive appropriate vitamin D3 (Vit.D3) supplementation and assessed the dose–response relationship between daily intake and path-VF risk, particularly in older adults. **Methods**: A total of 210 patients treated with kyphoplasty or PISF (2022–2023) were classified into a path-VF or control group. Daily oral Vit.D3 intake was categorised as Zero- (0 IU), Low- (<2000 IU), or High-Dose (≥2000 IU). Statistical analyses were performed for each dosage group, including subgroup analyses for patients aged ≥67.5 years. Vertebral BMD was estimated using mean Hounsfield Units (HU) from T11–L5. **Results**: Patients in the path-VF group received significantly lower Vit.D3 doses than controls (1431.4 ± 1055.7 vs. 2366.7 ± 1186.7 IU/day, $p < 0.001$). Low-dose supplementation was associated with a markedly increased risk of path-VF compared with high-dose in the overall cohort (OR = 6.5, $p = 0.003$) and in patients aged ≥67.5 years (OR = 8.6, $p = 0.008$). Logistic regression identified a threshold of 1900 IU/day (AUC = 0.805). Mean vertebral HU values were significantly lower in the path-VF group than in controls (71.9 ± 29.1 vs. 133.5 ± 52.6, $p < 0.001$), and no consistent HU gains were observed with increasing Vit.D3 dosage. **Conclusions**: Low-dose Vit.D3 supplementation was associated with increased path-VF risk, especially in patients aged >67.5 years. Patients without path-VF had received significantly higher doses, suggesting broader benefits of adequate Vit.D3 beyond bone density. A daily intake above 1900 IU may serve as a practical threshold for at-risk elderly patients.

Keywords: vertebral fragility; pedicle screw loosening; ageing population; vitamin D3 supplementation; posterior instrumented spinal fusion; spine surgery

1. Introduction

Vitamin D (Vit.D) deficiency is a well-recognised risk factor for impaired spinal health and is closely associated with pathological vertebral fragility (path-VF). It increases the risk of fragility fractures (FF) [1], delays postoperative recovery and physical rehabilitation [2], reduces spinal fusion success rates [3], and contributes to implant-related complications such as early pedicle screw loosening (PSL). Despite its clinical relevance, the risks of path-VF are often insufficiently assessed in clinical practice prior to posterior instrumented spinal fusion (PISF). Only 44% of spine surgeons perform preoperative bone mineral density (BMD) evaluations, and just 12% assess metabolic laboratory parameters, including 25-hydroxyvitamin-D (25(OH)D), parathyroid hormone, and calcium levels [4].

Although the above considerations support the role of Vit.D, perioperative supplementation in bone surgeries, especially in spine surgery, has shown inconsistent results. Some study reported improved fusion rates, symptom relief, and recovery despite small sample sizes [3]. Others, show no clear postoperative benefits and no consistent dose–response relationship [5,6]. Similar inconsistencies are seen in broader orthopedic research, often limited by heterogeneous designs and low methodological quality [7,8].

The biomechanical integrity of the vertebrae is maintained through dynamic bone remodelling, adapting to internal and external influences such as ageing, nutrition, biomechanical stress, menopause, chronic inflammatory conditions, and other systemic disorders [9,10]. Disruption of this osteogenic–osteoclastic balance significantly reduces BMD, predisposing vertebrae to fragility and increasing the risk of path-VF [11]. Vit.D is crucial for bone development and mechanical strength, facilitating calcium and phosphate metabolism [12,13]. Among available Vit.D supplements, vitamin D3 (Vit.D3) demonstrates superior efficacy in elevating serum 25(OH)D concentrations compared with vitamin D2 (Vit.D2) [14].

Existing international guidelines for Vit.D3 supplementation in adults vary widely in both age grouping and dosage and often provide ambiguous recommendations regarding target populations (typically limited to categories such as infants, children, adults, and pregnant or lactating women), initiation timing, and optimal dosage. Some countries make no age distinction for adults, while others introduce multiple age categories but recommend almost identical adequate intake levels [15–19]. Internationally [15–19], daily doses range from as low as 9 μg (360 IU) to as high as 100 μg (4000 IU). This discrepancy fosters subjective decision-making in clinical practice, frequently overlooking certain patient groups (particularly males) and leading to arbitrary dosing within this broad range.

This study was performed to evaluate Vit.D3 supplementation in spinal surgery patients and to determine whether those at risk of path-VF (including FF and early PSL following PISF) receive appropriate supplementation compared with those without such risk. In addition, this study sought to identify specific cut-off values for age and daily Vit.D3 dosage that may guide supplementation strategies. The findings may provide evidence to refine clinical guidelines for Vit.D3 supplementation, with the aim of reducing the incidence of path-VF and its associated complications in spinal surgery patients.

2. Materials and Methods

2.1. Patients

In this retrospective case–control study, we evaluated 210 patients who underwent spinal surgical treatments, including balloon kyphoplasty and PISF, in the thoracic and lumbar regions at a single spine centre between 2022 and 2023.

2.2. Definitions of Path-VF and Early PSL

For this study, the diagnostic criteria for path-VF were based on the framework established in a previous study [20], with adaptations to the present research context. A diagnosis of path-VF was considered if any of the following conditions were met, after histological exclusion of tumour-related fractures:

(1) cases requiring balloon kyphoplasty for path-VF,
(2) intraoperative use of cement-augmented pedicle screws during the first PISF, or
(3) occurrence of non-traumatic PSL within 6 months after the initial PISF in the absence of prior screw reinforcement.

The indications for PISF in this study included severe degenerative lumbar stenosis with instability, idiopathic scoliosis, advanced spondylolisthesis, and de novo lumbar scoliosis. Patients with spondylodiscitis or spinal tumours were excluded.

Among the available techniques for enhancing screw fixation in osteoporotic vertebrae, cement augmentation is regarded as the most widely used and effective [21,22]. Therefore, only cement-augmented screws were used in the present cohort, while other reinforcement options (e.g., expandable screws, specialised thread designs, or bioactive-coated implants) were excluded.

The decision to perform screw reinforcement was made by senior spine surgeons following thorough preoperative assessment. Consistent with earlier findings, early PSL (<6 months) is predominantly associated with low BMD and reduced bone quality [23], whereas later PSL (>1 year) is more often related to mechanical overload, adjacent segment degeneration, suboptimal implant positioning, or chronic low-grade infection [24–26]. Based on these considerations, a 6-month threshold was applied in this study to define early PSL.

PSL was diagnosed using computed tomography (CT) imaging based on either a radiolucent rim > 1 mm around the screw or signs of screw pull-out/cut-out [26]. To reduce radiation exposure and costs, CT was limited to patients with severe symptoms such as intense localised pain or significant activity restriction [27].

2.3. Grouping

Patients were classified into two cohorts: the path-VF group, comprising individuals diagnosed with path-VF, and the control group, comprising patients without evidence of path-VF. Preoperative demographic data, including age, sex, and daily Vit.D3 supplementation dosage, were recorded for all participants.

2.4. Categorisation of Vit.D3 Dosage

Data on vitamin D supplementation were retrieved from general practitioner medication records or, when unavailable, collected during preoperative patient interviews.

To assess the impact of daily Vit.D3 intake, patients were categorised into three dosage groups: Zero-Dose (0 IU/day), Low-Dose (<2000 IU/day), and High-Dose (≥2000 IU/day). Patients whose Vit.D3 supplementation dosage changed between the PISF and the 6-month follow-up were excluded from the analysis.

Based on our previous study [20], which identified 67.5 years as the optimal age threshold for predicting path-VF risk, analyses were performed for the overall cohort and further stratified into subgroups above and below this threshold to examine the relationship between Vit.D3 intake and path-VF risk.

2.5. Measurement of Vertebral Hounsfield Units (HU)

To validate the definition of path-VF used in this study and to confirm the robustness of the subsequent grouping, vertebral bone quality was assessed using preoperative CT-based HU measurements. Among the 210 patients, only 8 had dual-energy X-ray absorptiometry (DEXA) results available before surgery. Preoperative lumbar spine CT scans were retrospectively evaluated in 88 patients. HU values were measured from Th11 to L5 using elliptical region of interest placed in the cancellous bone between the upper and middle thirds of each vertebral body, excluding cortical areas. Regions containing vascular structures, Schmorl's nodes, sclerosis, or tumorous changes were excluded. For each patient, the mean HU value from Th11 to L5 was calculated and used in subsequent analyses.

2.6. Statistical Analysis

All statistical analyses were conducted using R software version 4.4.1, 14 June 2024 (The R Foundation for Statistical Computing, Vienna, Austria). Continuous variables are reported as mean ± standard deviation, and statistical significance was defined as a two-tailed *p*-value of <0.05.

To compare means of numeric variables, the data normality was assessed previously using the Shapiro–Wilk test and Kolmogorov–Smirnov test, and variance homogeneity was verified using Levene's test and the F-test. Due to non-normality, variance inhomogeneity, or limited sample size, group comparisons for age, daily Vit.D3 dosage, and HU values were performed using the Mann–Whitney U test. Effect sizes were reported as rank-biserial correlation coefficients (r), with $r > 0.3$ and $r > 0.5$ interpreted as medium and large effects, respectively.

Associations between Vit.D3 dosage categories and the risk of path-VF or path-VF with early PSL were examined using Fisher's exact test, yielding odds ratios (ORs) with corresponding 95% confidence intervals (CIs).

To further explore potential predictors, multiple logistic regression was performed, incorporating sex, age, and Vit.D3 dosage categories (Zero-, Low-, and High-Dose) as independent variables. Multicollinearity among predictors was evaluated using variance inflation factors (VIF). A VIF < 5 was considered acceptable. Receiver operating characteristic (ROC) curve analysis was used to identify potential dosage thresholds, with an area under the curve (AUC) of ≥0.8 interpreted as indicating excellent discriminative ability.

3. Results

3.1. Demographics of the Study Cohort

The study cohort comprised 210 patients with a mean age of 67.5 years (range 18.5–87.9 years), including 80 males and 130 females. Of these, 84 patients were classified into the path-VF group and 126 into the control group. Osteoporosis was pre-diagnosed in 42 patients using DEXA or quantitative CT, of whom 13 did not take Vit.D3, 20 received a low dose, and 9 received a high dose. In total, 53 patients in the cohort received Vit.D3 supplementation at varying doses. Detailed demographic characteristics are summarised in Table 1.

Table 1. Demographics of the involved patients.

		Age (Years)			
	n	**Min.**	**Mean**	**Max.**	**SD**
Total	210	18.5	67.5	87.9	15.4
Male	80	18.5	63.9	87.6	17.9
Female	130	23.1	69.7	87.9	13.1
Path-VF group	84	53.0	75.3	87.9	9.0
Male	22	53.0	74.0	87.0	10.6
Female	62	52.0	75.8	87.0	8.5
Control group	126	18.5	62.2	87.6	16.5
Male	58	18.5	60.0	87.0	18.7
Female	68	23.0	64.1	86.0	14.2
Zero Vit.D3-Suplement (0 IU/Day)	157	18.5	65.1	87.4	16.1
Low Vit.D3-Suplement (<2000 IU/Day)	33	53.0	75.4	87.7	9.2
High Vit.D3-Suplement (≥2000 IU/Day)	20	52.4	73.1	87.9	11.2
Diagnosed Osteoporosis	42	53.0	76.2	87.9	8.2

Table 1. *Cont.*

		Age (Years)			
	n	Min.	Mean	Max.	SD
Osteoporosis with zero Vit.D3-Suplement	13	63.0	73.5	85.2	6.8
Osteoporosis with low Vit.D3-Suplement	20	53.0	77.7	86.8	9.1
Osteoporosis with high Vit.D3-Suplement	9	68.5	79.0	87.9	7.9
Patients with Hounsfield units Value	88	31.9	69.3	87.7	12.7

Path-VF: pathological vertebral fragility, SD: Standard deviation.

3.2. HU Values in the Path-VF and Control Groups

As expected, HU measurements confirmed the validity of the applied path-VF definition and the derived grouping. The path-VF group showed significantly lower mean vertebral HU values than did the control group (71.9 ± 29.1 vs. 133.5 ± 52.6, $p < 0.001$, $r = 0.61$), consistent with reduced bone quality in patients meeting the path-VF criteria.

3.3. Differences in Daily Doses of Vit.D3 Between the Path-VF and Control Groups

Oral daily Vit.D3 supplementation doses were compared between the path-VF and control groups using the Mann–Whitney U test. Patients in the path-VF group received significantly lower daily doses than those in the control group (Table 2).

Table 2. Vit.D3 Doses in At-risk and Without-risk groups.

	n	Mean	SD	*p*	*r*
Path-VF group	35	1431.4	1055.7	<0.001 ***	0.36
Control group	18	2366.7	1186.7		

SD: standard deviation, *** $p < 0.001$.

Figure 1 illustrates the age distribution of Vit.D3 supplementation. Patients without Vit.D3 supplementation and without path-VF risk were spread across all age ranges. By contrast, those not receiving Vit.D3 but meeting the path-VF criteria for FF or early PSL were mainly observed from approximately 50 years of age onwards. The previously established age threshold for path-VF risk (67.5 years) [20] is indicated by a vertical dashed line. Among patients receiving Vit.D3, daily doses below 2000 IU were predominantly found in the path-VF group, particularly in individuals above the 67.5-year threshold. By comparison, only 6 of 33 patients in the control group fell into this low-dose category. Conversely, most patients receiving ≥ 2000 IU/day (12 of 20) were in the control group and showed no path-VF risk.

3.4. ORs of Oral Vit.D3 Dosages for Path-VF Risk

ORs for different oral Vit.D3 dosage categories and path-VF risk were calculated for the overall cohort ($n = 210$) and for the subgroup of patients aged >67.5 years (Figure 2), with diagnosed osteoporosis serving as a positive control.

As expected, osteoporosis was significantly associated with increased path-VF risk in both the overall cohort (OR: 14.8, 95% CI [5.7–45.7], $p < 0.001$) and the older subgroup (OR: 6.4, 95% CI [2.3–20.9], $p < 0.001$). The Vit.D3 dosage showed similar patterns in both analyses. Compared with patients taking Low-Dose Vit.D3, those in the Zero-Dose category had a significantly lower path-VF risk in the overall cohort (OR: 0.10, 95% CI [0.03–0.27], $p < 0.001$) and in the older subgroup (OR: 0.11, 95% CI [0.02–0.43], $p < 0.001$). This apparent lower risk in the Zero-Dose group than in the Low-Dose group will be further considered in the Discussion. Low-Dose supplementation was associated with a significantly higher path-VF risk than was High-Dose supplementation (overall OR: 6.5, 95% CI [1.6–28.9],

$p = 0.003$; older subgroup OR: 8.6, 95% CI [1.6–64.2], $p = 0.008$). Zero-Dose versus High-Dose showed no significant association with path-VF (OR not different from 1; both p-values > 0.05).

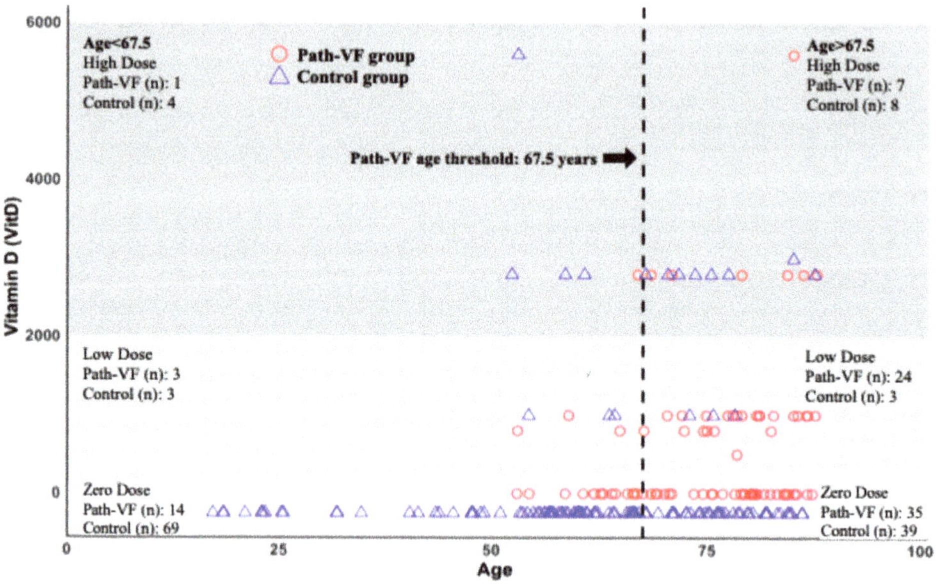

Figure 1. Distribution of daily vitamin D3 supplementation by age group and dosage category. Each dot represents an individual patient, with red circles indicating patients in the path-VF group and blue triangles indicating controls. The vertical dashed line marks the path-VF age threshold at 67.5 years. Vitamin D_3 supplementation is categorized into Zero Dose (0 IU/day), Low Dose (<2000 IU/day), and High Dose (≥2000 IU/day). Numbers of patients per subgroup are indicated for both path-VF and control groups.

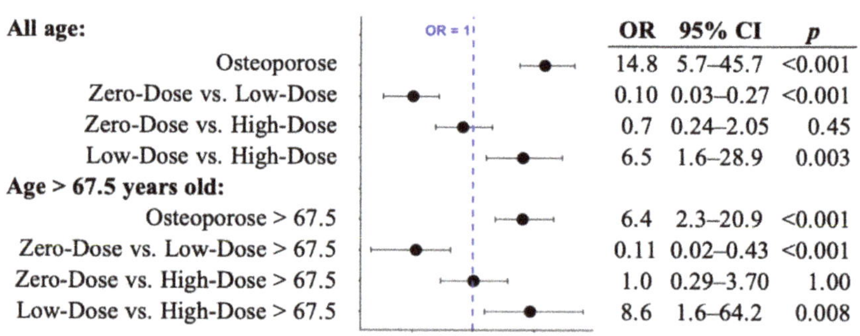

Figure 2. Forest plot of odds ratios (ORs) for path-VF risk across Vit.D3 dosage groups. ORs with 95% confidence intervals and p-values are shown for comparisons among Zero-, Low-, and High-Dose vitamin D_3 groups in the overall cohort and in patients aged over 67.5 years. ORs are displayed on a $\log_{10}$ scale.

Multiple logistic regression analysis assessed the associations between path-VF occurrence and age, sex, and daily Vit.D3 dosage (Zero-, Low-, and High-Dose). All predictors showed VIF values close to 1 (range: 1.00–1.07), indicating no evidence of multicollinearity. As shown in Table 3, female sex was positively but not significantly associated with path-VF risk ($\beta = 0.64$, $p > 0.05$). Higher daily Vit.D3 dosage was linked to a small yet statistically significant reduction in path-VF occurrence ($\beta = -0.001$, $p = 0.018$). Increasing age was significantly associated with elevated path-VF risk ($\beta = 0.08$, $p = 0.031$). ROC analysis for daily Vit.D3 dosage identified a threshold of 1900 IU/day, yielding an AUC of 0.805 (Figure 3), indicating good predictive accuracy.

Table 3. Multiple logistic regression.

	β	SE β	z	p	
(Intercept)	−4.34	2.94	−1.48	0.139	
Gender	0.64	0.92	0.69	0.490	
Vit.D3 Dose	−0.001	0.0004	−2.37	0.018	*
Age	0.08	0.04	2.15	0.031	*

SE: standard error, * $p < 0.05$.

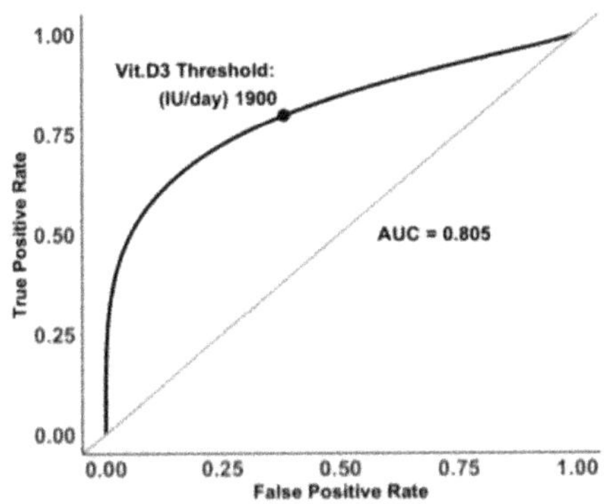

Figure 3. ROC curve identifying 1900 IU/day as the threshold of daily Vit.D3 intake for predicting path-VF (AUC = 0.805).

3.5. Effects of Different Vit.D3 Daily Doses on HU Values

Firstly, HU values in the path-VF group were significantly lower than in the control group ($p < 0.001$) (Figure 4A). The violin plots show that HU values for path-VF patients were concentrated below 100, whereas control patients displayed a broader distribution towards higher values. By contrast, patient age showed the opposite pattern (Figure 4B), with those in the path-VF group being older (74.6 ± 9.1 years) than those in the control group (63.7 ± 13.7 years, $p < 0.001$, $r = 0.42$).

We next examined the relationship between Vit.D3 dosage, HU values, and age. Mean HU values (Figure 5A) were 86.3 ± 37.9 (High-Dose, $n = 11$), 71.4 ± 27.4 (Low-Dose, $n = 16$), and 112.9 ± 55.7 (Zero-Dose, $n = 61$), with a statistically significant difference observed only between the Low-Dose and Zero-Dose groups ($p = 0.004$, $r = 0.55$). Corresponding mean ages (Figure 5B) were 70.3 ± 10.9, 76.9 ± 9.2, and 67.1 ± 13.2 years, respectively, with a significant difference again between the Low-Dose and Zero-Dose groups ($p = 0.006$, $r = 0.53$). All comparisons involving the High-Dose group showed no statistically significant differences, with small effect sizes ($r < 0.3$), suggesting that the limited sample size may have contributed to the lack of significance.

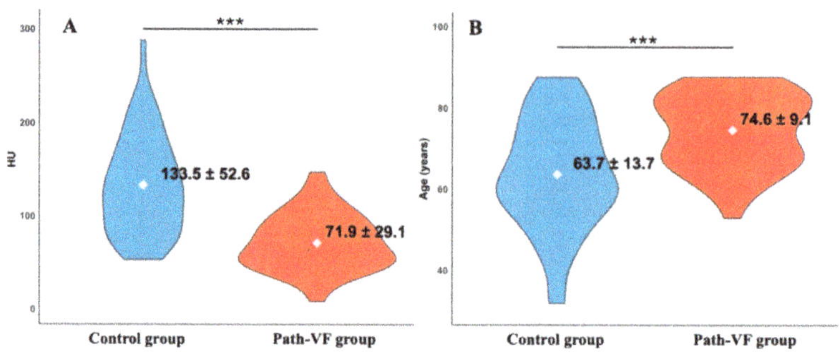

Figure 4. Violin plots comparing (**A**) vertebral HU values and (**B**) patient age between the control and path-VF groups. The path-VF group exhibited significantly lower HU and higher age (*** $p < 0.001$).

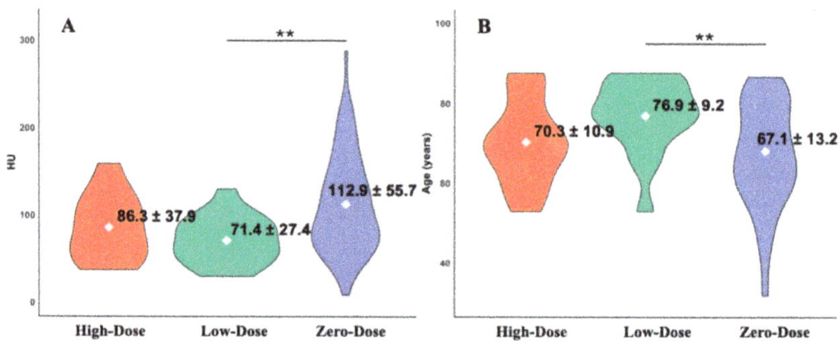

Figure 5. Violin plots comparing (**A**) vertebral HU values and (**B**) age among the High-, Low-, and Zero-Dose Vit.D_3 groups. The Low-Dose group showed significantly lower HU and higher age than the Zero-Dose group (** $p < 0.01$), while comparisons involving the High-Dose group did not reach statistical significance.

4. Discussion

Vit.D is a fat-soluble vitamin that plays a central role in regulating calcium, magnesium, and phosphorus metabolism. Serum 25(OH)D measurement is the standard method for assessing Vit.D status, with concentrations above 30 ng/mL generally regarded as sufficient [28]. Ageing, menopause, and reduced outdoor activity further exacerbate chronic Vit.D deficiency [29], increasing the risk of osteoporosis, path-VF with associated FF, and postoperative complications following instrumented spinal fusion [3].

4.1. Clinical Relevance in Spinal Surgery

In spinal surgery, Vit.D inadequacy is defined as serum 25(OH)D levels of 20–30 ng/mL, and deficiency as levels of <20 ng/mL [30]. While approximately 30% of the general population have levels below 20 ng/mL [31], the prevalence is markedly higher among patients requiring surgical treatment, with up to 73.6% for levels below 30 ng/mL and 36.8% for levels below 20 ng/mL [32]. Deficiency is linked to worse preoperative symptom severity, reflected in higher Japanese Orthopaedic Association, visual analogue scale, and Oswestry Disability Index (ODI) scores [28,33,34]. It is also associated with poorer postoperative recovery [2,35], longer fusion times [36], and lower fusion success rates [3].

Perioperative Vit.D3 supplementation has shown potential benefits in symptom relief and functional recovery, yet existing studies remain inconsistent regarding optimal dosage, timing, and patient selection [8]. Ko et al. used intramuscular injections of 100,000 IU perioperatively without specifying frequency [35], while Xu et al. observed improved fusion rates and reduced ODI scores after PISF, though without clear details on dosage or duration [37]. Waikakul et al. administered 600 IU/day of Vit.D2 for 10 days followed by 600 IU/day of Vit.D3 for maintenance in failed back surgery syndrome, noting symptomatic improvement despite the small sample size [33]. A meta-analysis reported no benefit for fractures, falls, or BMD, with no difference observed between doses above or below 800 IU/day [38]. These mixed findings align with broader orthopedic literature, where Vit.D3 supplementation shows limited or inconsistent effects on fracture healing and clinical outcomes, with positive results often linked to lower-quality studies or lacking dose–response clarity [6–8].

4.2. Global Variability and Clinical Uncertainty

International guidelines for Vit.D3 supplementation differ substantially in both dosage and age-group definitions. Some make no age distinctions, while others define multiple age brackets but recommend nearly identical adequate intake levels. Across all guidelines, the gap between the adequate intake and the upper level of intake (4000 IU/day) remains large. This complicates clinical decisions, particularly for spinal surgeons managing patients at risk of path-VF. For example, the United States recommends 600 IU/day for adults aged 19–70 years and 800 IU/day for those aged ≥71 years [15]. The European Food Safety Authority advises 600 IU/day for all adults and sets an upper level of intake of 4000 IU/day, while the German osteoporosis S3 guideline recommends 800 IU/day, advising against exceeding 2000–4000 IU/day [16,17]. The UK sets a range of 400–4000 IU/day for all adults without age subdivision [18]. South Korea recommends 400 IU/day for adults aged 19–49 years and 600 IU/day for those aged ≥50 years, with an upper limit of 4000 IU/day [19]. Japan recommends 360–4000 IU/day for all adults, subdivided into multiple age categories [39]. Such variability fosters subjective prescribing practices and underscores the lack of evidence-based dosing thresholds, a concern that is particularly relevant for spinal surgery patients.

4.3. Dose–Response Relationship in the Present Study

In this study, daily Vit.D3 intake showed a clear dose–response association with the risk of path-VF. Patients receiving supplementation at the lower end of guideline-recommended ranges had a substantially higher risk of path-VF. Consistent with this, patients in the path-VF group had significantly lower daily doses than those in the control group, with median values of 1431.4 IU versus 2366.7 IU, respectively (Table 2). This elevated risk for the Low-Dose group was evident in both the overall cohort and among patients above the identified age threshold of 67.5 years, with ORs indicating several-fold differences. The age distribution of supplementation in our cohort supports this interpretation because most patients in the path-VF group received around 1000 IU/day or less, particularly those above the threshold age, whereas higher-dose supplementation was more common among controls without path-VF. Based on this pattern, multiple logistic regression identified a threshold of approximately 1900 IU/day. One possible explanation is selection bias in supplementation practices; clinicians may preferentially initiate Vit.D3 at low doses without timely adjustment according to changes in the patient's condition or individual needs.

The consistent dose–response trend indicates that low-dose regimens may be inadequate for high-risk patients. Doses above the threshold may help reduce vertebral fragility—related complications. However, as the identified threshold of approximately 1900 IU/day is based on retrospective data, prospective studies are needed to validate its clinical significance. Results from the High-Dose group should also be interpreted with caution, as the low rank-biserial correlation coefficients ($r < 0.3$) reflect limited statistical power due to small sample size. Additionally, the unexpectedly lower risk observed in the Zero-Dose group warrants careful interpretation and will be addressed separately.

4.4. Interpretation of Zero-Dose Patient Outcomes

The observed ORs below 1 in the Zero-Dose group should be interpreted cautiously and are unlikely to reflect a true protective effect of no supplementation. A more likely explanation is 'healthy user' bias, where these patients may have better bone quality, fewer comorbidities, or higher physical activity, even at older ages [40,41].

Structural changes associated with ageing, such as Modic changes, endplate sclerosis, and intervertebral osteophyte fusion, may also contribute to increased vertebral stiffness and improved screw stability. Wagnac et al. demonstrated that large osteophytes can enhance vertebral rigidity and reduce fracture susceptibility [42], while Modic-related sclerosis has been shown to increase HU values and prevent cage subsidence [43,44].

The benefit in the Zero-Dose group likely reflects selection bias and structural adaptations, though this remains speculative without objective health data.

4.5. Effect of Vit.D3 on HU Values of Vertebrae

At this stage of the analysis, we further explored whether the increased risk observed in the Low-Dose group could be explained by lower vertebral BMD assessed through HU measurements, and whether HU values differed systematically across the three dosage categories (Zero, Low, High). As expected, HU values were significantly lower in patients with path-VF than in controls, confirming their role as a surrogate marker of bone fragility and screw stability [45].

When analysing HU values across dosage categories, we observed that patients receiving Low-Dose Vit.D3 indeed showed lower HU values and were older than those without supplementation, whereas patients on High-Dose Vit.D3 displayed intermediate HU values without statistical significance. This finding is consistent with earlier clinical trials showing that low daily doses of Vit.D3, typically below 800–1000 IU, fail to improve BMD at the lumbar spine or hip [38,46], and that even moderate doses around 900 IU did not yield significant BMD increases in postmenopausal women [47,48].

These results suggest that while low-dose supplementation may be insufficient to counteract age-related BMD decline, higher doses do not necessarily translate into measurable HU gains either. The significant difference in Vit.D3 intake between path-VF and control groups (Table 2) therefore indicates that the observed clinical association is more closely related to overall dose adequacy. The apparent benefit of sufficient supplementation is likely to involve additional mechanisms beyond direct increases in vertebral BMD, such as modulation of bone metabolism, muscle function, or inflammatory pathways.

4.6. Potential Mechanisms of Vit.D in Preventing Path-VF Risk

The protective association of Vit.D3 observed in this study is unlikely to be mediated solely through increases in vertebral BMD. Instead, several additional biological mechanisms may contribute to the reduced path-VF risk. Beyond its established skeletal effects, Vit.D is involved in diverse physiological processes, including immune regulation, cardiovascular function, endocrine balance, and metabolic pathways. It has also been reported to alleviate pain, improve mood, and influence recovery after surgery [49].

One important pathway is through muscle function. Vit.D enhances muscle strength and balance, thereby lowering fall risk, a key determinant of fracture occurrence. This effect is mediated by Vit.D receptors in muscle cells, which regulate protein synthesis and calcium uptake [50]. Age-related declines in Vit.D receptor expression may precede structural bone changes, but Vit.D-related muscle weakness (hypovitaminosis D myopathy) can be reversed with adequate supplementation [51]. Clinical evidence supports this indirect protective effect, with studies showing that Vit.D supplementation reduces fall rates in older adults [52].

Vit.D also modulates parathyroid hormone activity, which is central to bone metabolism. Persistent Vit.D deficiency can lead to secondary hyperparathyroidism, causing elevated bone turnover and cortical bone loss. Pfeifer et al. demonstrated that Vit.D3 combined with calcium supplementation reduces parathyroid hormone levels in elderly women and improves balance, thereby decreasing fracture risk [53].

Finally, Vit.D exerts immunomodulatory and anti-inflammatory effects. It reduces circulating proinflammatory cytokines such as interleukin-6, interleukin-8, and tumour necrosis factor, which are known to impair bone homeostasis and hinder surgical recovery [54]. AlGhamdi et al. showed that high-dose monthly Vit.D3 administration (80,000 IU, approximately 2666 IU/day) significantly decreased these cytokines [55]. Such effects may not only contribute to fracture prevention but also enhance postoperative recovery and reduce complications such as cage subsidence or PSL after spinal procedures.

Taken together, these pleiotropic actions of Vit.D3 reinforce its clinical relevance in spinal surgery patients, particularly when direct improvements in vertebral bone density are not consistently measurable.

5. Limitations

This study has several limitations. First, its retrospective design limits the ability to establish causality between Vit.D3 dosage and path-VF occurrence. Second, serum 25(OH)D levels were not routinely assessed, preventing correlation analyses between measured Vit.D status and clinical outcomes. Third, the sample size in the High-Dose group was relatively small, which may have reduced the statistical power to detect significant associations.

Finally, other confounding factors, such as comorbidities, nutritional status, or physical activity levels, were not systematically controlled and may have influenced the observed relationships. In particular, the absence of objective health-status indicators introduces a potential 'healthy user' bias in the Zero-Dose group, meaning that their apparently lower risk may partly reflect better baseline physiological reserve rather than a true protective effect of no supplementation.

6. Conclusions

This study found a clear dose–response relationship between daily Vit.D3 intake and path-VF risk. Patients with path-VF received significantly lower Vit.D3 doses than controls. The elevated risk observed in the Low-Dose group, particularly in those over 67.5 years, suggests that commonly recommended minimum doses may not provide sufficient protection. A threshold of approximately 1900 IU/day may be relevant for risk reduction in elderly patients.

These effects are unlikely to result solely from improvements in BMD but may instead reflect broader physiological benefits of adequate Vit.D3 availability, including contributions to muscle strength, metabolic balance, and reduced inflammation. Overall, these findings highlight the potential value of tailored Vit.D3 supplementation strategies in spinal surgery patients at elevated risk of vertebral fragility. Further prospective studies with larger cohorts and systematic monitoring of serum 25(OH)D levels are needed to define and validate clinically relevant dosing thresholds.

Author Contributions: Conceptualization, J.L.; methodology, J.L. and A.S.; software, J.L.; validation, J.L., A.S. and M.D.; formal analysis, J.L. and A.S.; investigation, J.L.; resources, B.K., S.K. and M.D.; data curation, J.L. and M.D.; writing—original draft preparation, J.L.; writing—review and editing, J.L., A.S., M.S., L.V., P.S. and M.D.; visualization, J.L.; supervision, M.S., L.V., P.S. and M.D.; project administration, M.D.; funding acquisition, M.D. All authors have read and agreed to the published version of the manuscript.

Funding: This research received no external funding.

Institutional Review Board Statement: The study was conducted in accordance with the Declaration of Helsinki and approved by the Institutional Review Board of RKH Orthopaedic Hospital Markgröningen (protocol code: 2023_04, approved on 15 October 2023, protocol code: 2025_NO_04, approved on 29 September 2025).

Informed Consent Statement: Informed consent was not required for this retrospective study using anonymized patient data, as approved by the institutional review board.

Data Availability Statement: The datasets generated and/or analysed during the current study are not publicly available due to institutional data ownership. The data are the property of RKH Orthopaedic Clinic Markgröningen, 71706 Markgröningen, Baden-Württemberg, Germany. Data may be made available upon reasonable request and with prior approval from the institution. Requests should be directed to the corresponding author.

Conflicts of Interest: The authors declare no conflicts of interest.

Abbreviations

The following abbreviations are used in this manuscript:

25(OH)D	25-hydroxyvitamin-D
AUC	Area under the curve
BMD	Bone mineral density
CI	Confidence intervals
CT	Computed tomography
DEXA	Dual-energy X-ray absorptiometry
FF	Fragility fractures
HU	Hounsfield units
ODI	Oswestry disability index
OR	Odds Ratio
Path-VF	Pathological vertebral fragility
PISF	Posterior instrumented spinal fusion
PSL	Pedicle screw loosening
ROC	Receiver operating characteristic curve
SD	Standard deviation
SE	Standard error
VF	Vertebral fragility
VIF	Variance inflation factors
Vit.D	Vitamin D
Vit.D2	Vitamin D2
Vit.D3	Vitamin D3

References

1. Maier, G.S.; Seeger, J.B.; Horas, K.; Roth, K.E.; Kurth, A.A.; Maus, U. The prevalence of vitamin D deficiency in patients with vertebral fragility fractures. *Bone Jt. J.* **2015**, *97*, 89–93. [CrossRef]
2. Xu, H.W.; Shen, B.; Hu, T.; Zhao, W.-D.; Wu, D.-S.; Wang, S.-J. Preoperative vitamin D status and its effects on short-term clinical outcomes in lumbar spine surgery. *J. Orthop. Sci.* **2020**, *25*, 787–792. [CrossRef]
3. Hu, M.H.; Tseng, Y.-K.; Chung, Y.-H.; Wu, N.-Y.; Li, C.-H.; Lee, P.-Y. The efficacy of oral vitamin D supplements on fusion outcome in patients receiving elective lumbar spinal fusion-a randomized control trial. *BMC Musculoskelet. Disord.* **2022**, *23*, 996. [CrossRef]
4. Dipaola, C.P.; Bible, J.E.; Biswas, D.; Dipaola, M.; Grauer, J.N.; Rechtine, G.R. Survey of spine surgeons on attitudes regarding osteoporosis and osteomalacia screening and treatment for fractures, fusion surgery, and pseudoarthrosis. *Spine J.* **2009**, *9*, 537–544. [CrossRef]

5. Donnally, C.J.; Sheu, J.I.; Bondar, K.J.; Mouhanna, J.N.; Li, D.J.; Butler, A.J.; Rush, A.J.; Gjolaj, J.P. Is There a Correlation Between Preoperative or Postoperative Vitamin D Levels with Pseudarthrosis, Hardware Failure, and Revisions After Lumbar Spine Fusion. *World Neurosurg.* **2019**, *130*, e431–e437. [CrossRef]
6. Slobogean, G.P.; Bzovsky, S.; O'HAra, N.N.; Marchand, L.S.; Hannan, Z.D.; Demyanovich, H.K.; Connelly, D.W.; Adachi, J.D.; Thabane, L.; Sprague, S.; et al. Effect of Vitamin D3 Supplementation on Acute Fracture Healing: A Phase II Screening Randomized Double-Blind Controlled Trial. *JBMR Plus* **2023**, *7*, e10705. [CrossRef] [PubMed]
7. Gatt, T.; Grech, A.; Arshad, H. The Effect of Vitamin D Supplementation for Bone Healing in Fracture Patients: A Systematic Review. *Adv. Orthop.* **2023**, *2023*, 6236045. [CrossRef] [PubMed]
8. Mayo, B.C.; Massel, D.H.; Yacob, A.; Narain, A.S.; Hijji, F.Y.; Jenkins, N.W.; Parrish, J.M.; Modi, K.D.; Long, W.W.; Hrynewycz, N.M.; et al. A Review of Vitamin D in Spinal Surgery: Deficiency Screening, Treatment, and Outcomes. *Int. J. Spine Surg.* **2020**, *14*, 447–454. [CrossRef] [PubMed]
9. Singh, S.; Sarma, D.K.; Verma, V.; Nagpal, R.; Kumar, M. From Cells to Environment: Exploring the Interplay between Factors Shaping Bone Health and Disease. *Medicina* **2023**, *59*, 1546. [CrossRef]
10. Castañeda, S.; Ceballos, C.N.; Jaeger, J.U.; Benadiba, C.d.M.; Martín, E.G.; Díaz-Guerra, G.M.; Alvarez-Galovich, L. Management of Vertebral Fragility Fracture in Older People: Recommendations from a Spanish Consensus of Experts. *Geriatrics* **2024**, *9*, 24. [CrossRef]
11. Al-Bari, A.A.; Al Mamun, A. Current advances in regulation of bone homeostasis. *FASEB Bioadv.* **2020**, *2*, 668–679. [CrossRef]
12. Demontiero, O.; Vidal, C.; Duque, G. Aging and bone loss: New insights for the clinician. *Ther. Adv. Musculoskelet. Dis.* **2012**, *4*, 61–76. [CrossRef] [PubMed]
13. Sornay-Rendu, E.; Duboeuf, F.; Chapurlat, R.D. Postmenopausal women with normal BMD who have fractures have deteriorated bone microarchitecture: A prospective analysis from The OFELY study. *Bone* **2024**, *182*, 117072. [CrossRef]
14. van den Heuvel, E.G.; Lips, P.; Schoonmade, L.J.; Lanham-New, S.A.; van Schoor, N.M. Comparison of the Effect of Daily Vitamin D2 and Vitamin D3 Supplementation on Serum 25-Hydroxyvitamin D Concentration (Total 25(OH)D, 25(OH)D2, and 25(OH)D3) and Importance of Body Mass Index: A Systematic Review and Meta-Analysis. *Adv. Nutr.* **2024**, *15*, 100133. [CrossRef]
15. Demay, M.B.; Pittas, A.G.; Bikle, D.D.; Diab, D.L.; Kiely, M.E.; Lazaretti-Castro, M.; Lips, P.; Mitchell, D.M.; Murad, M.H.; Powers, S.; et al. Vitamin D for the Prevention of Disease: An Endocrine Society Clinical Practice Guideline. *J. Clin. Endocrinol. Metab.* **2024**, *109*, 1907–1947. [CrossRef]
16. Gesellschafte, D.W.O. DVO-Leitlinie (2023) Leitlinie des Dachverbands der Deutschsprachigen Wissenschaftlichen Osteologischen Gesellschaften 2023—Prophylaxe, Diagnostik und Therapie der Osteoporose. Available online: https://register.awmf.org/assets/guidelines/183-001l_S3_Prophylaxe-Diagnostik-Therapie-der-Osteoporose_2023-11.pdf (accessed on 9 August 2025).
17. EFSA Panel on Nutrition; Novel Foods and FoodAllergens (NDA); Turck, D.; Bohn, T.; Castenmiller, J.; de Henauw, S.; Hirsch-Ernst, K.-I.; Knutsen, H.K.; Maciuk, A.; Mangelsdorf, I.; et al. Scientific opinion on the tolerable upper intake level for vitamin D, including the derivation of a conversion factor for calcidiol monohydrate. *EFSA J.* **2023**, *21*, e08145. [CrossRef]
18. National Institutes of Health; National Institute of Occupational Health. Vitamins and Minerals—Vitamin D. 2025. Available online: https://www.nhs.uk/conditions/vitamins-and-minerals/vitamin-d/ (accessed on 9 August 2025).
19. Kim, J.H.; Park, H.S.; Pae, M.; Park, K.H.; Kwon, O. Evidence and suggestions for establishing vitamin D intake standards in Koreans for the prevention of chronic diseases. *Nutr. Res. Pract.* **2022**, *16*, S57–S69. [CrossRef]
20. Li, J.; Strahl, A.; Kunze, B.; Krebs, S.; Stangenberg, M.; Viezens, L.; Strube, P.; Dreimann, M. Ageing and BMI in Focus: Rethinking Risk Assessment for Vertebral Fragility and Pedicle Screw Loosening in Older Adults. *J. Clin. Med.* **2025**, *14*, 5296. [CrossRef] [PubMed]
21. Boucas, P.; Mamdouhi, T.; Rizzo, S.E.; Megas, A. Cement Augmentation of Pedicle Screw Instrumentation: A Literature Review. *Asian Spine J.* **2023**, *17*, 939–948. [CrossRef] [PubMed]
22. Song, Z.; Zhou, Q.; Jin, X.; Zhang, J. Cement-augmented pedicle screw for thoracolumbar degenerative diseases with osteoporosis: A systematic review and meta-analysis. *J. Orthop. Surg. Res.* **2023**, *18*, 631. [CrossRef] [PubMed]
23. Weiser, L.; Huber, G.; Sellenschloh, K.; Viezens, L.; Püschel, K.; Morlock, M.M.; Lehmann, W. Insufficient stability of pedicle screws in osteoporotic vertebrae: Biomechanical correlation of bone mineral density and pedicle screw fixation strength. *Eur. Spine J.* **2017**, *26*, 2891–2897. [CrossRef]
24. Leitner, L.; Malaj, I.; Sadoghi, P.; Amerstorfer, F.; Glehr, M.; Vander, K.; Leithner, A.; Radl, R. Pedicle screw loosening is correlated to chronic subclinical deep implant infection: A retrospective database analysis. *Eur. Spine J.* **2018**, *27*, 2529–2535. [CrossRef] [PubMed]
25. Kim, J.B.; Park, S.-W.; Lee, Y.-S.; Nam, T.-K.; Park, Y.-S.; Kim, Y.-B. The Effects of Spinopelvic Parameters and Paraspinal Muscle Degeneration on S1 Screw Loosening. *J. Korean Neurosurg. Soc.* **2015**, *58*, 357–362. [CrossRef]
26. Marie-Hardy, L.; Pascal-Moussellard, H.; Barnaba, A.; Bonaccorsi, R.; Scemama, C. Screw Loosening in Posterior Spine Fusion: Prevalence and Risk Factors. *Glob. Spine J.* **2020**, *10*, 598–602. [CrossRef] [PubMed]

27. Galbusera, F.; Volkheimer, D.; Reitmaier, S.; Berger-Roscher, N.; Kienle, A.; Wilke, H.-J. Pedicle screw loosening: A clinically relevant complication. *Eur. Spine J.* **2015**, *24*, 1005–1016. [CrossRef]
28. Bajaj, A.; Shah, R.M.; Goodwin, A.M.; Kurapaty, S.; Patel, A.A.; Divi, S.N. The Role of Preoperative Vitamin D in Spine Surgery. *Curr. Rev. Musculoskelet. Med.* **2023**, *16*, 48–54. [CrossRef]
29. Khodabakhshi, A.; Davoodi, S.H.; Vahid, F. Vitamin D status, including serum levels and sun exposure are associated or correlated with bone mass measurements diagnosis, and bone density of the spine. *BMC Nutr.* **2023**, *9*, 48. [CrossRef]
30. Stoker, G.E.; Buchowski, J.M.; Bridwell, K.H.; Lenke, L.G.; Riew, K.D.; Zebala, L.P. Preoperative vitamin D status of adults undergoing surgical spinal fusion. *Spine* **2013**, *38*, 507–515. [CrossRef] [PubMed]
31. Rodriguez, W.J.; Gromelski, J. Vitamin d status and spine surgery outcomes. *ISRN Orthop.* **2013**, *2013*, 471695. [CrossRef]
32. Schmidt, T.; Ebert, K.; Rolvien, T.; Oehler, N.; Lohmann, J.; Papavero, L.; Kothe, R.; Amling, M.; Barvencik, F.; Mussawy, H. A retrospective analysis of bone mineral status in patients requiring spinal surgery. *BMC Musculoskelet. Disord.* **2018**, *19*, 53. [CrossRef]
33. Waikakul, S. Serum 25-hydroxy-calciferol level and failed back surgery syndrome. *J. Orthop. Surg.* **2012**, *20*, 18–22. [CrossRef]
34. Kim, T.H.; Yoon, J.Y.; Lee, B.H.; Jung, H.-S.; Park, M.S.; Park, J.-O.; Moon, E.-S.; Kim, H.-S.; Lee, H.-M.; Moon, S.-H. Changes in vitamin D status after surgery in female patients with lumbar spinal stenosis and its clinical significance. *Spine* **2012**, *37*, E1326–E1330. [CrossRef]
35. Ko, S.; Chae, S.; Choi, W.; Kwon, J.; Choi, J.Y. The effectiveness of vitamin D supplementation in functional outcome and quality of life (QoL) of lumbar spinal stenosis (LSS) requiring surgery. *J. Orthop. Surg. Res.* **2020**, *15*, 117. [CrossRef]
36. Ravindra, V.M.; Godzik, J.; Guan, J.; Dailey, A.T.; Schmidt, M.H.; Bisson, E.F.; Hood, R.S.; Ray, W.Z. Prevalence of Vitamin D Deficiency in Patients Undergoing Elective Spine Surgery: A Cross-Sectional Analysis. *World Neurosurg.* **2015**, *83*, 1114–1119. [CrossRef]
37. Xu, Y.; Zhou, M.; Liu, H.; Zhang, Q.; Hu, Z.; Zhang, N.; Ren, Y. Effect of 1,25-dihydroxyvitamin D3 on posterior transforaminal lumbar interbody fusion in patients with osteoporosis and lumbar disc degenerative disease. *Zhongguo Xiu Fu Chong Jian Wai Ke Za Zhi* **2014**, *28*, 969–972.
38. Bolland, M.J.; Grey, A.; Avenell, A. Effects of vitamin D supplementation on musculoskeletal health: A systematic review, meta-analysis, and trial sequential analysis. *Lancet Diabetes Endocrinol.* **2018**, *6*, 847–858. [CrossRef] [PubMed]
39. Ministry of Health, Labour and Welfare, Japan. Dietary Reference Intakes for Japanese. 2025. Available online: https://www.dobun.co.jp/scbookdata/stofcj2025.pdf (accessed on 9 August 2025). (In Japanese)
40. Albrecht, B.M.; Stalling, I.; Foettinger, L.; Recke, C.; Bammann, K. Adherence to Lifestyle Recommendations for Bone Health in Older Adults with and without Osteoporosis: Cross-Sectional Results of the OUTDOOR ACTIVE Study. *Nutrients* **2022**, *14*, 2463. [CrossRef] [PubMed]
41. Pinheiro, M.B.; Oliveira, J.; Bauman, A.; Fairhall, N.; Kwok, W.; Sherrington, C. Evidence on physical activity and osteoporosis prevention for people aged 65+ years: A systematic review to inform the WHO guidelines on physical activity and sedentary behaviour. *Int. J. Behav. Nutr. Phys. Act.* **2020**, *17*, 150. [CrossRef]
42. Wagnac, E.; Aubin, C.; Chaumoître, K.; Mac-Thiong, J.-M.; Ménard, A.-L.; Petit, Y.; Garo, A.; Arnoux, P.-J. Substantial vertebral body osteophytes protect against severe vertebral fractures in compression. *PLoS ONE* **2017**, *12*, e0186779. [CrossRef]
43. Liu, J.; Huang, B.; Hao, L.; Shan, Z.; Zhang, X.; Chen, J.; Fan, S.; Zhao, F. Association between Modic changes and endplate sclerosis: Evidence from a clinical radiology study and a rabbit model. *J. Orthop. Translat* **2019**, *16*, 71–77. [CrossRef] [PubMed]
44. Liu, J.; Ding, W.; Yang, D.; Wu, H.; Hao, L.; Hu, Z.; Fan, S.; Zhao, F. Modic Changes (MCs) Associated with Endplate Sclerosis Can Prevent Cage Subsidence in Oblique Lumbar Interbody Fusion (OLIF) Stand-Alone. *World Neurosurg.* **2020**, *138*, e160–e168. [CrossRef]
45. Zaidi, Q.; MacNeille, R.; Ramos, O.; Wycliffe, N.; Danisa, O.; İnCeoğlu, S.; Cheng, W. Predicting Pedicle Screw Pullout and Fatigue Performance: Comparing Lateral Dual-Energy X-Ray Absorptiometry, Anterior to Posterior Dual-Energy X-Ray Absorptiometry, and Computed Tomography Hounsfield Units. *Int. J. Spine Surg.* **2023**, *17*, 43–50. [CrossRef]
46. Reid, I.R.; Bolland, M.J.; Grey, A. Effects of vitamin D supplements on bone mineral density: A systematic review and meta-analysis. *Lancet* **2014**, *383*, 146–155. [CrossRef] [PubMed]
47. Jackson, R.D.; LaCroix, A.Z.; Gass, M.; Wallace, R.B.; Robbins, J.; Lewis, C.E.; Bassford, T.; Beresford, S.A.; Black, H.R.; Blanchette, P.; et al. Calcium plus vitamin D supplementation and the risk of fractures. *N. Engl. J. Med.* **2006**, *354*, 669–683. [CrossRef]
48. LeBoff, M.S.; Chou, S.H.; Murata, E.M.; Donlon, C.M.; Cook, N.R.; Mora, S.; Lee, I.-M.; Kotler, G.; Bubes, V.; Buring, J.E.; et al. Effects of Supplemental Vitamin D on Bone Health Outcomes in Women and Men in the VITamin D and OmegA-3 TriaL (VITAL). *J. Bone Miner. Res.* **2020**, *35*, 883–893. [CrossRef]
49. Ellison, D.L.; Moran, H.R. Vitamin D: Vitamin or Hormone. *Nurs. Clin. N. Am.* **2021**, *56*, 47–57. [CrossRef]
50. Bouillon, R.; Marcocci, C.; Carmeliet, G.; Bikle, D.; White, J.H.; Dawson-Hughes, B.; Lips, P.; Munns, C.F.; Lazaretti-Castro, M.; Giustina, A.; et al. Skeletal and Extraskeletal Actions of Vitamin D: Current Evidence and Outstanding Questions. *Endocr. Rev.* **2019**, *40*, 1109–1151. [CrossRef] [PubMed]

51. Glerup, H.; Mikkelsen, K.; Poulsen, L.; Hass, E.; Overbeck, S.; Andersen, H.; Charles, P.; Eriksen, E.F. Hypovitaminosis D myopathy without biochemical signs of osteomalacic bone involvement. *Calcif. Tissue Int.* **2000**, *66*, 419–424. [CrossRef]
52. Bischoff-Ferrari, H.A.; Dawson-Hughes, B.; Staehelin, H.B.; Orav, J.E.; E Stuck, A.; Theiler, R.; Wong, J.B.; Egli, A.; Kiel, D.P.; Henschkowski, J. Fall prevention with supplemental and active forms of vitamin D: A meta-analysis of randomised controlled trials. *BMJ* **2009**, *339*, b3692. [CrossRef] [PubMed]
53. Pfeifer, M.; Begerow, B.; Minne, H.W.; Abrams, C.; Nachtigall, D.; Hansen, C. Effects of a short-term vitamin D and calcium supplementation on body sway and secondary hyperparathyroidism in elderly women. *J. Bone Miner. Res.* **2000**, *15*, 1113–1118. [CrossRef]
54. Prietl, B.; Treiber, G.; Pieber, T.R.; Amrein, K. Vitamin D and immune function. *Nutrients* **2013**, *5*, 2502–2521. [CrossRef] [PubMed]
55. AlGhamdi, S.A.; Enaibsi, N.N.; Alsufiani, H.M.; Alshaibi, H.F.; Khoja, S.O.; Carlberg, C. A Single Oral Vitamin D3 Bolus Reduces Inflammatory Markers in Healthy Saudi Males. *Int. J. Mol. Sci.* **2022**, *23*, 11992. [CrossRef] [PubMed]

Journal of *Clinical Medicine*

MDPI

Article

Ageing and BMI in Focus: Rethinking Risk Assessment for Vertebral Fragility and Pedicle Screw Loosening in Older Adults

Jun Li [1,*], André Strahl [2], Beate Kunze [1], Stefan Krebs [1], Martin Stangenberg [3], Lennart Viezens [4], Patrick Strube [5] and Marc Dreimann [1]

1 Spine Center for Neuroorthopaedics, Spinal Cord Injuries, and Scoliosis, RKH Orthopaedic Clinic Markgröningen, 71706 Markgröningen, Germany; kunzbe01@rkh-gesundheit.de (B.K.); krebst01@rkh-gesundheit.de (S.K.); dreima01@rkh-gesundheit.de (M.D.)

2 Department of Psychosomatic Medicine and Psychotherapy, Centre for Internal Medicine, University Medical Center Hamburg-Eppendorf, 20246 Hamburg, Germany; a.strahl@uke.de

3 Department of Spinal Surgery and Neurosurgery, Tabea Hospital Hamburg, 22587 Hamburg, Germany; martin.stangenberg@artemed.de

4 Department of Trauma and Orthopaedic Surgery, Division of Spine Surgery, University Medical Center Hamburg-Eppendorf, 20246 Hamburg, Germany; l.viezens@uke.de

5 Department of Spine, German Center for Orthopaedics, Waldkliniken Eisenberg, 07607 Eisenberg, Germany; p.strube@waldkliniken-eisenberg.de

* Correspondence: jun.li@rkh-gesundheit.de

Abstract

Background/Objectives: Pathological vertebral fragility (path-VF) increases the risk of osteoporotic fractures and pedicle screw loosening (PSL) after posterior instrumented spinal fusion (PISF). While WHO body mass index (BMI) categories broadly identify risks related to underweight and obesity, fixed thresholds may inadequately reflect vertebral fragility risks among elderly patients, especially within the normal-weight range. This study investigates whether current BMI classifications sufficiently capture the risk of path-VF in older adults. **Methods**: This retrospective study included 225 patients who underwent kyphoplasty or PISF (2022–2023). Path-VF was defined by non-tumorous fractures, screw reinforcement, or PSL within six months without prior reinforcement. Patients were grouped into the path-VF (n = 94) and control (n = 131) groups. HU and BMI values, BMI-related ORs, and age trends were analysed, and a logistic regression was performed. **Results**: Mean HU values were significantly lower in the path-VF group (71.37 ± 30.50) than in controls (130.35 ± 52.53, $p < 0.001$). Path-VF females (26.26 ± 5.38) had a lower BMI than the control females (29.33 ± 5.98, $p = 0.002$); no difference was found in males. Normal-weight females showed a borderline risk for path-VF (OR 2.03, $p = 0.0495$). Obesity (OR_{male} 0.31/OR_{female} 0.37) and being male and overweight (OR 0.21) were protective (all $p < 0.05$). BMI declined with age in path-VF males ($p = 0.001$) but increased in the controls ($p = 0.023$). A logistic regression identified a BMI < 22.5 kg/m^2 and age > 67.5 years as significant risk thresholds. Notably, 20.2% of path-VF patients over 67.5 had a normal weight, suggesting a potentially overlooked subgroup. **Conclusions**: The current WHO lower limit for normal BMI (18.5 kg/m^2) may underestimate the risk of path-VF in patients older than 67.5 years, potentially overlooking 24.7% of cases. The results offer a new approach for clinicians to interpret BMI values at the lower end of the normal range (<22.5 kg/m^2) with caution in elderly patients undergoing spinal surgery.

Keywords: vertebral fragility; pedicle screw loosening; ageing population; body mass index (BMI); posterior instrumented spinal fusion; spine surgery

1. Introduction

Vertebral fragility (VF), characterised by reduced vertebral strength [1], significantly increases the risk of pathological fractures and early pedicle screw loosening (PSL) following posterior instrumented spinal fusion (PISF), even under normal physiological loading conditions [2]. VF, closely linked to osteoporosis and osteoporotic fractures [3], may progress asymptomatically and is influenced by multiple factors, including advanced age, obesity, previous fragility fractures, and anti-osteoporosis medications [4].

Successful outcomes after thoracic and lumbar PISF depend largely on vertebral biomechanics and patient-related factors, such as age, gender, nutrition, lifestyle, and body mass index (BMI) [5–7]. Although bone density measurement is standard for assessing VF, it is frequently omitted during preoperative planning [8]. Instead, the World Health Organisation (WHO) BMI classification is commonly applied to broadly evaluate nutritional status and surgical risk [9].

In spinal surgery, obesity and overweight status increase risks for conditions, such as spondylitis [10], and negatively impact outcomes by prolonging surgery duration, increasing blood loss, infection rates, and delayed healing [11–13]. Similarly, underweight patients often face complications related to malnutrition, poor bone quality, and reduced muscle mass, elevating the risk of hardware failure and impaired recovery [6,14,15]. Poor BMD, common among underweight individuals, also diminishes bone anchoring capacity and increases fracture susceptibility [16–18].

However, limited research has evaluated whether WHO BMI categories reliably predict postoperative complications specifically in ageing populations. Winter et al. [19] reported significantly increased mortality in elderly individuals (aged > 65) at a BMI < 23, while an elevated mortality among obese elderly individuals was seen only above a BMI of 33. Such findings raise questions about whether static BMI thresholds adequately reflect the nuanced health risks in elderly spinal surgery patients, particularly regarding pathological vertebral fragility.

To our knowledge, no prior research has specifically investigated whether the current WHO BMI classification accurately reflects the risk of pathological vertebral fragility (path-VF) in elderly patients, particularly whether a BMI within the 'normal weight' range of 18.5 to 24.9 kg/m^2 truly indicates no elevated risk. This study aims to address this gap.

2. Materials and Methods

2.1. Patients

This retrospective case-control study evaluated 225 patients treated at a single spine centre between 2022 and 2023, all of whom underwent their first balloon kyphoplasty or posterior instrumented spinal fusion (PISF) of the thoracic or lumbar spine. Preoperative demographic and BMI data were collected.

2.2. Inclusion and Exclusion Criteria

Inclusion Criteria:

Patients were included in the study if they presented with pathological vertebral fragility (path-VF), defined by non-tumorous pathological vertebral fractures necessitating balloon kyphoplasty, the requirement for intraoperative pedicle screw reinforcement during initial posterior instrumented spinal fusion (PISF), or non-traumatic pedicle screw loosening (PSL) within six months post-PISF without prior screw reinforcement. Both male and female patients were eligible, and no age limits were imposed for inclusion; however, while most participants were adults, individuals under 18 years old were only included if their surgical indication was severe spinal deformity (idiopathic scoliosis) and they had achieved full skeletal maturity at the time of surgery.

The path-VF group was defined based on a shared insufficiency of vertebral strength, resulting from factors such as low BMD, malnutrition, sarcopenia, and age-related decline [1,20]. The clinical manifestations ranged from fracture and screw reinforcement to early loosening, and the degree of fragility spanned from osteopenia to established osteoporosis, reflecting a spectrum of severity.

Surgical indications for PISF included the following:

(1) Severe degenerative spinal stenosis with instability;
(2) Idiopathic scoliosis;
(3) Spondylolisthesis;
(4) De novo lumbar scoliosis.

Exclusion Criteria:

Patients were excluded from the study if they had clinically suspected or confirmed spondylodiscitis, or if they presented with primary spinal tumours or spinal metastases originating from other malignancies.

2.3. Methodological Details of Screw Augmentation and Loosening Diagnosis

In this study, only cement-augmented screws were utilized, as this is the most established method for screw reinforcement; other techniques, such as expandable screws or bioactive coatings, were not included [21,22]. While subjective assessment might miss up to 31% of screws requiring augmentation in cases of low BMD, no overtreatment occurred in vertebrae with normal BMD, suggesting a low risk of overlooking true fragility [8]. A six-month threshold was applied to identify PSL related to bone fragility, thereby excluding later cases more likely attributable to mechanical overload or infection [23]. The diagnosis of PSL was confirmed via CT scans demonstrating a radiolucent rim greater than 1 mm or evidence of screw pull-out/cutting out [24]; these scans were performed only when postoperative symptoms, such as severe pain or limited mobility, indicated potential complications [25]. Finally, screw length was selected to reach the anterior third of the vertebral body without cortical breach, and the diameter was chosen to match the pedicle size for optimal fixation.

2.4. Measurement of Vertebral Hounsfield Unit (HU) Values

Given the strong correlation between vertebral HU values, BMD, and pedicle screw fixation stability [2,26], we retrospectively analysed mean HU values from vertebrae T11 to L5 on preoperative lumbar CT scans in 99 patients to validate risk grouping relative to bone quality. HU values were measured in elliptical regions of cancellous bone at the cephalad (middle) junction of each vertebral body from T11 to L5, excluding cortical bone, vascular tissue, Schmorl's nodes, cystic changes, severe endplate sclerosis, fractures, and tumours. Mean values across T11–L5 were utilised for statistical analysis.

2.5. Grouping and BMI Categories

Patients were classified into two groups: the path-VF group and those without (control group). According to the WHO BMI criteria, patients were divided into four weight categories: underweight (BMI < 18.5 kg/m^2), normal weight (BMI 18.5–24.9 kg/m^2), overweight (BMI 25.0–29.9 kg/m^2), and obese (BMI ≥ 30 kg/m^2) [9].

2.6. Statistical Analyses

Statistical analyses were performed using R software (version 4.4.1, The R Foundation for Statistical Computing, Vienna, Austria). Continuous variables are presented as mean $\pm$ standard deviation (SD), and statistical significance was defined as $p < 0.05$.

Student's t-test or Mann–Whitney U-test was used to compare age, BMI, and HU values between path-VF and control groups, depending on normality and variance homogeneity assessments. The Shapiro–Wilk test and the Kolmogorov–Smirnov test were used to assess normality, while Levene's test, Bartlett's test, and the F-test were applied to evaluate homogeneity of variances. Effect sizes were assessed using Cohen's d (d) for t-tests and rank-biserial correlation coefficient (r) for U-test. Thresholds for medium and large effects were set at >0.5 and >0.8 for d and >0.3 and >0.5 for r, respectively. Fisher's exact test calculated odds ratios (ORs) with 95% confidence intervals (CIs) for BMI categories associated with the occurrence of path-VF. Pearson's correlation test (coefficient: r_p) and Fisher's Z-test (coefficient Cohen's q: q) were used to examine BMI–age correlations between the path-VF and control groups. Additionally, binary logistic regression and receiver operating characteristic (ROC) curve analyses were conducted to evaluate the influence of gender, age, and BMI on the occurrence of path-VF and to identify threshold values for age and BMI. The area under the curve (AUC) was interpreted as fair if $0.7 \leq AUC < 0.8$ and excellent if $AUC \geq 0.8$ [27].

2.7. AI Statement

During the preparation of this manuscript, Trinka AI was used to assist with grammar and language editing. The corresponding author reviewed and revised the content afterward and takes full responsibility for the final version of the manuscript.

3. Results

3.1. Demographics of the Study Cohort

The study cohort consisted of 88 male and 137 female patients with an average age of 68.11 years (range: 17–92 years). One patient aged 17.28 years was not excluded due to severe scoliosis and confirmed skeletal maturity at the time of surgery. Treatment was consistent with adult protocols.

Detailed demographics are shown in Table 1.

Table 1. Demographics of the involved patients.

		Age			
	n	Min.	Mean	Max.	SD
Total	225	17	68.11	92	15.16
Male	88	17	65.26	92	17.78
Female	137	23	69.95	87	12.94
The path-VF group	94				
Male	26	53	75.72	87.4	9.83
Female	68	52	75.85	87	8.27
The control group	131				
Male	62	17	60.00	92	18.57
Female	69	23	64.13	86	14.09
Balloon Kyphoplasty (exclusive tumour)	33	58	78.27	87	8.68
1st PISF with reinforcement	47	53	74.77	86	8.21
1st PISF without reinforcement	141	17	63.38	92	16.25
2nd PISF due to PSL within six months	29	52	71.80	84	9.19

Path-VF: pathological vertebral fragility. PISF: posterior instrumented spinal fusion; PSL: pedicle screw loosening.

Patients in the path-VF group (all aged >50 years) were significantly older than those in the control group, for both males ($p < 0.001$, $d = 0.90$) and females ($p < 0.001$, $d = 1.01$). However, within the path-VF group, no significant age difference was observed between genders ($p > 0.05$, $d = 0.01$).

The distribution of BMI categories across the path-VF and control groups by gender is detailed in Table 2. Notably, the number of underweight patients was very small for both genders.

Table 2. BMI classification by gender and group.

Gender	BMI-Classification	Control (n)	Path-VF (n)	Total (n)
Female	Obesity	28	12	40
	Overweight	23	26	49
	Normal weight	16	29	45
	Underweight	2	1	3
Male	Obesity	17	6	23
	Overweight	28	8	36
	Normal weight	16	11	27
	Underweight	1	1	2

3.2. Differences in Vertebral HU Values Between the Path-VF and Control Groups

As illustrated in Figure 1, the mean HU value from vertebrae Th11 to L5 was significantly lower in the path-VF group (n = 52) compared to the control group (n = 47) (71.37 ± 30.50 vs. 130.35 ± 52.53, $p < 0.001$, $r = 0.58$), indicating reduced vertebral bone quality among patients with path-VF.

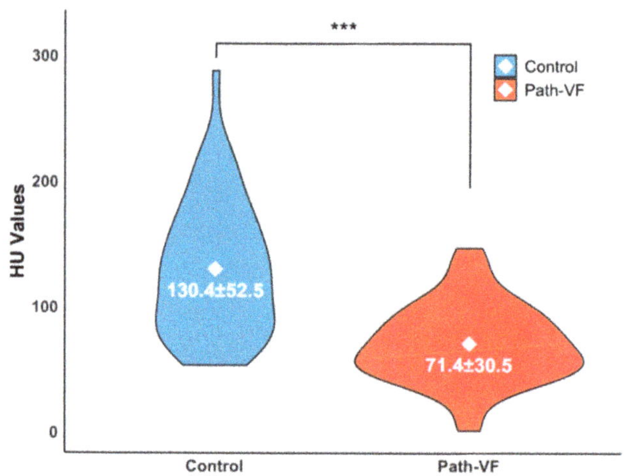

Figure 1. Violin plot of HU values of the path-VF and control groups. Mean ± SD, *** $p < 0.001$.

3.3. BMI Differences and Associations Between the Path-VF and Control Groups

In males, BMI differences between the path-VF (26.47 ± 5.46) and control (28.00 ± 4.52) groups were not significant ($p = 0.22$, $d = 0.32$). Conversely, females in the path-VF group had significantly lower BMIs (26.26 ± 5.38) compared to the control group (29.33 ± 5.98; $p = 0.002$, $d = 0.54$). The BMI distributions in the violin plot (Figure 2) suggest a shift toward lower BMI ranges in the path-VF group for both genders; however, this difference reached statistical significance only in females.

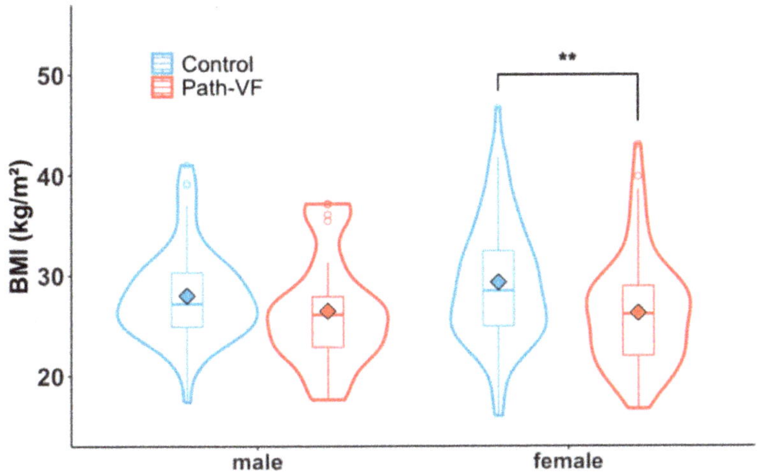

Figure 2. BMI of the path-VF and control groups in males and females. ** $p < 0.01$.

Obese males showed a significantly reduced risk of developing path-VF, with an OR of 0.31 (95% CI [0.11–0.82], $p = 0.024$). Being obese and female also demonstrated a protective effect, with an OR of 0.37 (95% CI [0.18–0.77], $p = 0.009$). In addition, overweight males had an even lower risk, with an OR of 0.21 (95% CI [0.09–0.50], $p < 0.001$). In contrast, normal-weight females were at significantly higher risk of path-VF, with an OR of 2.03 (95% CI [1.05–3.94], $p = 0.0495$) (Figure 3).

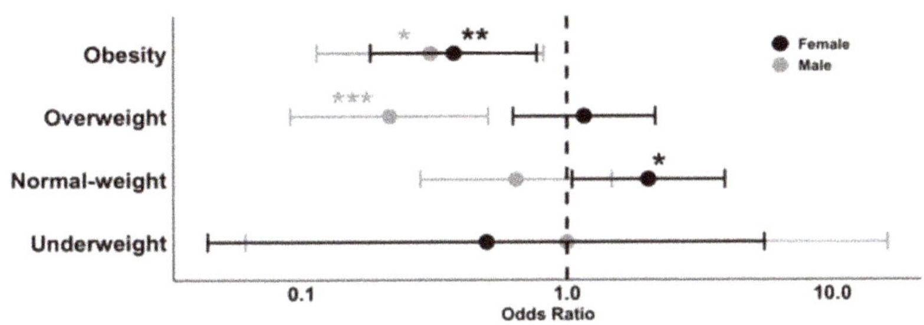

Figure 3. OR of BMI categories for the risk of path-V. * $p < 0.05$, ** $p < 0.01$, *** $p < 0.001$.

3.4. Age-Related Distributions of BMI

Furthermore, we explored the distribution trend of BMI in the path-VF and control groups with increasing age. In females (Figure 4A), no significant BMI–age correlations were observed (path-VF: $r_p = -0.05$, $p = 0.68$; control: $r_p = 0.12$, $p = 0.33$), and no crossover trend occurred ($p = 0.33$). Conversely, males (Figure 4B) showed significant BMI–age trends in the opposite direction: a significantly negative correlation in the path-VF group ($r_p = -0.59$, $p = 0.001$) and a positive correlation in the control group ($r_p = 0.29$, $p = 0.02$), with a significant crossover effect around age 70 ($p < 0.001$, $q = -0.98$).

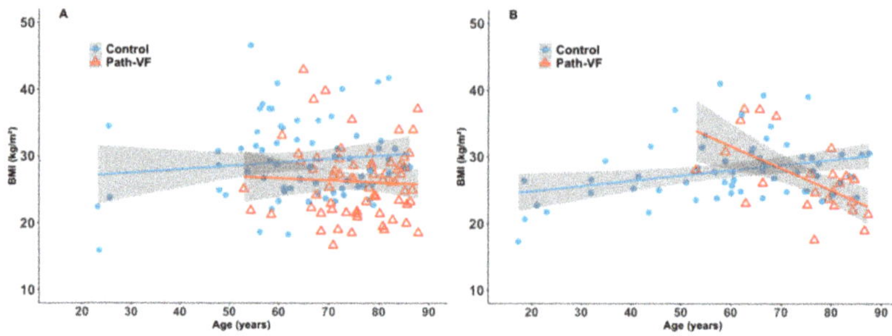

Figure 4. BMI distributions of the path-VF and control groups across ages. (**A**) Female patients; (**B**) male patients.

To identify age-specific BMI differences, patients were divided into eight age blocks for comparison (Figure 5). Females in the path-VF group had a significantly lower BMI compared to the control group at ages 50–59 (22.80 ± 5.12 (n = 3) vs. 31.87 ± 6.98 (n = 18), $p < 0.001$, $r = 0.47$, 70–79 (25.24 ± 4.22 (n = 28) vs. 28.74 ± 5.40 (n = 20), $p = 0.021$, $d = 0.74$) and 80+ (26.06 ± 4.90 (n = 25) vs. 31.34 ± 4.91 (n = 7), $p = 0.031$, $r = 0.42$). In males, a significantly lower BMI in the path-VF group was observed in the 70–79 (23.26 ± 3.60 (n = 5) vs. 28.41 ± 4.21 (n = 12), $p = 0.018$, $r = 0.58$) and 80+ age blocks (24.46 ± 3.59 (n = 13) vs. 27.26 ± 2.63 (n = 9), $p = 0.048$, $d = 0.86$) compared to the control group.

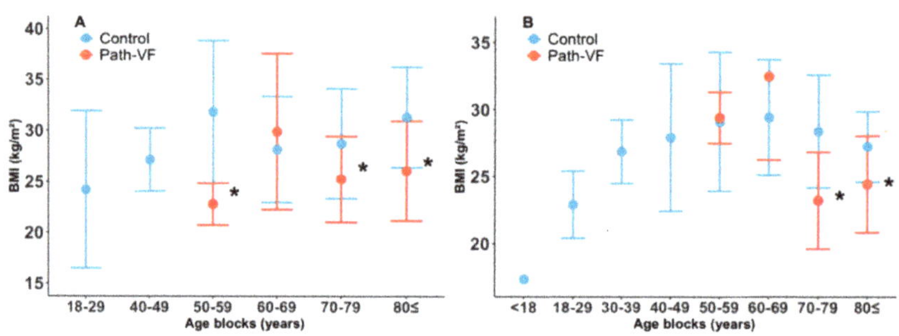

Figure 5. BMIs across age blocks of the path-VF and control groups. (**A**) Female patients; (**B**) male patients. * $p < 0.05$.

3.5. Binary Logistic Regression Analysis

Binary logistic regression analysis (Table 3) showed that age and BMI were significantly associated with the risk of path-VF. The female gender was associated with a higher risk, although this was not statistically significant ($\beta = 0.73$, $p = 0.054$), while a higher BMI was found to be significantly protective ($\beta = -0.10$, $p = 0.03$). Being of an advanced age also considerably increased this risk ($\beta = 0.41$, $p < 0.001$).

Table 3. Logistic regression for the risk of path-VF.

Predictor:	β	SE β	z Value	p
Constant	−5.03	1.20	−4.19	2.77×10^{-5} ***
Gender (Female)	0.73	0.38	1.93	0.054
Age	0.41	0.08	4.84	1.29×10^{-6} ***
BMI	−0.10	0.04	−2.17	0.03 *

SE: standard error; *: $p < 0.05$; ***: $p < 0.001$.

The ROC analysis (Figure 6) determined thresholds of 67.5 years for age (AUC = 0.804) and 22.5 kg/m^2 for BMI (AUC = 0.66). The whole logistic regression model showed excellent predictive performance (AUC = 0.85).

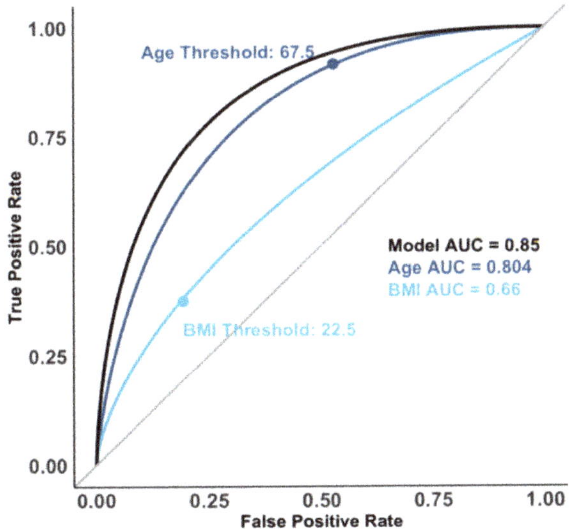

Figure 6. ROC curves of the logistic regression model with predictors of age and BMI for the risk of attending path-VF. AUC: area under the curve.

Ultimately, all 225 patients were plotted on an age versus BMI scatterplot, highlighting the normal BMI range and thresholds for age and BMI (Figure 7). An 'overlook zone' was identified within the normal BMI range, consisting of 19 patients over 67.5 years, all of whom were in the path-VF group. Notably, no patients from the control group were found in this zone. These patients accounted for 20.2% (19/94) of the path-VF group and represented 24.7% (19/77) of all patients older than 67.5 years, emphasising a potential overlooked risk in ageing patients with a normal BMI.

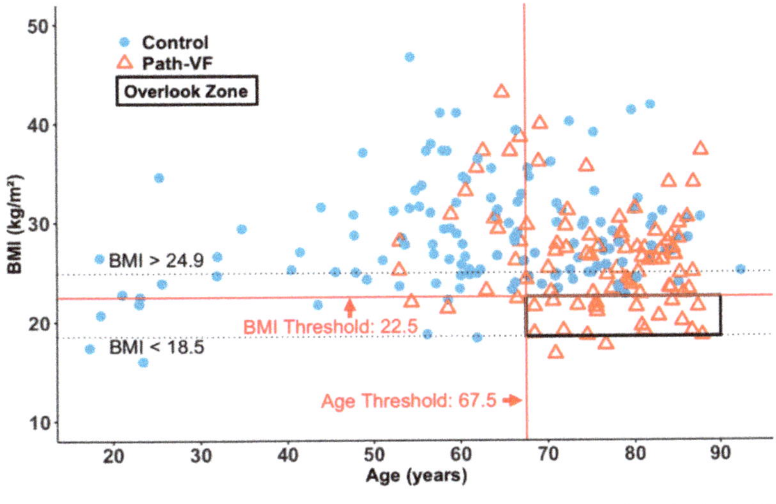

Figure 7. Age and BMI distribution highlighting the 'overlook zone' for the risk of path-VF. The area between the horizontal dashed lines represents the WHO-defined normal BMI range (18.5–24.9 kg/m^2).

The solid red line represents the BMI threshold of 22.5 kg/m^2, and the solid vertical line indicates the age threshold of 67.5 years. The black frame marks the 'Overlook Zone', in which all patients over 67.5 years with a BMI of 18.5–24.9 kg/m^2 showed path-VF.

4. Discussion

4.1. Protective Effects of Higher BMI in the Elderly

Recent evidence indicates that the relationship between BMI and health outcomes exhibits clear age-dependent patterns. Several studies suggest that in older adults, a BMI classified as "overweight" by WHO standards (>25 kg/m^2) may not be detrimental and can even confer protective effects in specific clinical contexts. For example, Huang et al., in a large cohort of hypertensive patients over 45 years of age, found that a BMI of 25 to 29.9 kg/m^2 was significantly associated with reduced all-cause mortality, whereas underweight (BMI < 18.5 kg/m^2) increased early mortality risk [28]. Similarly, a meta-analysis by Winter et al. reported that in individuals aged $\geq$ 65 years, a BMI below 22 kg/m^2 was associated with higher mortality, a trend not observed in younger populations [29]. Additionally, a retrospective analysis of 22,903 inpatients found that elderly individuals with a BMI > 25 kg/m^2 had a lower in-hospital mortality rate and shorter lengths of stay [30]. Collectively, these findings suggest the need to re-evaluate the clinical interpretation of BMI in older populations, as the current WHO classification may underestimate the risks associated with a low BMI and the potential benefits of a higher BMI in ageing individuals.

4.2. Age-Related Decline in Spinal Bone Strength

Secondly, the relationship between ageing and bone strength deterioration is well established. Numerous studies have demonstrated that BMD declines progressively with age, with the spine being particularly susceptible to age-related osteoporotic changes. Kamei et al. identified age 50 as a critical point for accelerated bone loss in women, particularly in the thoracic and lumbar regions, indicating an early risk of spinal osteoporosis in this group [31]. Szulc et al. observed site-specific reductions in BMD among 1040 adult men, with a significant loss in the lumbar spine. This was particularly evident in individuals without advanced facet joint arthrosis, supporting the sensitivity of spinal bone loss to age [32]. Rondanelli et al. found that the prevalence of osteoporosis in the lumbar spine and hip increased substantially with age. Although BMI was positively correlated with BMD, this association became weaker in older adults [33]. These findings highlight age as a key factor influencing osteoporosis and vertebral bone loss.

4.3. Impact of Underweight and Obesity on Spine Surgery Risk

BMI exhibits a U-shaped relationship with surgical outcomes, indicating increased postoperative complications for both underweight and morbidly obese patients [6,34].

Obese patients are reported at higher risk for postoperative complications, such as spondylodiscitis [10], surgical site infections, prolonged hospital stays, and increased readmission rates compared to those with a normal BMI [6,12,35]. Biomechanically, obesity adds stress to vertebral structures and surgical implants, potentially causing hardware failure and adjacent-segment degeneration [11]. However, some studies indicate that the impact of overweight and moderate obesity on spinal surgery outcomes may not always be significant or consistent [5,36].

On the other hand, recent studies have also highlighted significant risks associated with underweight in spinal surgery outcomes [15,18]. Underweight patients often face complications such as delayed wound healing due to malnutrition, increased infection risk, and slowed postoperative recovery [5]. Additionally, patients with a lower BMI typically exhibit poorer bone microarchitecture quality, elevating their susceptibility to fractures and PSL after PISF [37], thereby negatively impacting both their short-term recovery and long-term quality of life.

However, these studies mainly applied the standard WHO BMI classification [9], focusing predominantly on abnormal BMI categories [5,38]. Detailed analyses within the normal BMI range, which represents 85% of BMI distributions [39], and comprehensive age-specific evaluations remain lacking, despite conflicting evidence regarding risks at BMI extremes [18,36,40].

4.4. Rethinking BMI Thresholds in Vertebral Fragility Assessment

In this study, we initially confirmed the validity of our grouping criteria by verifying significantly lower vertebral HU values in the path-VF group, aligning with previous reports that HU values are strongly correlated with decreasing BMD and reliably predict PSL [41].

Notably, our analysis revealed distinct associations between BMI categories and path-VF risk compared to studies in the existing literature, which generally links abnormal BMI with increased vertebral fragility risk [5,38,39]. Specifically, we observed an elevated risk among normal-weight females, contrasting with a protective effect seen in overweight males and obese individuals. These findings suggest that traditional BMI classification might inadequately capture the nuanced relationship between body weight and vertebral health, particularly within the normal-weight range among older adults.

Our further analysis across age cohorts revealed distinct age–BMI patterns between groups. Specifically, a decreased BMI with an advanced age correlated with an increased likelihood of path-VF, particularly among elderly males, whereas females consistently exhibited a lower BMI across age categories. Interestingly, despite lower BMI values in the path-VF group, the mean BMI consistently remained within the normal-weight range, implying that standard BMI thresholds may underestimate vertebral fragility risk in elderly patients. This pattern aligns with the broader geriatric literature, highlighting an elevated mortality risk associated with a low/normal BMI in older populations [19].

A binary logistic regression reinforced these associations, indicating that an advanced age and the female gender independently increased the path-VF risk, while a higher BMI conferred protection specifically regarding path-VF, though not necessarily indicating overall health benefits. Indeed, overweight and obesity remain well-established risk factors for numerous perioperative and systemic complications [42]. The protective effect observed here could be explained by factors such as enhanced mechanical support from increased body mass and better overall nutritional status, which may contribute positively to bone quality [43,44].

Finally, our findings suggest a clinically relevant subgroup of elderly patients who, despite having a normal BMI, are at elevated risk for path-VF and could easily be overlooked under current WHO guidelines. This highlights the importance of re-evaluating BMI thresholds or supplementing BMI assessments with additional evaluations for bone fragility when planning spinal surgeries in older populations.

5. Limitations

This study has several limitations, starting with its single-centre design in one West-ern European country, which means the findings might reflect specific local surgical practices and patient profiles, potentially limiting their generalizability to other populations or healthcare systems. Furthermore, the absence of data on comorbidities, nutritional status, and various musculoskeletal indicators may have restricted a comprehensive analysis of all factors contributing to vertebral fragility. Finally, the 22.5 kg/m^2 BMI threshold, though derived from an ethnically diverse single-centre cohort, requires external validation through larger, population-specific studies to confirm its broader applicability.

6. Conclusions

Our findings suggest that the current WHO-defined lower limit of a normal BMI (18.5 kg/m^2) may be insufficient for assessing the risk of path-VF in patients older than 67.5 years. Relying solely on this threshold may result in the missed identification of approximately 24.7% of elderly patients at risk of early pedicle screw loosening due to path-VF. While we do not propose modifying the BMI classification itself, we recommend that spinal surgeons interpret BMI with greater caution in this population. Even patients classified as normal weight may require further evaluation for compromised bone integrity if their BMI lies at the lower end of the normal range.

Author Contributions: Conceptualization, J.L.; methodology, J.L. and A.S.; software, J.L.; validation, J.L., A.S. and M.D.; formal analysis, J.L. and A.S.; investigation, J.L.; resources, B.K., S.K. and M.D.; data curation, J.L. and M.D.; writing—original draft preparation, J.L.; writing—review and editing, J.L., A.S., M.S., L.V., P.S. and M.D.; visualization, J.L.; supervision, M.S., L.V., P.S. and M.D.; project administration, M.D.; funding acquisition, M.D. All authors have read and agreed to the published version of the manuscript.

Funding: This research received no external funding.

Institutional Review Board Statement: The study was conducted in accordance with the Declaration of Helsinki and approved by the Institutional Review Board of RKH Orthopaedic Hospital Markgröningen (protocol code 2025_NO_01, approved on 13 January 2025).

Informed Consent Statement: Informed consent was not required for this retrospective study using anonymized patient data, as approved by the institutional review board.

Data Availability Statement: The datasets generated and/or analysed during the current study are not publicly available due to institutional data ownership. The data are the property of RKH Orthopaedic Clinic Markgröningen, 71706 Markgröningen, Baden-Württemberg, Germany. Data may be made available upon reasonable request and with prior approval from the institution. Requests should be directed to the corresponding author.

Conflicts of Interest: The authors declare no conflicts of interest.

Abbreviations

The following abbreviations are used in this manuscript:

PSL	Pedicle screw loosening
PISF	Posterior instrumented spinal fusion
VF	Vertebral fragility
Path-VF	Pathological vertebral fragility
WHO	World Health Organization
BMI	Body mass index
HU	Hounsfield units
OR	Odds ratio
BMD	Bone mineral density
SD	Standard deviation
SE	Standard error
CI	Confidence intervals
ROC	Receiver operating characteristic curve
AUC	Area under the curve

d	Cohen's d
r	Rank-biserial correlation coefficient
r_p	Pearson's correlation test coefficient
q	Fisher's Z-test coefficient Cohen's q

References

1. Singh, S.; Sarma, D.K.; Verma, V.; Nagpal, R.; Kumar, M. From Cells to Environment: Exploring the Interplay between Factors Shaping Bone Health and Disease. *Medicina* **2023**, *59*, 1546. [CrossRef]
2. Zaidi, Q.; MacNeille, R.; Ramos, O.; Wycliffe, N.; Danisa, O.; İnceoğlu, S.; Cheng, W. Predicting Pedicle Screw Pullout and Fatigue Performance: Comparing Lateral Du-al-Energy X-Ray Absorptiometry, Anterior to Posterior Dual-Energy X-Ray Absorptiometry, and Computed Tomography Hounsfield Units. *Int. J. Spine Surg* **2023**, *17*, 43–50. [CrossRef]
3. Khan, A.A.; Slart, R.H.J.A.; Ali, D.S.; Bock, O.; Carey, J.J.; Camacho, P.; Engelke, K.; Erba, P.A.; Harvey, N.C.; Lems, W.F. Osteoporotic Fractures: Diagnosis, Evaluation, and Significance From the Interna-tional Working Group on DXA Best Practices. *Mayo Clin. Proc.* **2024**, *99*, 1127–1141. [CrossRef]
4. Robinson, W.A.; Carlson, B.C.; Poppendeck, H.; Wanderman, N.R.; Bunta, A.D.; Murphy, S.; Sietsema, D.L.; Daffner, S.D.; Edwards, B.J.; Watts, N.B. Osteoporosis-related Vertebral Fragility Fractures: A Review and Analysis of the American Orthopaedic Association's Own the Bone Database. *Spine* **2020**, *45*, E430–E438. [CrossRef]
5. Ottesen, T.D.; Galivanche, A.R.; Greene, J.D.; Malpani, R.; Varthi, A.G.; Grauer, J.N. Underweight patients are the highest risk body mass index group for perioperative adverse events following stand-alone anterior lumbar interbody fusion. *Spine J.* **2022**, *22*, 1139–1148. [CrossRef]
6. Bono, O.J.; Poorman, G.W.; Foster, N.; Jalai, C.M.; Horn, S.R.; Oren, J.; Soroceanu, A.; Ramachandran, S.; Purvis, T.E.; Jain, D.; et al. Body mass index predicts risk of complications in lumbar spine surgery based on surgical invasiveness. *Spine J.* **2018**, *18*, 1204–1210. [CrossRef]
7. Scaramuzzo, L.; Giudici, F.; Barone, G.; Pironti, P.; Viganò, M.; Ravier, D.; Minoia, L.; Archetti, M.; Zagra, A. Effect of Body Mass Index Percentile on Clinical and Radiographic Outcome and Risk of Complications after Posterior Instrumented Fusion for Adolescent Idiopathic Scoliosis: A Retrospective Cohort Study. *J. Clin. Med.* **2022**, *12*, 76. [CrossRef]
8. Oberthür, S.; Roch, P.J.; Klockner, F.; Jäckle, K.B.; Viezens, L.; Lehmann, W.; Sehmisch, S.; Weiser, L. Can You Feel it?—Correlation Between Intraoperatively Perceived Bone Quality and Objectively Measured Bone Mineral Density. *Glob. Spine J.* **2024**, *14*, 631–638. [CrossRef]
9. World Health Organization. Obesity and Overweight. Available online: https://www.who.int/news-room/fact-sheets/detail/obesity-and-overweight (accessed on 1 May 2025).
10. Schoof, B.; Stangenberg, M.; Mende, K.C.; Thiesen, D.M.; Ntalos, D.; Dreimann, M. Obesity in spontaneous spondylodiscitis: A relevant risk factor for severe disease courses. *Sci. Rep.* **2020**, *10*, 21919. [CrossRef]
11. Chen, X.T.B.; Shahrestani, S.; Ballatori, A.M.B.; Ton, A.B.; Buser, Z.; Wang, J.C. The Influence of Body Mass Index in Obese and Morbidly Obese Patients on Complications and 30- and 90-day Readmissions Following Lumbar Spine Fusion. *Spine* **2021**, *46*, 965–972. [CrossRef]
12. Malik, A.T.; Tamer, R.; Yu, E.; Kim, J.; Khan, S.N. The Impact of Body Mass Index (BMI) on 30-day Outcomes Following Posterior Spinal Fusion in Neuromuscular Scoliosis. *Spine* **2019**, *44*, 1348–1355. [CrossRef]
13. Burgstaller, J.M.; Held, U.; Brunner, F.; Porchet, F.; Farshad, M.; Steurer, J.; Ulrich, N. The Impact of Obesity on the Outcome of Decompression Surgery in Degener-ative Lumbar Spinal Canal Stenosis: Analysis of the Lumbar Spinal Outcome Study (LSOS): A Swiss Prospective Multicenter Cohort Study. *Spine* **2016**, *41*, 82–89. [CrossRef]
14. Sun, W.; Zhou, J.; Sun, M.; Qin, X.; Qiu, Y.; Zhu, Z.; Xu, L. Low body mass index can be predictive of bracing failure in patients with adolescent idiopathic scoliosis: A retrospective study. *Eur. Spine J.* **2017**, *26*, 1665–1669. [CrossRef]
15. Alsoof, D.; Johnson, K.; McDonald, C.L.; Daniels, A.H.; Cohen, E.M. Body Mass Index and Risk of Complications After Posterior Lumbar Spine Fusion: A Matched Cohort Analysis Investigating Underweight and Obese Patients. *J. Am. Acad. Orthop. Surg.* **2023**, *31*, e394–e402. [CrossRef]
16. Kim, J.G.; Hong, J.-Y.; Park, J.; Park, S.-M.; Han, K.; Kim, H.-J.; Yeom, J.S. Risk of fracture according to temporal changes of low body weight changes in adults over 40 years: A nationwide population-based cohort study. *BMC Public Health* **2023**, *23*, 948. [CrossRef]
17. Park, S.-M.; Park, J.; Han, S.; Jang, H.-D.; Hong, J.-Y.; Han, K.; Kim, H.-J.; Yeom, J.S. Underweight and risk of fractures in adults over 40 years using the nationwide claims database. *Sci. Rep.* **2023**, *13*, 8013. [CrossRef]
18. Nakajima, K.; Miyahara, J.; Ohtomo, N.; Nagata, K.; Kato, S.; Doi, T.; Matsubayashi, Y.; Taniguchi, Y.; Kawamura, N.; Higashikawa, A.; et al. Impact of body mass index on outcomes after lumbar spine surgery. *Sci. Rep.* **2023**, *13*, 7862. [CrossRef]

19. Winter, J.E.; MacInnis, R.J.; Wattanapenpaiboon, N.; Nowson, C.A. BMI and all-cause mortality in older adults: A meta-analysis. *Am. J. Clin. Nutr.* **2014**, *99*, 875–890. [CrossRef]
20. Al-Barghouthi, A.; Lee, S.; Solitro, G.F.; Latta, L.; Travascio, F. Relationships Among Bone Mor-phological Parameters and Mechanical Properties of Cadaveric Human Vertebral Cancellous Bone. *JBMR Plus* **2020**, *4*, e10351. [CrossRef]
21. Boucas, P.; Mamdouhi, T.; Rizzo, S.E.; Megas, A. Cement Augmentation of Pedicle Screw Instru-mentation: A Literature Review. *Asian Spine J.* **2023**, *17*, 939–948. [CrossRef]
22. Song, Z.; Zhou, Q.; Jin, X.; Zhang, J. Cement-augmented pedicle screw for thoracolumbar degenera-tive diseases with osteoporosis: A systematic review and meta-analysis. *J. Orthop. Surg. Res.* **2023**, *18*, 631. [CrossRef]
23. Ohtori, S.; Inoue, G.; Orita, S.; Yamauchi, K.; Eguchi, Y.; Ochiai, N.; Kishida, S.; Kuniyoshi, K.; Aoki, Y.; Nakamura, J.; et al. Comparison of Teriparatide and Bisphosphonate Treatment to Reduce Pedicle Screw Loosening After Lumbar Spinal Fusion Surgery in Postmenopausal Women With Osteoporosis From a Bone Quality Perspective. *Spine* **2013**, *38*, E487–E492. [CrossRef]
24. Marie-Hardy, L.; Pascal-Moussellard, H.; Barnaba, A.; Bonaccorsi, R.; Scemama, C. Screw Loosen-ing in Posterior Spine Fusion: Prevalence and Risk Factors. *Global Spine J.* **2020**, *10*, 598–602. [CrossRef]
25. Galbusera, F.; Volkheimer, D.; Reitmaier, S.; Berger-Roscher, N.; Kienle, A.; Wilke, H.-J. Pedicle screw loosening: A clinically relevant complication? *Eur. Spine J.* **2015**, *24*, 1005–1016. [CrossRef]
26. Oh, B.H.; Kim, J.Y.; Lee, J.B.; Hong, J.T.; Sung, J.H.; Than, K.D.; Lee, H.J.; Kim, I.S. Screw Insertional Torque Measurement in Spine Surgery: Correlation With Bone Mineral Density and Hounsfield Unit. *Neurospine* **2023**, *20*, 1177–1185. [CrossRef]
27. Carter, J.V.; Pan, J.; Rai, S.N.; Galandiuk, S. ROC-ing along: Evaluation and interpretation of re-ceiver operating characteristic curves. *Surgery* **2016**, *159*, 1638–1645. [CrossRef]
28. Huang, Y.; Peng, J.; Wang, W.; Zheng, X.; Qin, G.; Xu, H. Age-Dependent Association Between Body Mass Index and All-Cause Mortality Among Patients with Hypertension: A Longitudinal Population-Based Cohort Study in China. *Clin. Epidemiol.* **2023**, *15*, 1159–1170. [CrossRef]
29. Winter, J.E.; MacInnis, R.J.; Nowson, C.A. The Influence of Age the BMI and All-Cause Mortali-ty Association: A Meta-Analysis. *J. Nutr. Health Aging.* **2017**, *21*, 1254–1258. [CrossRef]
30. Woolley, C.; Thompson, C.; Hakendorf, P.; Horwood, C. The Effect of Age upon the Interrelation-ship of BMI and Inpatient Health Outcomes. *J. Nutr. Health Aging* **2019**, *23*, 558–563. [CrossRef]
31. Kamei, T.; Aoyagi, K.; Matsumoto, T.; Ishida, Y.; Iwata, K.; Kumano, H.; Murakami, Y.; Kato, Y. Age-Related Bone Loss: Relationship between Age and Regional Bone Mineral Density. *Tohoku J. Exp. Med.* **1999**, *187*, 141–147. [CrossRef]
32. Szulc, P.; Marchand, F.; Duboeuf, F.; Delmas, P. Cross-sectional assessment of age-related bone loss in men: The MINOS study. *Bone* **2000**, *26*, 123–129. [CrossRef]
33. Rondanelli, M.; Gasparri, C.; Perdoni, F.; Riva, A.; Petrangolini, G.; Peroni, G.; Faliva, M.A.; Naso, M.; Perna, S. Bone Mineral Density Reference Values in 18- to 95-Year-Old Population in Lombardy Region, Italy. *Am. J. Men's Health* **2022**, *16*, 15579883221119363. [CrossRef]
34. Henderson, R.M. The bigger the healthier: Are the limits of BMI risk changing over time? *Econ. Hum. Biol.* **2005**, *3*, 339–366. [CrossRef]
35. Park, J.; Han, S.; Park, S.-M.; Hwang, Y.; Park, J.; Han, K.; Suh, D.H.; Hong, J.-Y. Weight changes after smoking cessation affect the risk of vertebral fractures: A nation-wide population-based cohort study. *Spine J.* **2024**, *24*, 867–876. [CrossRef]
36. Chan, C.T.; A Rees, C. Association between body mass index and posterior spine fusion among patients with adolescent idiopathic scoliosis. *PLoS ONE* **2023**, *18*, e0286001. [CrossRef]
37. Mi, B.; Zhang, J.; Jiang, K.; Meng, H.; Shan, L.; Hao, D. Weight-adjusted waist index is a potential early predictor of degraded bone microarchitecture: A cross-sectional study of the national health and nutrition examination survey 2007–2008. *J. Orthop. Surg.* **2024**, *32*, 10225536241268827. [CrossRef]
38. Kim, J.; Lee, S.; Kim, S.S.; Lee, J.-P.; Kim, J.S.; Jung, J.G.; Yoon, S.J.; Kim, K.P.; Park, C.-K.; Kim, Y.-H. Association between body mass index and fragility fracture in postmenopausal women: A cross-sectional study using Korean National Health and Nutrition Examination Survey 2008-2009 (KNHANES IV). *BMC Women Health* **2021**, *21*, 60. [CrossRef]
39. Park, J.; Han, S.; Jang, H.-D.; Shin, G.; Han, K.; Hong, J.-Y. Underweight as a risk factor for vertebral fractures in the South Korean population. *Spine J.* **2023**, *23*, 877–884. [CrossRef]
40. Gleeson, M.M.; Solomito, M.J.; Kostyun, R.O.; Esmende, S.; Makanji, H. Low Body Mass Index Patients Undergoing an Anterior Lumbar Fusion May Have an Increased Risk of Perioperative Complications. *Int. J. Spine Surg.* **2023**, *17*, 787–793. [CrossRef]
41. Schreiber, J.J.; Anderson, P.A.; Hsu, W.K. Use of computed tomography for assessing bone mineral density. *Neurosurg. Focus* **2014**, *37*, E4. [CrossRef]
42. Katsevman, G.A.; Daffner, S.D.; Brandmeir, N.J.; Emery, S.E.; France, J.C.; Sedney, C.L. Complexities of spine surgery in obese patient populations: A narrative review. *Spine J.* **2020**, *20*, 501–511. [CrossRef]

43. El Maghraoui, A.; Sadni, S.; El Maataoui, A.; Majjad, A.; Rezqi, A.; Ouzzif, Z.; Mounach, A. Influence of obesity on vertebral fracture prevalence and vitamin D status in postmenopausal women. *Nutr. Metab.* **2015**, *12*, 44. [CrossRef]
44. Bae, K.; Han, S.; Han, K.; Park, J.; Hong, J.-Y.; Choi, S.H. Is Overweight Protective Against Fracture Occurrence? Age and Site-Dependent Different Association Between Body Mass Index and the Incidence of Hip and Vertebral Fractures. *Glob. Spine J.* 2025, *online ahead of print*. [CrossRef]

Journal of
Clinical Medicine

MDPI

Article

Ligamentotaxis Effect of Lateral Lumber Interbody Fusion and Cage Subsidence

Ryosuke Tomio

Department of Neurosurgery, Honjo Neurosurgery and Spine Surgery Clinic, Saitama 367-0030, Japan; tomy0807@hotmail.com; Tel.: +(81)-0495-23-9156

Abstract

Background/Objectives: Lateral lumbar interbody fusion (LLIF) has gained popularity as an effective technique for indirect decompression through ligamentotaxis. Despite the perceived importance of using appropriately sized cages for achieving optimal decompression, comprehensive reports on cage size and its impact on indirect decompression are limited. This study aimed to assess the ligamentotaxis effect by measuring the "backward bulging" length in pre- and postoperative MRIs and examining its correlation with cage size and subsidence. **Methods**: T2 images of 270 patients with lumbar herniated disc and/or lumbar spondylolisthesis (June 2022 to March 2025) were analyzed for 530 intervertebral spaces. Data on gender, age, length of hospital stay, preoperative and postoperative lumbar JOA scores, and the level of the disease were collected. Measurements included backward bulging length, intervertebral height, and cage subsidence. Statistical analysis was performed using StatMate. Surgical procedures involved oblique lateral interbody fusion (OLIF) to minimize impact on the iliopsoas and lumbar plexus. Trial cages starting from 8 mm were sequentially inserted, with confirmation through lateral fluoroscopy. Posterior fixation was performed using percutaneous pedicle screws. **Results**: Analysis of 530 intervertebral spaces revealed that 70% could accommodate a cage 3 mm or larger than the preoperative intervertebral height. Significant backward bulging shortening (3 mm or more) occurred in 339 spaces, predominantly with larger cages. Only 8.8% of cases (14/159) with a large backward bulging shortening had an intervertebral height extension of 3 mm or less. On the other hand, a large reduction in backward bulging was observed in 91.3% of cases (339/371) with an intervertebral height extension of 3 mm or more. Postoperative cage subsidence was observed in 9.2% (49/530) of all intervertebral spaces and 8.6% (32/371) in spaces where a cage larger than 3 mm was used. There was no statistically significant difference between these two groups. **Conclusions**: To achieve a sufficient ligamentotaxis effect, it is necessary to select a cage size that allows for an intervertebral height increase of at least 3 mm compared to the preoperative measurement.

Keywords: LLIF; OLIF; ligamentotaxis; indirect decompression; cage subsidence

1. Introduction

Lateral lumbar interbody fusion (LLIF) has become popular. LLIF is a surgical technique that offers advantages in terms of bone fusion rates and infection rates, and enables anterior fixation while preserving posterior structures such as the paraspinal muscles, spinous processes, laminae, and facet joints. In addition, indirect decompression by ligamentotaxis is effective for spinal stenosis, and it is considered particularly effective for decompressing pressure on the dural sac from the front, such as in cases of protruded hernia or lumbar spondylolisthesis [1–7]. If one were to point out the drawbacks of this surgical technique, they would include the risk of injury to abdominal organs, such as the intestines or to the aorta, when performed by surgeons not well versed in the procedure. Additionally, since anterior fixation of the vertebral body can be achieved without accessing the spinal canal from the posterior side, a separate posterior skin incision is required if direct decompression becomes necessary. Furthermore, because anterior fixation is typically performed in the lateral decubitus position, intraoperative repositioning from lateral to prone is necessary to perform percutaneous pedicle screw placement. At our institution, over the past three years, more than 300 cases of this surgical technique have been performed without a single major complication. Indirect decompression by LLIF provides a decompressive effect by stretching extensible structures such as the intervertebral disc and the flexible ligamentum flavum. Expanding the intervertebral height is also expected to have the effect of enlarging the intervertebral foramen. However, despite the belief that achieving an indirect decompression effect through ligamentotaxis requires the use of an appropriately sized cage, detailed reports on cage size and the indirect decompression have been limited [8,9]. Generally, the use of larger cages raises concerns about the risk of cage subsidence. The objective of this study is to identify the appropriate cage size and the extent of intervertebral height increase necessary to achieve sufficient indirect decompression. In this study, the ligamentotaxis effect was estimated by the measurement of the backward bulging length in MRI, pre- and post-operation. The relationships between cage size and backward bulging shortening, cage size and cage subsidence were examined.

2. Materials and Methods

2.1. Study Design

This is single-center, retrospective study. Materials are T2 images of 270 patients from June 2022 to March 2025, and 530 intervertebral spaces with spinal stenosis by herniated disc or spondylolisthesis. The inclusion criteria consisted of all cases and all intervertebral levels in which OLIF was performed for neurological symptoms caused by either central-type lumbar disc herniation or lumbar spondylolisthesis. Cases in which OLIF was performed solely for correction of lumbar alignment, such as scoliosis or kyphosis, without neurological symptoms due to anterior elements (e.g., intervertebral disc or posterior longitudinal ligament) compressing the dural sac, were excluded. The disc herniations included in this study were all extensive protruded hernias involving medial protrusion, and did not include paramedian small hernias, such as those treatable by simple herniotomy or endoscopy. Cases with only mild disc bulging and minimal posterior compression from discs were also not included in this study. Additionally, cases with sequestration herniation were not included in this study.

Data on gender, age, length of hospital stay, preoperative and postoperative lumbar JOA scores [10], and the level of the disease were collected. The present study and data collection were approved by the ethics committee of the Honjo Neurosurgery and Spine surgery clinic. StatMate 5 (Nihon 3B Scientific Inc., Niigata, Japan) was used for statistical analysis. Two-thirds of all surgical cases were performed by the author, while the remaining one-third was handled by another surgeon. All data collection and analysis was conducted solely by the author.

2.2. Measurements of Results

The measurement objects were the backward bulging length and the intervertebral height extension length. The definition for the backward bulging is the maximum posterior bulging length from the posterior surface of the vertebral body located forward at the level of the intervertebral disc (Figure 1).

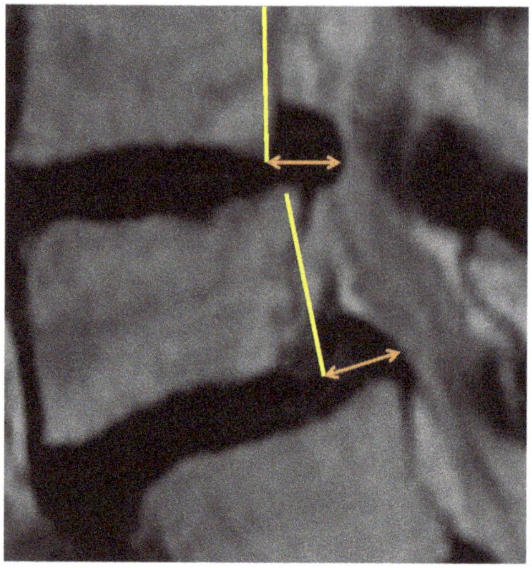

Figure 1. Definition of the "backward bulging" is posterior bulging length (orange arrow) from the posterior surface of the vertebral body (yellow line) at the level of the intervertebral disc.

If this backward bulging shortening was larger than 3 mm, we defined it as large shortening. We also measured the intervertebral height extension and divided it into these 3 groups: less than 3 mm, more than 3 mm, and 4 mm (Figure 2).

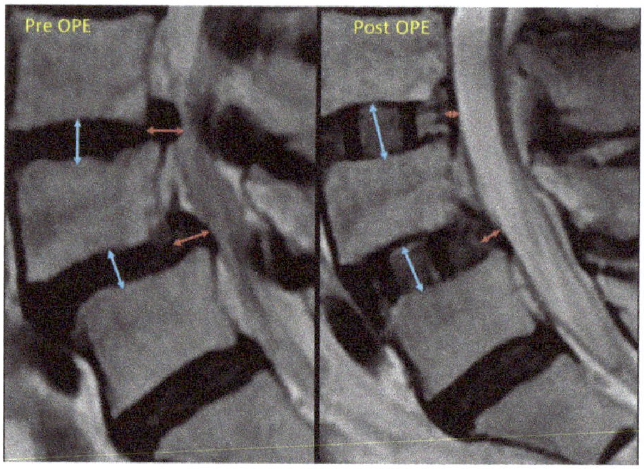

Figure 2. This is the schema of the "backward bulging" length measurement. The red arrow indicates the backward bulging length. We measured the difference between pre- and post-operation measurements. If this backward bulging shortening exceeded 3 mm, we defined it as significant shortening. The blue arrow indicates the "intervertebral height". Post-operation, this height equals the size of the cage. We also measured the difference as the "intervertebral height extension". These measurements were then divided into three groups: less than 3 mm, more than 3 mm, and 4 mm.

The occurrence of cage subsidence and its relationship with cage size were also investigated postoperatively. The follow-up period ranged from a minimum of 3 months to a maximum of 24 months. In this study, cases with a subsidence of 1/4 or more of the cage height were classified as having subsidence. The incidence of cage subsidence was examined between intervertebral spaces where a cage larger than 3 mm compared to the preoperative intervertebral height was used and those where it was not used.

2.3. Surgical Procedures

In order to minimize the impact on the iliopsoas and lumbar plexus, we perform oblique lateral interbody fusion (OLIF), prepsoaps approach. Set up in the right lateral decubitus position, muscle dissection and access were performed layer by layer under direct observation. Reaching the lateral aspect of the intervertebral disc by pulling the psoas muscle dorsally, a guide wire is inserted into the disc. After confirming through lateral fluoroscopy that the wire is positioned at near the center of the lateral aspect of the intervertebral disc, an access device is inserted to expand the surgical field. After clearing the disc space, trial cages are sequentially inserted, starting from 8 mm, to assess whether they are in the appropriate position and to confirm the fitting sensation. The cage size was determined based on the feel during trial cage insertion, ensuring that an appropriate size was selected without causing undue pressure. After inserting the appropriately sized cage, each muscle layer is sutured with fascia, and subcutaneous and skin closure is performed, concluding the lateral decubitus position procedure. Subsequently, a change in position to the prone position is carried out, and posterior fixation is performed using percutaneous pedicle screws.

3. Results

3.1. Patient Etiology

Out of 270 patients, 159 were male and 111 were female. The average age was 71.9 years (range 30–90), with a median age of 74 years. The youngest patient was 30 years old, and the oldest was 90 (Table 1). There were 201 cases of extensive protruded hernias involving medial protrusion and 121 cases of spondylolisthesis. In 52 cases, disc herniation was accompanied by spondylolisthesis at the affected intervertebral level. Most cases were affected by extensive protruded hernias or spondylolisthesis, leading to spinal canal stenosis.

Table 1. Patients etiology and Results.

All cases: n	270
Male: female	159:111
Age: average (median, range)	72.0 (74, 30–90)
Cases with extensive protruded hernia: n	201
Cases with spondylolisthesis: n	121
L1/2 level: n	2
L2/3 level: n	86
L3/4 level: n	200
L4/5 level: n	238
Hospital stay days: average (median, range)	9.6 (9, 4–28)
Preoperative lumbar JOA score: average (median, range)	14.4 (15, 0–27)
Postoperative lumbar JOA score: average (median, range)	23.6 (24, 8–29)
All intervertebral spaces: n	530
≥3 mm larger cage inserted: % (n)	70% (371/530)
<3 mm larger cage inserted: % (n)	30% (159/530)

Table 1. *Cont.*

Intervertebral spaces with large shortening of the BB length(≧3 mm): n	353
≥3 mm larger cage inserted: % (n)	96.0% (339/353)
<3 mm larger cage inserted: % (n)	4.0% (14/353)
Large BB shortening rate: % (n)	
<3 mm intervertebral height extension	8.8% (14/159)
≥3 mm intervertebral height extension	91.3% (339/371)
≥4 mm intervertebral height extension	92.0% (229/249)
Cases which required additional direct decompression: % (n)	6.3% (17/270)
Cage subsidence rate of all intervertebral spaces: % (n)	9.2% (49/530)
Cage subsidence rate where ≥3 mm larger cage was used: % (n)	8.6% (32/371)
Cage subsidence rate where <3 mm larger cage was used: % (n)	10.7% (17/159)

BB: backward bulging.

Regarding the levels involved, there were two cases at L1/2, eighty-six cases at L2/3, two hundred cases at L3/4, and two hundred thirty-eight cases at L4/5. The average hospital stay for the cases was 9.6 days. The average preoperative lumbar JOA score was 14.4 (median 15), and it improved to an average of 23.6 (median 24) postoperatively.

3.2. Results of Backward Bulging Shortening and Cage Subsidence

Among all 530 intervertebral spaces, in 371 intervertebral spaces (70%), a cage 3 mm or larger than the preoperative intervertebral height could be inserted. In the remaining 159 intervertebral spaces (30%), cages of equal or less than 3 mm greater than the preoperative intervertebral height were inserted.

Among all 530 intervertebral spaces, significant shortening of the backward bulging length (3 mm or more) was observed in 353 intervertebral spaces. Among these, 339 intervertebral spaces were those where a cage 3 mm or larger than the preoperative intervertebral height was inserted. In only 14 intervertebral spaces, cages with a height less than 3 mm greater than the preoperative intervertebral height were inserted, but significant shortening of the backward bulging length was observed.

Only 8.8% of cases (14/159) with a large backward bulging shortening had an intervertebral height extension of 3 mm or less. On the other hand, a large reduction in backward bulging was observed in 91.4% of cases (339/371) with an intervertebral height extension of 3 mm or more, and in 92.0% of cases (229/249) with an intervertebral height extension of 4 mm or more.

These results suggest that the indirect decompression is likely to be obtained by a cage larger than 3 mm compared to the preoperative intervertebral height ($p < 0.05$). There was no statistically significant difference observed between cases using a cage larger by 3 mm or more compared to preoperative intervertebral height and cases using a cage larger by 4 mm or more.

In total, 17 patients (6.3%) required additional direct decompression in this series. In 14 cases, it was revealed that, in addition to the effects of an extensive protruded hernia or lumbar spondylolisthesis, there was significant bony lateral recess stenosis and ligamentum flavum hypertrophy. Therefore, direct decompression was performed simultaneously with LLIF. In three cases, symptoms did not sufficiently improve after LLIF through indirect decompression, so direct decompression was added. In all three cases, symptoms improved with direct decompression.

Postoperative cage subsidence was observed in 9.2% (49/530) of all intervertebral spaces, 8.6% (32/371) in spaces where a cage larger than 3 mm was used, and 10.7% (17/159) in spaces where smaller cages (not larger than 3 mm) were utilized. There was no statistically significant difference between these two groups. Among the cases that exhibited cage subsidence, there were no instances that required additional direct decompression after the initial surgery. In two cases, persistent low back pain was observed due to vertebral compression fractures caused by cage subsidence. Both patients had osteoporosis, with a young adult mean (YAM) of 70% or lower as measured by DEXA. Among the 107 cases treated after August 2024, 14 patients (13.1%) were diagnosed with osteoporosis based on DEXA. Of these fourteen patients, three patients (21.4%4) experienced cage subsidence.

3.3. Two Example of the Cases

Showcasing the measurement results of two representative cases, example case 1 (Figure 3) shows spinal stenosis with disc hernia and kyphosis L2-5. The backward bulging shortenings are all large (>3 mm) in these three intervertebral spaces (L2-5). Intervertebral height extension lengths are all quite large (>4 mm).

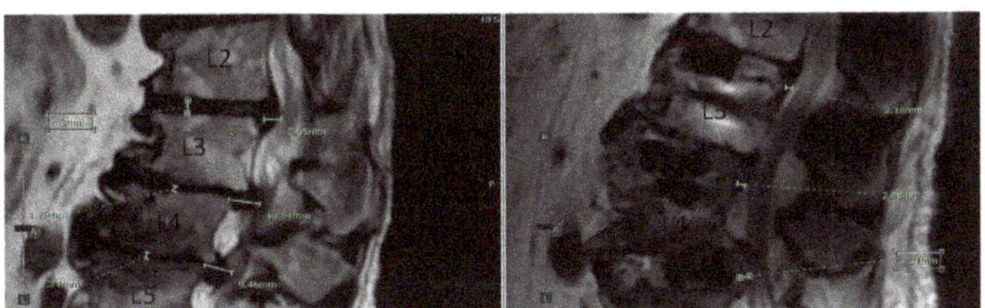

Figure 3. Example case 1, spinal stenosis with disc hernia and kyphosis. Backward bulging shortenings are all large in these 3 intervertebral spaces. Intervertebral height extension lengths are all large.

Example case 2 (Figure 4) reveals spondylolisthesis L4/5 with disc hernia L3/4. The backward bulging shortenings are large in L4/5 (>3 mm), but small in L3/4 (<3 mm). Intervertebral height extension lengths are more than 3 mm.

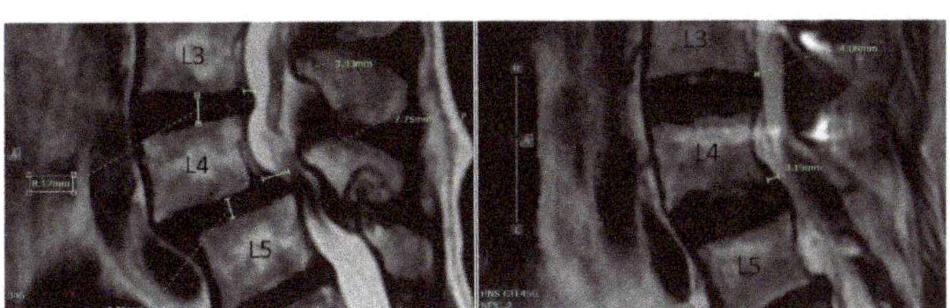

Figure 4. Example case 3, spondylolisthesis with disc hernia. Backward bulging shortenings are large in L 4/5, but small in L3/4. Intervertebral height extension lengths are more than 3 mm.

4. Discussion

These are multiple factors related to indirect decompression failure. Yngsakmongkol et al. reported several risk factors [2]. Low postoperative disc height is considered a risk. Except in cases of cage subsidence, the postoperative intervertebral height usually becomes the same as the height of the cage. The present results demonstrate that using a cage that is 3 mm or larger than the original intervertebral height yields a greater ligamentotaxis effect. By increasing the intervertebral height, soft tissues such as the intervertebral disc and the posterior longitudinal ligament are stretched vertically, resulting in a reduction in posterior compression. Since this ligamentotaxis effect also applies to central-type disc herniations, it can help decompress nerve compression caused by large disc herniations that protrude extensively into the spinal canal. In cases of lumbar spondylolisthesis, increasing the intervertebral height also reduces the anteroposterior displacement between vertebral bodies, thereby alleviating nerve compression. For foraminal stenosis, expansion of the intervertebral height directly enlarges the intervertebral foramen in the vertical direction.

In cases of spinal canal stenosis, if the cause is hypertrophied but soft ligamentum flavum or bulging of the intervertebral disc, symptom improvement can be expected through the indirect decompression effect achieved by restoring intervertebral height. However, when bony stenosis of the lateral recess is present or the ligamentum flavum has hardened due to calcification, the indirect decompression effect is less likely to be effective. Furthermore, in cases where the facet joints have undergone bony fusion, it is difficult to achieve sufficient intervertebral height extension, making the indirect decompression effect similarly unlikely.

Cage subsidence has been reported as a risk factor for indirect decompression failure. It is speculated that subsidence leads to a loss of vertebral height, weakening the ligamentotaxis effect and diminishing the enlargement of the intervertebral foramina. The occurrence of cage subsidence is believed to be influenced by various factors, including osteoporosis, intraoperative intervertebral manipulation, cage size, and other related factors. The assessment of bone quality, such as preoperative bone density, is considered important. While it is generally believed that using larger cages increases the likelihood of cage subsidence, this study did not observe a statistically significant difference. Among the series of surgical procedures from intervertebral disc curettage to cage insertion, the most likely to cause endplate injury is the technique of penetrating the disc tissue from the left to the right side near the vertebral endplate using instruments such as a Cobb spinal elevator in combination with a hammer or the technique of forcefully inserting a trial cage into the intervertebral space. Most endplate injuries that lead to cage subsidence are thought to occur during these steps. Therefore, these procedures should be performed carefully, with fluoroscopic confirmation of the instrument's position and angle. Additionally, during the insertion of the trial cage or LLIF cage, the intervertebral space must be adequately cleared of disc material. If disc tissue remains unevenly, the cage may not be inserted at an appropriate angle, increasing the risk of vertebral endplate injury and subsequent cage subsidence. Attention must also be paid to facet joint bony fusion. When posterior bony fusion is present, even if a larger cage is inserted with the expectation of achieving indirect decompression, the intervertebral height may not expand due to the fusion, potentially resulting in cage subsidence. Therefore, it is important to evaluate preoperative CT scans, particularly sagittal views, to confirm the presence or absence of facet joint fusion. In the present series, cage subsidence occurred in 9.2% of all treated intervertebral levels; however, no cases required additional direct decompression due to a diminished indirect decompression effect. Nevertheless, in cases where cage subsidence led to vertebral body deformation, prolonged low back pain was observed, indicating the need for caution regarding cage subsidence.

As a result, in our case series, there were only three cases that required additional direct decompression and eleven cases that required direct decompression simultaneously with LLIF. The majority of cases, other than the 14 instances that required direct decompression, have shown symptom improvement and a favorable postoperative course without the need for direct decompression. Indirect decompression is thought to work by reducing anterior–posterior protrusion by stretching soft tissues such as the intervertebral disc, posterior longitudinal ligament, and ligamentum flavum vertically. Therefore, in cases where there is primarily bony spinal canal stenosis, the effects of indirect decompression are not realized. Furthermore, in cases of significant ligamentum flavum hypertrophy or lateral recess stenosis, even if indirect decompression occurs, it may not provide sufficient decompressive effects on the nerve roots. Instead, the elongation of the intervertebral height could stretch the nerve roots, potentially worsening symptoms such as neuralgia. Therefore, in cases of bony spinal canal stenosis, lateral recess stenosis, or significant ligamentum flavum hypertrophy, it is considered necessary to combine direct decompression with the procedure.

The results of this study indicate that using a cage with a height 3 mm or more greater than the original intervertebral height is effective in achieving a favorable ligamentotaxis effect on imaging. Based on these findings, selecting a cage size that allows an increase of 3 mm or more in intervertebral height is considered effective. The decision to use a cage that is 3 mm or more larger is made based on factors such as the sensation during the insertion of the trial cage into the intervertebral space, bone density, facet joint bony fusion, and overall safety considerations. It is also important to evaluate preoperatively using CT images whether the cage can be inserted safely and without undue force, based on the insertion angle and its spatial relationship with the iliac crest. We use a larger cage only when it is deemed fitting and can be done safely in a comprehensive manner.

Moreover, the primary purpose of using a larger cage is to expand the intervertebral height. Therefore, in patients whose vertebral endplates are not flat but have a concave, curved shape centrally, it is not necessarily required to add an additional 3 mm to the preoperatively measured intervertebral height. In cases where the endplate contour is curved and degenerative changes have caused the rims of the upper and lower vertebral bodies across the disc space to be in close contact, sufficient intervertebral height expansion can be achieved with a minimal-height cage—as long as the inserted cage adequately supports both lateral rims of the vertebral bodies. Indeed, the fact that a significant ligamentotaxis effect was observed in 8.8% of cases even with cages that were not substantially larger than the preoperative intervertebral height (i.e., +3 mm or less) is likely attributable to the reasons mentioned above. In other words, to safely achieve an intervertebral height expansion of more than 3 mm, it is essential to thoroughly assess factors such as the vertebral bone morphology on preoperative CT images, the degree of endplate sclerosis, and the extent of residual intervertebral disc tissue.

The limitation of this study is that the follow-up period varied among cases, ranging from 3 months to 1 year. Therefore, the results regarding the risk of cage subsidence may change as the follow-up period is extended in the future.

5. Conclusions

To achieve a sufficient ligamentotaxis effect, it is necessary to select a cage size that allows for an intervertebral height increase of at least 3 mm compared to the preoperative measurement. The risk of cage subsidence associated with the use of larger cages will require further investigation through longer-term follow-up.

Funding: This research received no external funding.

Institutional Review Board Statement: The study was conducted in accordance with the Declaration of Helsinki and approved by the Institutional Review Board of the Honjo Neurosurgery and Spine Surgery Clinic (protocol code 2023-002, 21 July 2023) for studies involving humans.

Informed Consent Statement: In this study, we adopted an opt-out approach by disclosing the details of the research in advance on a website and providing patients with the opportunity to decline participation.

Data Availability Statement: Data in this article is available upon request to interested researchers.

Conflicts of Interest: The author declares no conflicts of interest.

Abbreviations

The following abbreviations are used in this manuscript:

LLIF	Lateral lumbar interbody fusion
OLIF	Oblique lateral interbody fusion
JOA	Japanese Orthopedic Association
BB	Backward bulging

References

1. Albanese, V.; Raich, A.L.; Dettori, J.R.; Sherry, N.; Balsano, M.; Barbagallo, G.M.V. Lumbar Lateral Interbody Fusion (LLIF): Comparative Effectiveness and Safety versus PLIF/TLIF and Predictive Factors Affecting LLIF Outcome. *Evid. Based Spine Care J.* **2014**, *5*, 28–37. [CrossRef] [PubMed]
2. Malham, G.M.; Parker, R.M.; Goss, B.; Blecher, C.M. Clinical results and limitations of indirect decompression in spinal stenosis with laterally implanted interbody cages: Results from a prospective cohort study. *Eur. Spine J.* **2015**, *24* (Suppl. 3), 339–345. [CrossRef] [PubMed]
3. Malham, G.M.; Ellis, N.J.; Parker, R.M.; Blecher, C.M.; White, R.; Goss, B.; Seex, K.A. Maintenance of Segmental Lordosis and Disc Height in Standalone and Instrumented Extreme Lateral Interbody Fusion (XLIF). *Clin. Spine Surg.* **2017**, *30*, E90–E98. [CrossRef] [PubMed]
4. Malham, G.M.; Ellis, N.J.; Parker, R.M.; Seex, K.A. Clinical outcome and fusion rates after the first 30 extreme lateral interbody fusions. *Sci. World J.* **2012**, *2012*, 246989. [CrossRef] [PubMed]
5. Mobbs, R.J.; Phan, K.; Malham, G.; Seex, K.; Rao, P.J. Lumbar interbody fusion: Techniques, indications and comparison of interbody fusion options including PLIF, TLIF, MI-TLIF, OLIF/ATP, LLIF and ALIF. *J. Spine Surg.* **2015**, *1*, 2–18. [PubMed]
6. Ozgur, B.M.; Aryan, H.E.; Pimenta, L.; Taylor, W.R. Extreme Lateral Interbody Fusion (XLIF): A novel surgical technique for anterior lumbar interbody fusion. *Spine J.* **2006**, *6*, 435–443. [CrossRef] [PubMed]
7. Phan, K.; Rao, P.J.; Scherman, D.B.; Dandie, G.; Mobbs, R.J. Lateral lumbar interbody fusion for sagittal balance correction and spinal deformity. *J. Clin. Neurosci.* **2015**, *22*, 1714–1721. [CrossRef] [PubMed]
8. Nakashima, H.; Kanemura, T.; Satake, K. Unplanned Second-Stage Decompression for Neurological Deterioration Caused by Central Canal Stenosis after Indirect Lumbar Decompression Surgery. *Asian Spine* **2019**, *13*, 584–591. [CrossRef] [PubMed]
9. Yingsakmongkol, W.; Jitpakdee, K.; Kerr, S. Successful Criteria for Indirect Decompression with Lateral Lumbar Interbody Fusion. *Neurospine* **2022**, *19*, 805–815. [CrossRef] [PubMed]
10. Fujiwara, A.; Kobayashi, N.; Saiki, K.; Kitagawa, T.; Tamai, K.; Saotome, K. Association of the Japanese Orthopaedic Association score with Oswestry Disability Index, Roland-Morris Disabilitiy Questionnaire, and short-form. *Spine* **2003**, *28*, 1601–1607. [CrossRef] [PubMed]

Journal of
Clinical Medicine

MDPI

Article

Impact of the Disc Vacuum Phenomenon on Surgical Outcomes in Lumbar Spinal Stenosis: A Comparative Study between Endoscopic Decompression and Minimally Invasive Oblique Lateral Interbody Fusion

Hyung Rae Lee [1], Kun Joon Lee [2], Seung Yup Lee [1] and Jae Hyuk Yang [1,*]

1 Department of Orthopedic Surgery, Korea University Anam Hospital, Seoul 02855, Republic of Korea; drhrleeos@gmail.com (H.R.L.); yup1019@naver.com (S.Y.L.)
2 College of Medicine, Korea University, Seoul 02855, Republic of Korea; slcjohn@daum.net
* Correspondence: kuspine@gmail.com; Tel.: +82-2-920-3549; Fax: +82-2-920-8555

Abstract: Objective: This study investigated the influence of the vacuum phenomenon (VP) on surgical outcomes in patients with lumbar spinal stenosis, comparing minimally invasive oblique lateral interbody fusion (MIS OLIF) and endoscopic decompression. **Methods**: A cohort of 110 patients diagnosed with lumbar spinal stenosis underwent either endoscopic decompression or MIS OLIF. Patients were classified into two groups based on the presence or absence of the VP on preoperative CT scans, non-VP (n = 42) and VP (n = 68). Radiologic and clinical outcomes, including back and leg pain assessed using the visual analogue scale (VAS), the Oswestry Disability Index (ODI), and the EuroQol-5 Dimension (Eq5D), were compared pre- and postoperatively over a 2-year follow-up period. **Results**: Preoperatively, the VP group exhibited significantly greater leg pain ($p = 0.010$), while no significant differences were observed in back pain or the ODI between the groups. In the non-VP group, decompression and fusion yielded similar outcomes, with decompression showing a better ODI score at 1 month ($p = 0.018$). In contrast, in the VP group, patients who underwent fusion showed significantly improved long-term leg pain outcomes compared to those who underwent decompression at both 1-year ($p = 0.042$) and 2-year ($p = 0.017$) follow-ups. **Conclusions**: The VP may indicate segmental instability and may play a role in the persistence of radiculopathy. Fusion surgery appears to offer better long-term relief in patients with the VP, whereas decompression alone is a viable option in non-VP cases. These findings suggest that the VP may be a useful factor in guiding surgical decision-making.

Keywords: vacuum phenomenon; lumbar spinal stenosis; endoscopic decompression; MIS OLIF; surgical outcomes

1. Introduction

Lumbar spinal stenosis is prevalent in the ageing population and often necessitates surgical intervention when conservative treatments fail [1–3]. Traditionally, spinal surgeons rely on two main surgical options, spinal decompression and fusion [4]. However, recent advancements in minimally invasive techniques, particularly endoscopic decompression, have revived interest in decompression alone, offering benefits such as reduced surgical times and a quicker recovery [4–8]. Despite these advancements, the decision between decompression and fusion remains challenging, particularly in the presence of factors indicating instability, such as isthmic spondylolisthesis, dynamic instability, and facet diastasis [1,4,8]. In this context, the disc vacuum phenomenon (VP), which is indicative of instability at the disc level, has attracted considerable attention [6,9–16]. While traditionally associated with the management of back pain through procedures such as cement discoplasty, emerging research suggests that the VP may also serve as a key factor in determining the necessity for fusion surgery [9,17].

The VP is characterized by the accumulation of gas within the intervertebral disc, typically appearing as a radiolucent area on plain radiographs or as hypodense regions on CT scans [14–16]. Previous studies have demonstrated a correlation between the VP and increased back pain, as well as greater instability, particularly when vertical motion exceeds a certain threshold on dynamic radiographs [12,18,19]. The VP reflects disc instability, making it an essential consideration in surgical planning, particularly in cases where conservative treatments have failed to address symptoms. While these findings highlight the potential importance of the VP in surgical decision-making, the question remains as to whether the VP alone warrants fusion surgery or whether decompression could be equally effective.

There is no consensus on whether the VP should be considered a definitive indication for fusion akin to conditions such as isthmic spondylolisthesis [1,4]. Additionally, the long-term comparative outcomes of fusion versus decompression in patients with the VP have not been thoroughly investigated. While the VP is often viewed as a marker of instability, there are cases where patients with the VP can undergo endoscopic decompression alone and achieve favourable outcomes without fusion, suggesting that the VP does not always necessitate fusion surgery. This highlights the importance of evaluating each case individually, balancing the potential instability indicated by the VP against the benefits of a less invasive decompression procedure. Endoscopic decompression and MIS OLIF (minimal invasive oblique lateral interbody fusion) are effective surgical options; however, they operate based on different principles. MIS OLIF achieves indirect decompression by restoring disc height, which can alleviate symptoms without directly decompressing neural elements [20–23]. Over time, this approach may facilitate biological remodelling, potentially reversing degenerative changes and stabilizing the spine [20]. In contrast, endoscopic decompression directly targets neural elements but does not result in arthrodesis [2,5].

Therefore, this study aimed to compare the radiological and clinical outcomes of endoscopic decompression and MIS OLIF in patients with lumbar spinal stenosis, focusing on the presence and implications of the VP.

2. Materials and Methods

2.1. Study Design and Patients

This cohort study was approved by the Institutional Review Board (IRB No. 2024AN0320, approval date 2024-07-15). This study was conducted following the ethical principles of the Declaration of Helsinki and adhered to the Strengthening the Reporting of Observational Studies in Epidemiology guidelines to ensure transparency and rigour in the presentation of observational research [24]. The study population comprised patients diagnosed with single-level central lumbar stenosis, with or without foraminal stenosis, who underwent MIS OLIF or endoscopic decompression between January 2019 and June 2022. The patient selection process is illustrated in Figure 1. Initially, 164 patients with single-level central lumbar spine stenosis, with or without foraminal stenosis, were screened for inclusion and treated with MIS OLIF or endoscopic decompression. Patients included in the study presented with symptoms of neurogenic claudication and/or sciatica due to central stenosis or severe leg pain due to foraminal stenosis. The decision to proceed with surgical treatment was made after discussions with the patients, particularly when they did not achieve satisfactory symptom relief from conservative treatments, such as medication or nerve blocks. To meet the insurance criteria, patients undergoing decompression were required to have received at least 6 weeks of conservative treatment, and those undergoing fusion surgery needed a minimum of 3 months of conservative management. The diagnosis of lumbar stenosis was based on clinical symptoms compatible with radiological findings on MRI, where central or foraminal stenosis was observed. The inclusion criteria were restricted to single-level surgeries, meaning only patients requiring surgery at a single lumbar level were included in the study. The exclusion criteria were as follows: patients who had undergone previous surgery on the affected segment (n = 11); those with infections, trauma, or tumours affecting the lumbar spine (n = 23); and patients who underwent MIS OLIF concurrently with open or endoscopic decompression (n = 2). After applying these exclusion criteria, 128 patients were eligible for further analysis. An additional 18 patients were excluded due to loss of follow-up or incomplete electronic medical records and radiographic data, resulting in a final cohort of 110 patients. These 110 patients were subsequently categorized into two groups based on the presence of the VP in the disc space at the surgical level, as observed on CT scans. The non-VP and VP groups comprised 42 and 68 patients, respectively.

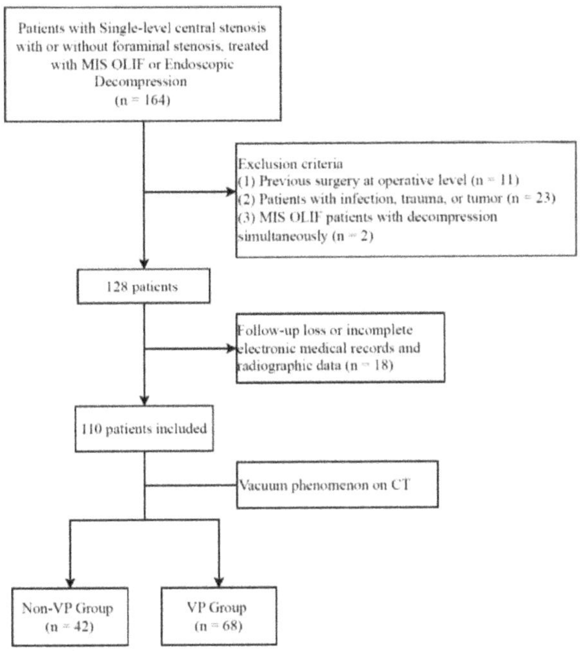

Figure 1. Patient selection flow chart. The figure outlines the process of including and excluding patients from the study cohort, from the initial screening to the final categorization into VP and non-VP groups.

2.2. Surgical Procedures

The surgical procedures included biportal endoscopic interlaminar decompression and MIS OLIF.

Endoscopic decompression was performed via the interlaminar approach using the biportal endoscopic technique [2,25]. This procedure involves the creation of two small portals, one for the endoscope and another for the surgical instruments. Decompression was achieved by resecting the ligamentum flavum and performing a partial laminotomy. When necessary, the hypertrophic facet joints were trimmed to relieve nerve compression. The biportal approach allows adequate visualization and decompression of neural elements while minimizing soft tissue disruption. This procedure was performed by one of the authors (H.R.L). The MIS OLIF was performed with the patient in the lateral decubitus position [20,26,27]. An oblique approach was used to access the disc space anteriorly, avoiding the psoas muscle and reducing the risk of lumbar plexus injury. The intervertebral disc was removed, and an interbody cage was inserted to restore disc height and spinal alignment. Subsequently, percutaneous pedicle screw fixation was performed using a posterior approach to provide additional stability to the surgical segments. The OLIF procedures were conducted by only one senior author (J. H. Y.) to ensure consistency in the surgical technique across patients.

2.3. Data Collection and Radiologic Assessments

Demographic characteristics such as age, sex, American Society of Anesthesiologists (ASA) classification, height, weight, body mass index (BMI), bone mineral density (BMD), and medical history (including hypertension, diabetes mellitus, and smoking status) were extracted from the patients' electronic medical records. Additionally, details regarding the type and specific level of surgery were documented. Radiological measurements were performed to assess the structural characteristics of the lumbar spine. Instability in spondylolisthesis (ISL) was evaluated using plain and dynamic lateral lumbar radiography. Preoperative MRI axial cuts were used to assess the degree of central stenosis and graded according to the Schizas classification [28]. The presence and extent of the VP were determined through preoperative CT scans [11,14]. Based on the percentage of the disc space occupied by a vacuum (V), the VP was classified into four grades as follows: Grade 0 (no VP), Grade 1 (V < 20%), Grade 2 (20% ≤ V < 80%), and Grade 3 (V ≥ 80%), as illustrated in Figure 2. Additionally, endplate sclerosis was noted [22]. Quantitative measurements included anterior disc height (ADH), posterior disc height (PDH), foraminal height, and foraminal area. These measurements were obtained from preoperative CT scans using the region of interest (ROI) measurement function in a picture archiving and communication system (PetaVision for Clinics, 3.1, Korea University Anam Hospital, Seoul, Republic of Korea).

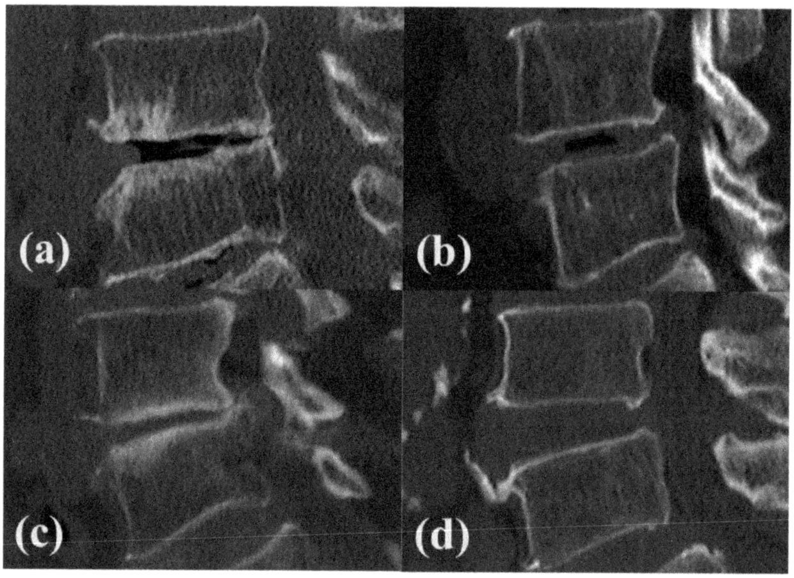

Figure 2. Illustration of the vacuum phenomenon (VP) and an endplate sclerosis assessment. The CT sagittal view shows the presence of the air in the disc space, indicating the VP. The most prominent VP cut was used for evaluation. Based on the ratio of the VP area to the disc area, the grades were categorized as follows: <20% as Grade 1, 20–80% as Grade 2, and >80% as Grade 3. Endplate sclerosis was noted when more than 20% of the vertebral endplate exhibited sclerotic changes. The VP with endplate sclerosis is shown in (**a**), the VP without endplate sclerosis in (**b**), non-VP with endplate sclerosis in (**c**), and non-VP without endplate sclerosis in (**d**).

2.4. Clinical Outcome Measures

Clinical outcomes were evaluated preoperatively and at multiple postoperative time points for up to 2 years, including 1 month, 6 months, 1 year, and 2 years. The outcomes measured were back pain using the visual analogue scale (VAS), leg pain VAS, the Oswestry Disability Index (ODI), and the EuroQol-5 Dimension (Eq5D). These patient-reported outcome measures were collected to assess the effectiveness of surgical interventions in both the VP and non-VP groups.

2.5. Statistical Analyses

Statistical analyses were performed using the SPSS software (version 26.0; IBM Corp., Armonk, NY, USA). Continuous variables were expressed as mean ± standard deviation (SD), and categorical variables were presented as numbers and percentages. The Shapiro–Wilk test was used to assess the normality of continuous variables [29]. For comparisons between the VP and non-VP groups, an independent t-test was used for continuous variables, and the Chi-squared test or Fisher's exact test was used for categorical variables, as appropriate. Repeated measures analysis of variance was used for normally distributed continuous variables to evaluate the clinical outcomes between decompression and fusion surgeries within each group, with post hoc pairwise comparisons performed using the Bonferroni correction. Statistical significance was set at $p < 0.05$.

Quantitative variables, including ADH, PDH, foraminal height, and foraminal area, as well as the VP grade, were independently measured by two spine surgeons who had completed their fellowship training. The surgeons were blinded to each other's assessments and the patient groups. To ensure the reliability of the measurements, interobserver and intraobserver variabilities were calculated using the intraclass correlation coefficient (ICC).

3. Results

3.1. Demographic and Clinical Characteristics

Of the 110 patients, 42 were classified as non-VP and 68 were classified as VP. The VP group was slightly older (70.4 ± 9.0 vs. 67.5 ± 11.2 years, $p = 0.203$) with a similar male-to-female ratio ($p = 0.165$). ASA classification, height, weight, BMI, BMD, and the prevalence of hypertension, diabetes mellitus, and smoking were comparable between the groups ($p > 0.05$). The proportion of patients who underwent decompression or fusion was similar in both groups ($p = 0.556$). Additionally, there was no significant difference in the operative locations between the groups, with most surgeries performed at L4–5 ($p = 0.616$) (Table 1).

Table 1. Comparison of demographic characteristics between VP and non-VP groups.

	Non-VP	VP	p Value
	(n = 42)	(n = 68)	
Age, years	67.5 ± 11.2	70.4 ± 9.0	0.203
Sex, M:F	19:23	40:28	0.165
ASA classification			
2	21 (60.0%)	24 (52.2%)	0.569
3	14 (40.0%)	21 (45.7%)	
4	0 (0.0%)	1 (2.2%)	
Height, cm	159.8 ± 5.7	157.2 ± 7.3	0.137
Weight, kg	62.5 ± 11.3	60.7 ± 8.5	0.208
BMI (kg/m^2)	24.5 ± 2.4	24.6 ± 3.3	0.975
BMD, T-score	−1.2 ± 1.8	−1.5 ± 1.4	0.702
HTN, n	15 (35.7%)	21 (30.9%)	0.599
DM, n	7 (16.7%)	17 (25.0%)	0.304
Smoking, n	5 (11.9%)	11 (16.2%)	0.537
Operation type			0.556
Decompression	23 (54.8%)	32 (47.1%)	
Fusion	19 (45.2%)	36 (52.9%)	
Location			
L1–2	0 (0.0%)	1 (1.5%)	0.616
L2–3	1 (2.4%)	6 (8.8%)	
L3–4	5 (11.9%)	9 (13.2%)	
L4–5	31 (73.8%)	44 (64.7%)	
L5–S1	5 (11.9%)	8 (11.8%)	

VP, vacuum phenomenon; ASA, American Society of Anesthesiologists physical status classification; BMD, bone mineral density; HTN, hypertension; DM, diabetes mellitus.

3.2. Imaging Characteristics

The Schizas grade, which reflects the severity of central stenosis, showed no significant difference ($p = 0.773$). In the VP group, the VP grades were classified as Grade 1 (39.7%), Grade 2 (42.6%), and Grade 3 (17.6%). Endplate sclerosis was significantly more prevalent in the VP group (48.5% vs. 14.3%, $p = 0.001$). Although ISL was slightly more frequently experienced in patients within the VP group (8.8% vs. 4.8%), this difference was not significant ($p = 0.425$). The VP group exhibited a shorter ADH (7.6 ± 2.8 mm vs. 9.7 ± 2.9 mm) and PDH (3.8 ± 1.4 mm vs. 5.5 ± 1.9 mm) (both $p < 0.001$), but foraminal measurements in terms of foraminal height and area showed no significant differences ($p > 0.05$) (Table 2). The reliability of these measurements was assessed using the ICC, which demonstrated excellent interobserver and intraobserver agreement. For ADH, the interobserver reliability using the ICC was 0.85 and the intraobserver reliability was 0.88. PDH had an interobserver reliability of 0.82 and an intraobserver reliability of 0.87. Similarly, the foraminal height and area had an interobserver reliability of 0.83 and 0.84 and an intraobserver reliability of 0.89 and 0.86. Furthermore, the VP grading showed the highest reliability, with an interobserver reliability of 0.96 and intraobserver reliability of 0.98.

Table 2. Comparison of imaging characteristics between VP and non-VP groups.

	Non-VP (n = 42)	VP (n = 68)	*p* Value
Schizas grade, n			0.773
B	2	3	
C	23	41	
D	18	24	
VP grade, n			
0	42 (100.0%)		
1		27 (39.7%)	<0.001 *
2		29 (42.6%)	
3		12 (17.6%)	
Endplate sclerosis, n	6 (14.3%)	33 (48.5%)	0.001 *
ISL, n	2 (4.8%)	6 (8.8%)	0.425
CT measurements			
ADH, mm	9.7 ± 2.9	7.6 ± 2.8	<0.001 *
PDH, mm	5.5 ± 1.9	3.8 ± 1.4	<0.001 *
RFH, mm	11.6 ± 2.9	10.9 ± 2.5	0.262
RFA, mm^2	67.0 ± 22.5	61.4 ± 21.1	0.222
LFH, mm	11.8 ± 2.8	12.2 ± 9.4	0.762
LFA, mm^2	66.2 ± 21.0	64.5 ± 18.4	0.673

VP, vacuum phenomenon; ISL, isthmic spondylolisthesis; ADH, anterior disc height; PDH, posterior disc height; RFH, right foraminal height; RFA, right foraminal area; LFH, left foraminal height; LFA, left foraminal area. * p value < 0.05.

3.3. Clinical Outcomes

In the preoperative assessment, the VP group (n = 68) demonstrated a greater mean leg pain on the VAS (5.3 ± 2.1) than that of the non-VP group (n = 42), which had a mean leg pain VAS score of 4.4 ± 1.8 ($p = 0.010$). However, no significant differences were observed between the two groups in terms of back pain ($p = 0.55$), the ODI ($p = 0.335$), or the Eq5D scores ($p = 0.856$). At the 2-year follow-up, there were no significant differences between the VP and non-VP groups in any of the assessed clinical outcomes, including back pain ($p = 0.948$), leg pain ($p = 0.422$), the ODI score ($p = 0.085$), and the Eq5D score ($p = 0.449$) (Table 3).

When comparing the clinical outcomes between decompression and fusion within the non-VP group (Table 4), no significant differences were observed in back pain, leg pain, and the ODI and Eq5D scores across all assessed time points. However, at the 1-month follow-up, the fusion group had a significantly higher ODI score (44.3 ± 15.6) than that of the decompression group (33.0 ± 13.9), with a p value of 0.018. No other significant differences were noted between the two groups in the longer term.

Table 3. Clinical measures preoperatively and at the final follow-up for VP and non-VP groups.

	Total (n = 110)	Non-VP (n = 42)	VP (n = 68)	p Value
Preoperative				
Back pain	6.5 ± 2.3	6.3 ± 2.5	6.7 ± 2.0	0.55
Leg pain	4.8 ± 2.0	4.4 ± 1.8	5.3 ± 2.1	0.010 *
ODI score	61.1 ±15.8	59.7 ± 15.9	62.5 ± 15.9	0.335
Eq5D score	15.4 ± 3.1	15.4 ± 3.3	15.4 ± 2.8	0.856
2 years				
Back pain	2.3 ± 1.9	2.3 ± 2.0	2.3 ± 1.9	0.948
Leg pain	1.4 ± 1.5	1.3 ± 1.4	1.6 ± 1.6	0.422
ODI score	29.8 ± 17.2	25.8 ± 17.5	32.6 ± 16.6	0.085
Eq5D score	9.1 ± 3.3	8.8 ± 3.5	9.4 ± 3.2	0.449

VP, vacuum phenomenon; ODI, Oswestry Disability Index; Eq5D, EuroQol-5 Dimension. * p value < 0.05.

Table 4. Comparison of clinical outcomes between decompression and fusion in non-VP patients.

	Decompression (n = 23)	Fusion (n = 19)	p Value
Back Pain VAS			
Preoperative	6.6 ± 2.0	6.4 ± 2.2	0.738
1 Month	2.7 ± 1.5	2.7 ± 2.0	0.9
6 Months	2.0 ± 1.6	2.2 ± 2.0	0.751
1 Year	2.3 ± 1.8	2.2 ± 1.7	0.832
2 Years	2.1 ± 1.8	2.6 ± 2.3	0.499
Leg Pain VAS			
Preoperative	4.0 ± 2.1	4.7 ± 1.9	0.293
1 Month	1.9 ± 1.4	1.9 ± 2.2	0.974
6 Months	1.5 ± 1.7	1.0 ± 1.4	0.29
1 Year	1.1 ± 1.0	1.0 ± 1.2	0.684
2 Years	1.3 ± 1.1	1.3 ± 1.7	0.964
Oswestry Disability Index			
Preoperative	61.6 ± 17.5	64.6 ± 12.5	0.55
1 Month	33.0 ± 13.9	44.3 ± 15.6	0.018 *
6 Months	24.4 ± 10.3	31.9 ± 17.6	0.135
1 Year	23.0 ± 12.0	29.8 ± 17.1	0.22
2 Years	22.5 ± 14.4	29.8 ± 20.4	0.242
EuroQol-5 Dimension			
Preoperative	14.8 ± 3.4	15.2 ± 2.9	0.695
1 Month	9.7 ± 2.6	10.8 ± 2.9	0.24
3 Months	8.5 ± 2.5	9.0 ± 3.0	0.595
6 Months	8.0 ± 1.8	9.2 ± 3.3	0.235
1 Year	8.2 ± 2.4	9.5 ± 4.5	0.35

VAS, visual analogue scale; VP, vacuum phenomenon. * p value < 0.05.

In the VP group (Table 5), patients who underwent fusion (n = 36) showed significantly better outcomes in terms of leg pain at both the 1-year ($p = 0.042$) and 2-year ($p = 0.017$) follow-ups than those who underwent decompression (n = 32). Although the fusion group had lower ODI scores at various time points, these differences were not statistically significant. Similarly, the groups had no significant differences in back pain or Eq5D scores throughout the follow-up period. These results are illustrated in Figure 3, which presents the trends in the clinical outcomes (back pain, leg pain, and ODI and Eq5D scores) over time, comparing decompression and fusion within the VP and non-VP groups. There were no major complications observed in either group. In the endoscopic decompression group, no revision surgeries were required. One case of revision due to hematoma occurred in the non-VP group. Additionally, incidental durotomies were noted in one patient from the non-VP group and two patients from the VP group. During OLIF surgery in the VP group, an iliac vein branch injury occurred, but it was successfully repaired intraoperatively by a vascular surgeon without further complications. No revision surgeries were required in the OLIF group.

Table 5. Comparison of clinical outcomes between decompression and fusion in the VP group.

	Decompression (n = 32)	Fusion (n = 36)	*p* Value
Back Pain VAS			
Preoperative	6.7 ± 2.1	7.0 ± 1.6	0.499
1 Month	2.5 ± 1.5	3.5 ± 1.9	0.02
6 Months	2.5 ± 2.2	2.5 ± 1.3	0.973
1 Year	2.3 ± 1.6	2.8 ± 1.3	0.24
2 Years	2.7 ± 2.5	2.0 ± 1.2	0.27
Leg Pain VAS			
Preoperative	5.2 ± 2.2	5.2 ± 2.1	1
1 Month	2.2 ± 1.8	2.7 ± 1.3	0.355
6 Months	1.7 ± 1.6	1.8 ± 1.7	0.664
1 Year	1.9 ± 1.5	1.3 ± 1.5	0.042 *
2 Years	2.1 ± 1.8	1.2 ± 1.4	0.017 *
Oswestry Disability Index			
Preoperative	59.7 ± 13.8	60.0 ± 12.7	0.939
1 Month	38.5 ± 17.2	46.4 ± 10.2	0.028
6 Months	32.3 ± 20.7	36.2 ± 12.6	0.382
1 Year	28.7 ± 17.4	34.4 ± 13.1	0.196
2 Years	34.4 ± 21.7	31.0 ± 11.0	0.52
EuroQol-5 Dimension			
Preoperative	15.1 ± 2.3	15.4 ± 2.7	0.726
1 Month	10.0 ± 2.7	11.3 ± 2.3	0.079
6 Months	9.9 ± 3.8	9.9 ± 1.9	0.967
1 Year	9.0 ± 3.3	9.7 ± 2.0	0.423
2 Years	9.6 ± 4.3	9.2 ± 2.2	0.723

VAS, visual analogue scale; VP, vacuum phenomenon. * p value < 0.05.

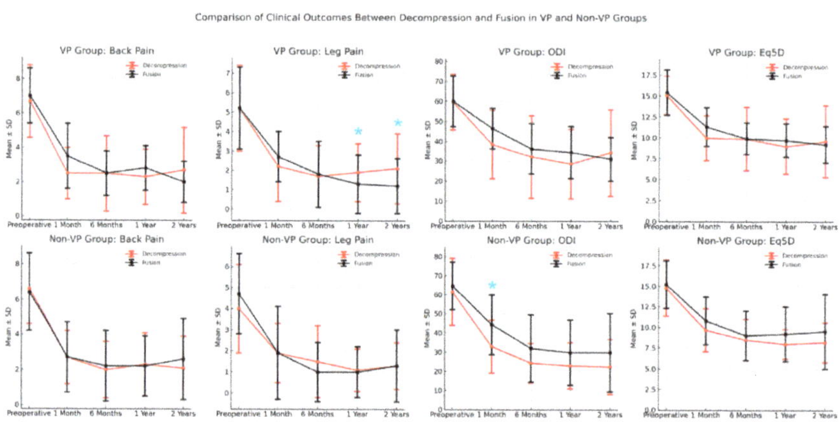

Figure 3. Comparison of clinical outcomes (back pain, leg pain, ODI, Eq5D) over time between decompression and fusion subgroups within the VP and non-VP groups. The blue asterisks (*) indicate points where $p < 0.05$.

4. Representative Cases

Figure 4 illustrates four representative cases comparing VP and non-VP patients treated with either endoscopic decompression or MIS OLIF. In Figure 4a, a patient with severe L4-5 stenosis and no evidence of the VP on CT underwent endoscopic decompression. In Figure 4b, a patient with Grade 2 VP at L4-5 also underwent endoscopic decompression. Figure 4c shows a case of degenerative spondylolisthesis at L4-5 without the VP, where the patient was treated with MIS OLIF. Lastly, in Figure 4d, a patient with Grade 2 VP at L4-5 underwent MIS OLIF for fusion. The red arrow indicates non-VP, while the yellow arrow marks the presence of the VP on the CT scans.

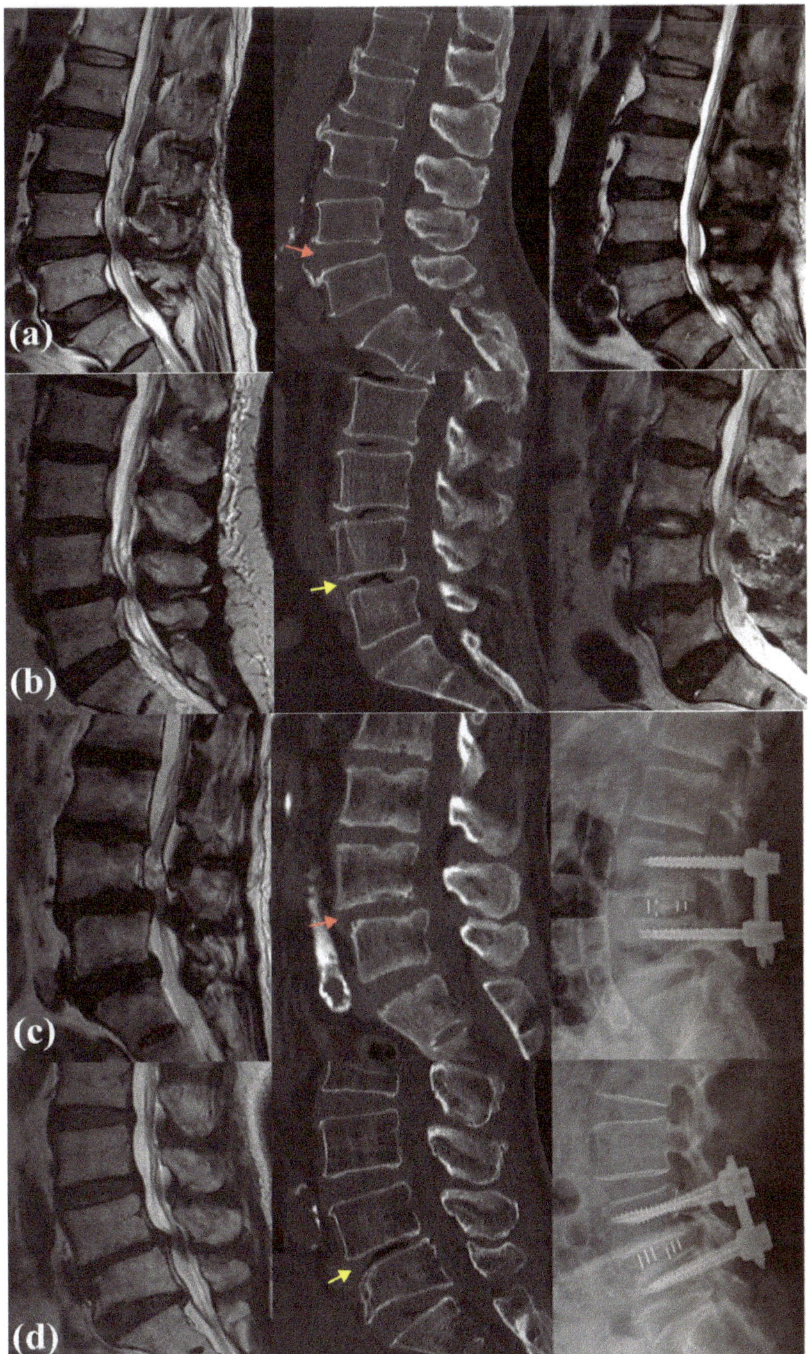

Figure 4. Comparative cases of patients with and without the VP undergoing endoscopic decompression and OLIF. (**a**) Preoperative MRI shows severe L4-5 stenosis with no VP observed on CT (non-VP,

indicated by red arrow). Postoperative MRI confirms adequate decompression following endoscopic decompression. (**b**) Preoperative MRI shows severe L4-5 stenosis, with Grade 2 VP detected on CT (VP sign indicated by yellow arrow). Postoperative MRI confirms adequate decompression following endoscopic decompression. (**c**) Preoperative MRI reveals severe stenosis at L4-5 due to degenerative spondylolisthesis (DSL), but no significant VP sign is observed on CT (non-VP, indicated by red arrow). MIS OLIF was performed at L4-5. (**d**) Preoperative MRI shows severe stenosis at L4-5, with Grade 2 VP confirmed on CT (VP sign indicated by yellow arrow). MIS OLIF was performed at L4-5.5.

5. Discussion

This study highlights the significant role of the disc VP in influencing the surgical outcomes of patients with lumbar spinal stenosis. Our study demonstrated that the patients in the VP group experienced more severe preoperative leg pain than those in the non-VP group. This aligns with the existing literature that associates the VP with advanced degenerative changes and segmental instability, typically resulting in increased back pain and disability [6,9]. However, our study further revealed that the VP not only correlates with these symptoms but also has a profound impact on radiculopathy. Patients with the VP who underwent fusion had better long-term outcomes in terms of leg pain than those who underwent decompression alone, suggesting that the instability caused by the VP extends beyond the disc and affects the nerve roots, thereby exacerbating radiculopathy. This supports the notion that the VP is a critical factor in determining the appropriate surgical approach, particularly when considering the potential benefits of fusion for stabilizing the spine and alleviating nerve irritation [11].

The underlying mechanisms by which the VP contributes to radiculopathy and leg pain likely involve several factors. Instability, driven by the presence of the VP, is a key contributor. Gas accumulation within the disc space, a characteristic of the VP, indicates significant disc degeneration, which in turn leads to micromovement in the affected spinal segment [8,30,31]. These micromovements can result in abnormal mechanical loading and increased stress on adjacent neural structures, particularly the nerve roots [11]. Mechanical irritation of the nerve roots may directly cause radicular symptoms that manifest as leg pain. Additionally, the instability and micromovements associated with the VP can induce a pro-inflammatory state within the disc and surrounding tissues [32]. This inflammatory response is mediated by the release of cytokines and other inflammatory mediators that can further irritate the nerve roots and contribute to the chronicity and severity of radiculopathy [32,33]. These combined mechanical and biochemical factors underscore the significance of the VP in the pathophysiology of radiculopathy in lumbar spinal stenosis.

Despite the known associations between the VP and increased back pain or higher ODI scores reported in previous studies [6,12,19,34], our study did not find a significant relationship between the VP and these outcomes. One possible explanation is that chronic back pain in these patients may have been present for an extended period, leading to a level of pain and disability that was less responsive to surgical interventions such as fusion. While previous studies often highlight a strong correlation between the VP and worsened back pain or ODI scores [6,9–12,17,19,34], our findings suggest that the severity of the VP does not necessarily equate to more severe back pain preoperatively. This could be because although the VP may suggest instability, decompression alone may still be a feasible option in cases where the disc height has significantly decreased [4,6,8]. Thus, it is essential to consider an individual patient's pain profile and the extent of disc degeneration when deciding on a suitable surgical approach. In addition to the VP, which indicates a level of instability that may benefit from fusion, our study found a higher incidence of endplate sclerosis in the VP group. This sclerosis likely contributes to a more favourable environment for fusion, particularly with techniques like OLIF [11,17,20,22]. Endplate sclerosis provides a solid bony interface, essential for safely inserting an OLIF cage and restoring disc height [20–22]. This suggests that the higher incidence of endplate sclerosis in the VP group could influence the decision to perform fusion rather than decompression.

However, our study challenges the notion that a higher VP grade is associated with increased back pain, as suggested by Ohyama et al. [34], who reported a direct correlation between the VP grade and back pain severity. Our findings indicate that the presence of the VP does not always translate into severe back pain, nor does it guarantee a poor surgical outcome. This highlights the need for a better understanding of the VP and its impact on clinical symptoms, suggesting that the VP may not be a poor indicator of surgical outcomes, as previously reported [10,11,19,34].

In contrast, in the absence of the VP, the differences in outcomes between decompression and fusion were minimal. This finding is consistent with previous studies suggesting that fusion may not be necessary in patients without the VP, where decompression alone might suffice [4,7,21,35]. Moreover, our results showed that at the 1-month follow-up, patients in the non-VP group who underwent decompression had significantly better ODI scores than those in the VP group who underwent fusion. This suggests that in cases without the VP, the less invasive nature of decompression combined with its ability to relieve neural compression directly can lead to better immediate outcomes and faster recovery [7,8,35]. These observations underscore the potential of the VP as a guideline for surgical decision-making, although it is not an absolute indication for fusion. This suggests that in the absence of the VP, decompression may be preferable, sparing the additional risks and recovery times associated with fusion [4,7,36,37].

The ongoing debate between fusion and decompression in the management of lumbar spinal stenosis is well documented. Traditionally, factors such as patient age, instability, and the degree of degenerative change have guided this decision [4,7,8,22,30,35,36]. Fusion is often favoured in cases of severe arthritic changes, instability, or listhesis, aiming to achieve solid arthrodesis and prevent further degeneration [4,36,37]. However, decompression alone is effective in patients without significant instability or those at a higher risk for complications associated with fusion [4,7,8]. Our study adds to this body of evidence by demonstrating that the VP, indicative of disc degeneration and instability, could be a valuable factor in guiding this choice. Specifically, our findings suggest that fusion may be more beneficial in patients with the VP, whereas those without the VP could potentially achieve outcomes similar to those opting for decompression alone.

Moreover, the VP and disc height relationship should not be overlooked, particularly in the context of minimally invasive procedures such as OLIF. OLIF is known for its ability to restore disc height and achieve indirect decompression, making it a suitable option for patients with the VP [20–22] in whom maintaining or restoring disc height is crucial. Conversely, in cases where the disc height is already significantly reduced, other factors such as ligamentum flavum hypertrophy and central canal stenosis become more critical, potentially influencing the decision to perform direct decompression [4]. These considerations highlight the need for a nuanced approach when selecting the appropriate surgical intervention, considering the presence of the VP and the overall spinal environment and pathologies.

Our study had some limitations. First, the relatively small sample size, particularly when subgrouping patients into the VP and non-VP groups, may limit the generalizability of our findings. This sample size constraint could influence the robustness of our results and therefore, further studies with larger cohorts are needed to validate these findings and strengthen their applicability in broader clinical practise. Secondly, although we used MIS OLIF and endoscopic decompression as representative surgical techniques, these methods may not fully capture the outcomes of traditional open fusion or decompression surgeries, respectively. Although MIS OLIF and endoscopic decompression are currently increasingly favoured owing to their minimally invasive nature [2,5,23], they may not be directly comparable to other more conventional procedures. This limits the applicability of the results to all fusion and decompression surgeries. However, the growing adoption of these minimally invasive approaches in clinical practise underscores the relevance of our study in addressing current surgical trends [23]. Finally, while our study identifies the VP as a potential factor in deciding between decompression and fusion, it does not provide a definitive algorithm for surgical decision-making. To develop such a strategy, it would be necessary to integrate and validate additional measures of instability, such as the degree of listhesis, facet joint cystic changes, and dynamic radiographic findings. Further research could use our findings to inform future guidelines, with the VP being one of the important factors in the overall assessment of instability.

6. Conclusions

Although the presence of the VP should not be viewed as an absolute indication for fusion, it may play a considerable role in determining surgical outcomes, particularly leg pain and radiculopathy. Our findings suggest that the presence of the VP may be related to leg pain recurrence when fusion is not performed. Further large cohort studies or randomized controlled trials are required to confirm our findings and thoroughly explore the implications of the VP in spinal surgery.

Author Contributions: Conceptualization: J.H.Y. and H.R.L.; data curation and formal analysis: H.R.L. and K.J.L.; investigation: K.J.L. and S.Y.L.; supervision: J.H.Y.; writing—original draft: K.J.L. and H.R.L.; writing—review and editing: all authors. All authors have read and agreed to the published version of the manuscript.

Funding: This research received no external funding.

Institutional Review Board Statement: This retrospective cohort study was approved by the Institutional Review Board of the Korea University Anam Hospital (IRB No. 2024AN0320, approval date 15 July 2024) and adhered to the ethical guidelines of the World Medical Association Declaration of Helsinki.

Informed Consent Statement: Patient consent was waived due to the retrospective nature of the study.

Data Availability Statement: The datasets used and/or analyzed in the current study are available from the corresponding author upon reasonable request.

Conflicts of Interest: The authors declare no conflicts of interest.

References

1. Katz, J.N.; Zimmerman, Z.E.; Mass, H.; Makhni, M.C. Diagnosis and management of lumbar spinal stenosis: A review. *JAMA* **2022**, *327*, 1688–1699. [CrossRef] [PubMed]
2. Park, J.; Ahn, D.-K.; Choi, D.-J. Treatment concept and technical considerations of biportal endoscopic spine surgery for lumbar spinal stenosis. *Asian Spine J.* **2024**, *18*, 301–323. [CrossRef]
3. Kasai, Y.; Paholpak, P.; Wisanuyotin, T.; Sukitthanakornkul, N.; Hanarwut, P.; Chaiyamoon, A.; Iamsaard, S.; Mizuno, T. Incidence and skeletal features of developmental cervical and lumbar spinal stenosis. *Asian Spine J.* **2023**, *17*, 240–246. [CrossRef] [PubMed]
4. Schönnagel, L.; Caffard, T.; Zhu, J.; Tani, S.; Camino-Willhuber, G.; Amini, D.A.; Haffer, H.; Muellner, M.; Guven, A.E.; Chiapparelli, E.; et al. Decision-making algorithm for the surgical treatment of degenerative lumbar spondylolisthesis of L4/L5. *Spine* **2024**, *49*, 261–268. [CrossRef] [PubMed]
5. Chin, B.Z.; Yong, J.H.; Wang, E.; Sim, S.I.; Lin, S.; Wu, P.H.; Hey, H.W.D. Full-endoscopic versus microscopic spinal decompression for lumbar spinal stenosis: A systematic review & meta-analysis. *Spine J.* **2024**, *24*, 1022–1033. [CrossRef] [PubMed]
6. Camino-Willhuber, G.; Schönnagel, L.; Caffard, T.; Zhu, J.; Tani, S.; Chiapparelli, E.; Arzani, A.; Shue, J.; Duculan, R.; Bendersky, M.; et al. Severe intervertebral vacuum phenomenon is associated with higher preoperative low back pain, ODI, and indication for fusion in patients with degenerative lumbar spondylolisthesis. *Clin. Spine Surg.* **2024**, *37*, E1–E8. [CrossRef] [PubMed]
7. Joaquim, A.F.; Milano, J.B.; Ghizoni, E.; Patel, A.A. Is there a role for decompression alone for treating symptomatic degenerative lumbar spondylolisthesis?: A systematic review. *Clin. Spine Surg.* **2016**, *29*, 191–202. [CrossRef] [PubMed]
8. Moliterno, J.; Veselis, C.A.; Hershey, M.A.; Lis, E.; Laufer, I.; Bilsky, M.H. Improvement in pain after lumbar surgery in cancer patients with mechanical radiculopathy. *Spine J.* **2014**, *14*, 2434–2439. [CrossRef]
9. Camino-Willhuber, G.; Vildoza, S.; Martinez, E.; Canestrari, L.; Holc, F.; Oh, M.; Bhatia, N.; Lee, Y.P.; Bianchi, H.; Bendersky, M. Intervertebral vacuum phenomenon—prevalence and severity CT-scan analysis in patients older than 50 years: A retrospective cohort study. *Acta Radiol.* **2024**, *65*, 56–61. [CrossRef]
10. Camino-Willhuber, G.; Schönnagel, L.; Chiapparelli, E.; Amoroso, K.; Tani, S.; Caffard, T.; Arzani, A.; Guven, A.E.; Verna, B.; Zhu, J.; et al. Association between lumbar intervertebral vacuum phenomenon severity and posterior paraspinal muscle atrophy in patients undergoing spine surgery. *Eur. Spine J.* **2024**, *33*, 1013–1020. [CrossRef]

11. Kanna, R.M.; Hajare, S.; Thippeswamy, P.B.; Shetty, A.P.; Rajasekaran, S. Advanced disc degeneration, bi-planar instability and pathways of peri-discal gas suffusion contribute to the pathogenesis of intradiscal vacuum phenomenon. *Eur. Spine J.* **2022**, *31*, 755–763. [CrossRef] [PubMed]
12. Ekşi, M.Ş.; Özcan-Ekşi, E.E.; Akkaş, A.; Orhun, Ö.; Arslan, H.N.; Zarbizada, M.; Küçüksüleymanoğlu, D.; Pamir, M.N.; Benzel, E.C. Intradiscal vacuum phenomenon and spinal degeneration: A cross-sectional analysis of 219 subjects. *Curr. Med. Res. Opin.* **2022**, *38*, 255–263. [CrossRef] [PubMed]
13. Cianci, F.; Ferraccioli, G.; Ferraccioli, E.S.; Gremese, E. Comprehensive review on intravertebral intraspinal, intrajoint, and intradiscal vacuum phenomenon: From anatomy and physiology to pathology. *Mod. Rheumatol.* **2021**, *31*, 303–311. [CrossRef]
14. Murata, K.; Akeda, K.; Takegami, N.; Cheng, K.; Masuda, K.; Sudo, A. Morphology of intervertebral disc ruptures evaluated by vacuum phenomenon using multi-detector computed tomography: Association with lumbar disc degeneration and canal stenosis. *BMC Musculoskelet. Disord.* **2018**, *19*, 164. [CrossRef]
15. Yanagawa, Y.; Ohsaka, H.; Jitsuiki, K.; Yoshizawa, T.; Takeuchi, I.; Omori, K.; Oode, Y.; Ishikawa, K. Vacuum phenomenon. *Emerg. Radiol.* **2016**, *23*, 377–382. [CrossRef] [PubMed]
16. Morishita, K.; Kasai, Y.; Uchida, A. Clinical symptoms of patients with intervertebral vacuum phenomenon. *Neurologist* **2008**, *14*, 37–39. [CrossRef] [PubMed]
17. Camino Willhuber, G.; Bendersky, M.; De Cicco, F.L.; Kido, G.; Duarte, M.P.; Estefan, M.; Petracchi, M.; Gruenberg, M.; Sola, C. Development of a new therapy-oriented classification of intervertebral vacuum phenomenon with evaluation of intra- and interobserver reliabilities. *Glob. Spine J.* **2021**, *11*, 480–487. [CrossRef]
18. Buttiens, A.; Simko, M.; Van Goethem, J. Vacuum phenomenon in the lumbar spine: Pilot study for accuracy of magnetic resonance imaging. *J. Belg. Soc. Radiol.* **2023**, *107*, 83. [CrossRef] [PubMed]
19. Tsukamoto, M.; Morimoto, T.; Kobayashi, T.; Muranaka, K.; Yoshihara, T.; Maeda, K.; Sonohata, M.; Kasai, Y.; Otani, K.; Mawatari, M. The relationship between traction spurs, Modic change, vacuum phenomenon, and segmental instability of the lumbar spine. *Sci. Rep.* **2022**, *12*, 9939. [CrossRef]
20. Chen, P.Q.; Zeng, Z.Y.; Zhao, X.; Fan, S.Y.; Wu, H.F.; Yu, W.; Zhang, J.Q.; Song, Y.X.; Fan, S.W.; Fang, X.Q.; et al. Application of oblique lateral interbody fusion in the treatment of lumbar intervertebral disc degeneration in patients with Modic change and endplate sclerosis. *Zhongguo Gu Shang* **2023**, *36*, 29–37. [CrossRef]
21. Iwasaki, M.; Hayase, H.; Takamiya, S.; Yamazaki, K. Preoperative dorsal disc height is a predictor of indirect decompression effect through oblique lateral interbody fusion in lumbar degenerative stenosis. *Medicine* **2022**, *101*, e31020. [CrossRef] [PubMed]
22. Liu, J.; Ding, W.; Yang, D.; Wu, H.; Hao, L.; Hu, Z.; Fan, S.; Zhao, F. Modic changes (MCs) associated with endplate sclerosis can prevent cage subsidence in oblique lumbar interbody fusion (OLIF) stand-alone. *World Neurosurg.* **2020**, *138*, e160–e168. [CrossRef] [PubMed]
23. Chang, S.Y.; Kang, D.H.; Cho, S.K. Innovative developments in lumbar interbody cage materials and design: A comprehensive narrative review. *Asian Spine J.* **2024**, *18*, 444–457. [CrossRef] [PubMed]
24. Sanmarchi, F.; Bucci, A.; Nuzzolese, A.G.; Carullo, G.; Toscano, F.; Nante, N.; Golinelli, D. A step-by-step researcher's guide to the use of an AI-based transformer in epidemiology: An exploratory analysis of ChatGPT using the STROBE checklist for observational studies. *J. Public Health* **2023**, 1–36. [CrossRef] [PubMed]
25. Kaen, A.; Park, M.K.; Son, S.-K. Clinical outcomes of uniportal compared with biportal endoscopic decompression for the treatment of lumbar spinal stenosis: A systematic review and meta-analysis. *Eur. Spine J.* **2023**, *32*, 2717–2725. [CrossRef]
26. Jun, L.; Zou, T.; Wei, J.J.; Huo, T.; Min, W.; Wei, C.; Zhao, H. Comparison of the effects between oblique lateral interbody fusion (OLIF) and minimally invasive transforaminal interbody fusion (MIS-TLIF) in the treatment of adult degenerative lumbar scoliosis. *J. Orthop.* **2024**, *58*, 58–65. [CrossRef]
27. Scheufler, K.-M. *OLIF Technique (Oblique Lumbar Interbody Fusion)*; Minimally Invasive Spine Intervention; Springer: Berlin/Heidelberg, Germany, 2023; pp. 253–261.
28. Ko, Y.J.; Lee, E.; Lee, J.W.; Park, C.Y.; Cho, J.; Kang, Y.; Ahn, J.M. Clinical validity of two different grading systems for lumbar central canal stenosis: Schizas and Lee classification systems. *PLoS ONE* **2020**, *15*, e0233633. [CrossRef]
29. Wei, J. The adoption of repeated measurement of variance analysis and Shapiro-Wilk test. *Front. Med.* **2022**, *16*, 659–660. [CrossRef]
30. Zuckerman, S.L.; Devin, C.J. Pseudarthrosis of the cervical spine. *Clin. Spine Surg.* **2022**, *35*, 97–106. [CrossRef] [PubMed]
31. Goel, A. Is the symptom of cervical or lumbar radiculopathy an evidence of spinal instability? *J. Craniovertebr. Junction Spine* **2018**, *9*, 81–82. [CrossRef]
32. Shamji, M.F.; Guha, D.; Paul, D.; Shcharinsky, A. Systemic inflammatory and Th17 immune activation among patients treated for lumbar radiculopathy exceeds that of patients treated for persistent postoperative neuropathic pain. *Neurosurgery* **2017**, *81*, 537–544. [CrossRef] [PubMed]
33. Sutovsky, J.; Benco, M.; Sutovska, M.; Kocmalova, M.; Pappova, L.; Miklusica, J.; Frano, A.; Kurca, E. Cytokine and chemokine profile changes in patients with lower segment lumbar degenerative spondylolisthesis. *Int. J. Surg.* **2017**, *43*, 163–170. [CrossRef] [PubMed]
34. Ohyama, S.; Aoki, Y.; Inoue, M.; Nakajima, T.; Sato, Y.; Sato, M.; Yoh, S.; Takahashi, H.; Nakajima, A.; Kotani, T.; et al. Effect of preoperative severity and location of lumbar intervertebral disc vacuum phenomenon on surgical outcomes after single-level transforaminal lumbar interbody fusion. *World Neurosurg.* **2023**, *173*, e727–e737. [CrossRef] [PubMed]

35. Hallett, A.; Huntley, J.S.; Gibson, J.N.A. *Foraminal Stenosis and Single-Level Degenerative Disc Disease: A Randomized Controlled Trial Comparing Decompression with Decompression and Instrumented Fusion*; LWW: Philadelphia, PA, USA, 2007.
36. Leufvén, C.; Nordwall, A. Management of chronic disabling low back pain with 360 degrees fusion. Results from pain provocation test and concurrent posterior lumbar interbody fusion, posterolateral fusion, and pedicle screw instrumentation in patients with chronic disabling low back pain. *Spine* **1999**, *24*, 2042–2045. [CrossRef]
37. Herkowitz, H.N.; Sidhu, K.S. Lumbar spine fusion in the treatment of degenerative conditions: Current indications and recommendations. *J. Am. Acad. Orthop. Surg.* **1995**, *3*, 123–135. [CrossRef] [PubMed]

Journal of
Clinical Medicine

MDPI

Article

Comparing Clinical Outcomes of Microdiscectomy, Interspinous Device Implantation, and Full-Endoscopic Discectomy for Simple Lumbar Disc Herniation

Chien-Ching Lee [1,2], Ruey-Mo Lin [3], Wei-Sheng Juan [4], Hao-Yu Chuang [4,5], Hung-Lin Lin [6], Cheng-Hsin Cheng [4,7,*,†] and Chun-Hsu Yao [8,9,10,11,*,†]

1 Department of Anesthesia, An Nan Hospital, China Medical University, Tainan 70965, Taiwan
2 Department of Medical Sciences Industry, Chang Jung Christian University, Tainan 71101, Taiwan
3 Department of Orthopedics, An Nan Hospital, China Medical University, Tainan 70101, Taiwan
4 Department of Neurosurgery, An Nan Hospital, China Medical University, Tainan 70965, Taiwan
5 Department of Neurosurgery, China Medical University Beigang Hospital, Yunlin 65152, Taiwan
6 Department of Neurosurgery, China Medical University Hospital, Taichung 40447, Taiwan
7 Graduate Institute of Medical Sciences, Chang Jung Christian University, Tainan 71101, Taiwan
8 Department of Biomedical Imaging and Radiological Science, China Medical University, Tainan 70965, Taiwan
9 School of Chinese Medicine, China Medical University, Tainan 70965, Taiwan
10 Biomaterials Translational Research Center, China Medical University Hospital, Taichung 40447, Taiwan
11 Department of Biomedical Informatics, Asia University, Taichung 41354, Taiwan
* Correspondence: u701018.tw@yahoo.com.tw (C.-H.C.); chyao@mail.cmu.edu.tw (C.-H.Y.);
Tel.: +886-6-3553111 (C.-H.C.); Fax: +886-4-22081447 (C.-H.Y.)
† These authors contributed equally to this work.

Abstract: Background/Objectives: The treatment for lumbar disc herniation (LDH) is surgical discectomy. This surgery may enhance spinal instability and exacerbate disc degeneration. The most common treatment options include microdiscectomy (MD), interspinous process device (IPD) implantation, and percutaneous endoscopic lumbar discectomy (PELD). As few studies have compared these three procedures, this study focused on collecting data on the clinical, functional, and imaging outcomes of surgery for symptomatic LDH. **Methods**: This is a retrospective, transverse, and analytical study, with a total of 383 patients who received operations for symptomatic LDH between 2018 and 2022. Medical information from the charts of these patients was collected. The results were followed up on for a minimum of one year by collecting responses from several questionnaires and clinical data, including patients' scores on the visual analogue scale (VAS), Oswestry Disability Index (ODI), and symptomatic improvement score (SIS), as well as wound size, blood loss, hospital stay, postoperative disc change, and complications. **Results**: At the end of data collection, the VAS and ODI scores all showed significant improvement following these three procedures ($p < 0.01$). The SISs were all ranked as good (8.1, 8.5, and 7.9) post-surgery. PELD was a minimally invasive procedure that resulted in the smallest wound size (0.82 cm), minimal blood loss (21 mL), and a short hospital stay (4.2 days). A substantial pre-/postoperative change in disc height was noted in the MD (−17%) and PELD (−15%) groups. The complication rates were similar among the three groups (3%, 5%, and 5.6%). **Conclusions**: IPD implantation and PELD yielded outcomes comparable to those of conventional MD for symptomatic relief and functional recovery. Although the complication rates were similar, the postoperative complications were quite different from those of the other procedures. PELD resulted in rapid recovery and minimal invasion, and IPD implantation showed a good ability to preserve disc height and spinal stability; however, the clinical relevance of these findings in disc degeneration remains controversial.

Keywords: degenerative disc disease; discectomy endoscopic; interspinous process devices; lumbar disc herniation; microdiscectomy; percutaneous endoscopic lumbar discectomy

1. Introduction

The increasing ageing population has encountered substantial challenges in spinal medical care. Lumbar disc herniation (LDH) is a critical spinal disease primarily treated with surgical decompression [1]. The symptoms of LDH may present as radicular signs, neurogenic claudication, and low back pain, and they frequently occur in individuals over 50 years of age [2]. The options for the management of LDH include conservative treatment (such as epidural steroid/morphine injections), surgical decompression with microdiscectomy (MD), the implantation of an interspinous process device (IPD), and percutaneous endoscopic lumbar discectomy (PELD) [3]. **Surgical decompression is indicated if conservative treatments fail** [4–6]. Definitive decisions regarding surgical methods for simple LDH remain controversial [7–9]. Since Caspar and Yasargil developed the method of surgical discectomy with microscopic assistance in 1977, MD has become the gold standard technique for LDH [10–13]. Recently, some studies have stated that the disruption of the paravertebral muscles in the subperiosteal approach and the destruction of the lamina may induce spinal instability and failed-back syndrome [14,15]. A randomized controlled study showed no significant differences in functional outcomes and recovery times between open and minimally invasive MD [16,17]. IPDs have been used for decades and may be designed as a static or dynamic component according to the material, manufacturing, and design [7,18–22]. In 1986, a hard dynamic stabilized system was created to decrease postoperative spinal instability with an interspinous mass and reduce the angle of extension; tension bands were used to fix the implanted graft in the adjacent spinous processes [23]. The considerable indications of application are extensive and can treat spinal canal stenosis, symptomatic facet syndrome for low back pain, discogenic pain, radiculopathy by disc herniation, and an unstable spine [18,19,24,25]. This technique is reversible in cases of recurrent or persistent low back pain. The stabilization system was removed and replaced with a rigid fixation system. In 1997, Minns first presented an interspinous silicone implant for dynamic lumbar stabilization [26]. Since then, an increasing number of soft dynamic system products have been created for lumbar degenerative disc surgery [9,27]; however, their associated use with conventional MD is controversial, requiring a more evidenced database [22,25]. This, combined with its non-specific and 'useful-for-all' characteristics, has made its use debatable among spinal operators [8,25]. PELD with a 1 cm incision has been widely performed for LDH and the stenosis of the spinal canal [28]. Its advantages include minimal wounds, less destruction, less blood loss, and a short operative time [29,30]. However, in endoscopic percutaneous spine surgery with one small linear incision, its unidirectional axis and working channel limit the operative view and decompressive area [31]. Several reports have found similar clinical outcomes in terms of the safety and effectiveness of PELD and MD procedures in the management of LDH [32,33]; however, analyses and reviews focusing on the comparison of MD, IPD implantation, and PELD have not yet been widely reported. Therefore, this study tried to estimate the clinical and functional outcomes of these three different methods for the management of LDH.

2. Materials and Methods

In total, 383 patients (average age, 59.9 years; range, 18–82 years) who received spine surgery for symptomatic LDH between January 2018 and December 2022 were selected for evaluation. The inclusion criteria were symptoms of persistent and severe radiculopathy caused by LDH, **failure of conservative treatment** for 3–6 months, confirmation of diagnosis with spine magnetic resonance imaging (MRI), treatment of a patient by a conventional discectomy of the MD/IPD/PELD procedures, and a follow-up of 1 year. The exclusion criteria included the revelation of an objective neurological deficit via clinical evaluation; revelation of other associated pathological problems such as tumours, infection, spine fracture, spondylosis, spinal stenosis, and facet syndrome via imaging studies (MRI or X-ray); and a history of previous spine surgery.

Clinical Data Collection

The data analysis of the variables in this study was divided into four steps. First, basic data were collected from the patients' medical records, such as age, sex, cigarette use, body mass index (BMI), surgical spinal level, and type of operation. Second, data were obtained from the medical charts of patients who received operations, including wound size, surgical time, amount of bleeding, admission days, and postoperative complications with or without further re-intervention, if any, together with the time period from the first surgery to the next intervention.

Thirdly, a radiographic assessment was conducted. For all cases studied, a lateral upright lumbar radiograph was obtained before and 6 months after the operations. To evaluate disc differences, the intervertebral disc height (IDH) was calculated preoperatively/postoperatively using Dabbs' method [34,35]. The IDH was recorded as the average sum at the height of the anterior (A) and posterior (B) edge of the disc. The calculated formula was ((A + B)/2) (Figure 1). Average IDH values were compared among the three groups. Furthermore, the correlation between the clinical outcomes and changes in postoperative IDH was evaluated. All of the imaging calculations were performed by the same radiologist.

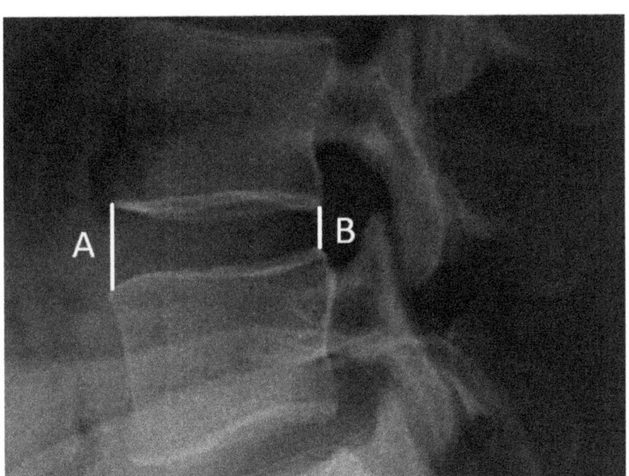

Figure 1. Measurement of disc height. Calculation of disc height via Dabbs' method (A + B/2).

Finally, the final clinical response after surgical intervention was evaluated using consistent surveys frequently used in spinal surgical evaluation. The questionnaires included the Oswestry Disability Index (ODI) to estimate the degree of disability and the visual analogue scale (VAS) to record the pain strength. The VAS score was assessed from 0 (no pain) to 10 (worst pain) using a millimetre rule. The data of the ODI are presented as a percentage from 0 to 100% and recorded with standardized measurements. Questionnaires were collected for both the preoperative status and postoperative follow-up. A symptomatic improvement score (SIS) was also designed to better understand the symptomatic improvement before and after surgery to a greater degree. Satisfaction with the surgery ranged from 0 to 10 on the SIS by the patients' self-judgement or a caretaker's inference (0–2: poor; 3–5: satisfactory; 6–8: good; and 9–10: excellent).

3. Results

The average age of the patients was 59.9 (59.8% male and 40.2% female). Of the patients, 200 underwent conventional MD, 76 underwent IPD implantation, and 107 underwent PELD. The baseline data and clinical profiles of these three groups revealed no statistically significant differences according to their p-values (>0.05). The data of the VAS, ODI, and SIS were also recorded. The data showed that the VAS and ODI scores improved meaningfully in all three groups after operation ($p < 0.01$) (Table 1). The satisfaction of patients was scored using the SIS and was 8.1, 8.5, and 7.9 out of 10 for MD, IPD, and PELD, respectively ($p > 0.05$). The operative spinal levels are listed in Table 1.

Table 1. Baseline clinical characteristics and demographic data.

	MD	IPD	PELD
Age (y/o)	58.1 ± 17.43	53.5 ± 14.10	53.5 ± 15.55
Male/female	121/79	42/34	66/41
Smoking (%)	35%	25%	21%
BMI	31.8 ± 4.36 *	28.4 ± 5.67 *	27.5 ± 4.22 *
Preop./postop. VAS *	8.22/1.39 *	7.35/1.89 *	8.35/1.34 *
Preop./postop. ODI (%)	75.4/18.7 *	73.5/16.3	71.2/12.4 *
SIS	8.1	8.5	7.9
Op. Level (N)			
L1/2	3	2	
L2/3	12	7	5
L3/4	22	10	6
L4/5	91	57	59
L5/S1	72	0	37

BMI: body mass index; IPD: interspinous process device; MD: microdiscectomy; N: number; ODI: Oswestry Disability Index; PELD: percutaneous endoscopic lumbar discectomy; SIS: symptom improvement score; VAS: visual analogue scale; and * p-value < 0.001.

According to our medical records, the mean operative times were 126.35 ± 38.5, 171.59 ± 56.98, and 127.92 ± 47.64 min in the MD, IPD, and PELD groups, respectively, as shown in Table 2. The average operative time in the IPD patients was significantly longer than in the MD and PELD patients ($p < 0.001$). Nevertheless, the operative blood loss (21 ± 23.13 mL) and length of hospital stays (4.2 ± 2.35 days) in the PELD patients were significantly lower than those in the MD patients (73.1 ± 102.25 mL and 5.5 ± 3.59 days, respectively) and IPD group (164.74 ± 180.75 mL and 6.97 ± 4.22 days, respectively). The operative wound sizes were similar in the MD and IPD groups. The PELD group demonstrated the smallest wound size (average of 0.82 mm). The IDH was measured separately for each surgical lumbar level, both preoperatively and postoperatively. The IDH decreased postoperatively in the MD (−17%) and PELD (−15%) groups. In contrast, the mean IDH in the IPD group increased by 3%.

Table 2. Operative record information.

	MD	IPD	PELD
Operative time (mins)	126.35 ± 38.5	171.59 ± 56.98	127.92 ± 47.64
Blood loss (mL) *	73.1 ± 102.25	164.74 ± 180.75	21 ± 23.13
Wound size (cm)	5.89 ± 3.76	6.74 ± 2.86	0.82 ± 0.76
Hospital stays (days)	5.5 ± 3.59	6.97 ± 4.22	4.2 ± 2.35
Medical cost (NT$) *	32,845 ± 3458	150,984 ± 8354	107,304 ± 5748
Preop./postop. disc height (mm)	10.2/8.43 *	9.12/9.35	8.23/7.03 *
Change in IDH (%)	−17%	+3%	−15%
Complication rate (%)	4%	5.2%	7.5%

IDH: intervertebral disc height; IPD: interspinous process device; MD: microdiscectomy; PELD: percutaneous endoscopic lumbar discectomy; and * p-value < 0.001.

The total complication rate was 4% (n = 8), 5.2% (n = 4), and 7.5% (n = 8) for the MD, IPD, and PELD groups, respectively (Table 2). No difference was noted among the three groups. Surgical infection (SI) is a common complication in spinal surgery. Four patients each from the MD and IPD groups underwent debridement and antibiotic treatment for postoperative infections. No infections were observed in the PELD group. Residues/recurrences of lumbar herniated discs were present in three patients of the MD group and four patients of the PELD group. No secondary operations were performed for recurrent disc rupture in the IPD group.

Neural damage (drop foot) may be encountered in spine surgery. In this study, it occurred in only one patient in the MD group due to nerve traction. The patient recovered completely after six months of rehabilitation and medication. The PELD group presented four cases of dural tears, whereas no incidental durotomy happened in the other groups. Four patients with dural openings in the PELD group underwent open surgery for dural repair. In our review, six patients in the MD group, one in the IPD group, and three in the PELD group underwent fusion surgery due to spinal instability within 1 year of the follow-up. The specific data for secondary surgery are listed in Table 3.

Table 3. Cause of secondary operation for three studied groups.

	MD	IPD	PELD
SI	4	4	-
Recurrent rupture disc	3	-	4
Drop foot	1	-	-
Dura tear	-	-	4
Spine instability	6	1	3

IPD: interspinous process device; MD: microdiscectomy; PELD: percutaneous endoscopic lumbar discectomy; and SI: surgical infection.

4. Discussion

In most circumstances, patients were in favour of a minimally invasive approach to surgical intervention because of its fast postoperative recovery times [36,37]. Whether minimally invasive spinal surgery (MISS) can offer better clinical results compared to traditional spine operations has long been a concern for spine operators [38]. Therefore, there is a growing interest in less invasive therapeutic solutions as alternatives to lumbar fusion. Other types of implants with lower local aggressiveness, such as IPDs, are also included in this context [39]. PELD is a recently developed MISS technique. Reports from case series have revealed satisfactory clinical outcomes in the management of LDH [15,40–42]. Thus far, few reports have compared the operative outcomes of patients undergoing PELD,

IPD implantation, and open MD. Hence, this study attempted to understand the clinical outcomes of these three popular spine procedures for symptomatic LDH.

The collected results showed that the PELD, IPD, and MD groups all achieved great progress in their postoperative VAS and ODI scores. In this retrospective study, the data revealed that MD, PELD, and IPD implantation can reach satisfactory and similar clinical results at a 1-year follow-up. In particular, PELD showed faster postoperative recovery, which was reflected in fewer hospital days and less operative bleeding with limited wound size ($p < 0.01$). All three groups achieved high levels of satisfaction. While PELD and IPD implantation may have higher initial costs, their suitability depends on the patient's condition. Microdiscectomy is generally the most cost-effective option for disc herniation. Both immediate surgical costs and long-term recovery expenses should be considered when choosing the best treatment [43]. The conventional MD procedure remained an efficient and well-recovered procedure in our series.

The PELD procedure presents a similar interlaminar approach to MD [26,35]. This distinguishing feature requires endoscopic procedures to take advantage of MD [23,35]. Nevertheless, this MISS technique necessitates a great learning curve for young beginners [36]; skilled and well-trained surgeons may produce different clinical outcomes. Several reports have shown that the operative time for endoscopic surgery is longer than that for MD [25,37]. In our data, the average operative time was similar for the MD and PELD groups (126.35 min and 127.92 min), demonstrating that PELD has no benefits with regard to shortening the operative time; however, IPD implantation resulted in the longest operative time, more blood loss, and larger wound size, which may be caused by the larger operative area approach and instrument implantation. In the consideration of surgical procedures, the creation of a working area, operative hemostasis, and implant adjustment are time-intensive. The period of hospital admission in the PELD group was significantly shorter than that for the other two groups, **possibly** indicating that patients who underwent spinal endoscopic surgery were able to undergo rapid exercise, rehabilitation, walking, and an earlier return to daily work. These issues are very critical, particularly for young patients who are willing to return to their work earlier and older people who have a better quality of life. Our study showed that patients receiving an IPD paid higher admission fees than those receiving MD and PELD techniques. This may be related to the health insurance system of Taiwan, where this study was conducted.

There was no difference in the total complication rate among all of the groups in our study ($p > 0.05$). Four instances of SI occurred in the MD and IPD groups, whereas no such complications were found in the PELD group. These infectious complications were treated with surgical debridement, cleaning, and antibiotic injections, with good recovery. The data demonstrate the benefit of a minimally invasive procedure in decreasing wound-related problems. The rate of a recurrent disc is a substantial concern for endoscopic spine procedures, with a possibility ranging from 0 to 6.9% [44–46]. Patients that received the PELD procedure are considered as being at a higher risk of re-ruptured disc herniation owing to the restricted flexibility in management and the limited operative field. Although the recurrent rates in the conventional MD and PELD groups were similar at the 1-year follow-up, studies with longer periods are required to validate this observation. Therefore, it is noteworthy that there were no secondary operations for recurrent ruptured discs in the IPD group. IPD implantation helps to reduce spinal extension motion and disc/facet joint stresses [47]. This may be one of the reasons for its lower recurrence rates; however, it has special complications, such as implant dislocation, malposition, or fracture of the spinal process [48].

In the MD group, there was one case of foot drop immediately after the operation due to nerve traction. The patient received steroids and underwent rehabilitation without surgical intervention. The neurological deficiency recovered well after six months of treatment. There were no postoperative neurological deficits in the PELD or IPD group of the present study.

A total of 27% of patients who undergo discectomy present postdiscectomy syndrome or failed-back syndrome, requiring a second surgery within 10 years of the first intervention [48,49]. One possible solution with which to avoid postdiscectomy syndrome is to perform lumbar fusion instrumented with pedicle screws during surgical discectomy. Unsatisfactory long-term pain relief after lumbar MD occurred in 8–25% of examined patients [50,51]. Segmental instability is a critical issue that contributes to failed-back syndrome. Extensive operative techniques and bony destruction during MD may increase the possibility of secondary segmental instability [52]. In our series, six cases (3%) in the MD group and three (2.8%) in the PELD group underwent spinal fusion operation within a follow-up of 1 year due to spinal instability. Only one patient (1.3%) in the IPD group underwent a secondary fusion operation. The purpose of an IPD is to keep segmental stability, preserve the focal segment mobility, and minimize the degenerative effects of adjacent segments. This may have resulted in lower postoperative segmental instability [53].

This study had a few limitations, including a relatively small number of samples and a short follow-up period. Hence, more randomized controlled and prospective studies with designs for the PELD and IPD procedures are necessary to confirm our findings. Additionally, only patients with LDH were discussed, whereas those with spinal stenosis or mild-to-moderate spinal instability were excluded. Therefore, there are no reasons to suppose that the conclusions of this research are reasonable for current surgical decisions for LDH patients.

5. Conclusions

The PEID and IPD procedures yielded comparable outcomes to traditional MD for pain improvement and clinical outcomes 1 year postoperation. In addition, PELD enables shorter hospital stays and faster recovery in the immediate postoperative period. Although an IPD leads to a prolonged operative time, more bleeding, and extended hospital stays, its long-term patient satisfaction is similar to that of other procedures. The subsequent effects of a limited range of motion and decreased disc pressure are a concern. The MD technique is an effective and efficient operation for symptomatic LDH. As this was a retrospective study with only 1 year of follow-up, more randomized controlled and prospective trials would be required to validate our observations.

6. Limitation

This study's small sample size limits the generalizability of the results. A larger cohort would provide more reliable data on the efficacy and safety of the treatments. Additionally, the one-year follow-up may not be long enough to capture long-term outcomes or complications. A longer follow-up would better assess treatment durability and late complications.

Future research with more cases and extended follow-up is needed to fully evaluate these procedures' long-term effectiveness and safety.

Author Contributions: Data curation, C.-C.L., H.-Y.C. and H.-Y.C.; Validation, C.-C.L.; Supervision, C.-C.L., H.-Y.C., H.-L.L. and C.-H.C.; Resources, W.-S.J.; Investigation, W.-S.J.; Methodology, H.-L.L.; Software, C.-H.C.; Visualization, C.-H.C.; Writing—original draft, R.-M.L., W.-S.J., H.-Y.C., W.-S.J. and C.-H.C.; Writing—review & editing, C.-H.C. and C.-H.Y. All authors have read and agreed to the published version of the manuscript.

Funding: This work was supported by the Tainan Municipal An-Nan Hospital, China Medical University (ANHRF111-49), and China Medical University (CMU111-S-03, CMU112-S-02).

Institutional Review Board Statement: This study was conducted in accordance with the Declaration of Helsinki and approved by the Ethics Committee of Affiliated Hospital of China Medical University (protocol code CMUH105-REC2-099 and 2024-10-18).

Informed Consent Statement: Informed consent was obtained from all subjects involved in this study.

Data Availability Statement: The original contributions presented in the study are included in the article, further inquiries can be directed to the corresponding authors.

Conflicts of Interest: The authors declare no conflicts of interest.

References

1. Phan, K.; Rao, P.J.; Ball, J.R.; Mobbs, R.J. Interspinous process spacers versus traditional decompression for lumbar spinal stenosis: Systematic review and meta-analysis. *J. Spine Surg.* **2016**, *2*, 31–40. [CrossRef]
2. Machado, G.C.; Ferreira, P.H.; Harris, I.A.; Pinheiro, M.B.; Koes, B.W.; van Tulder, M.; Rzewuska, M.; Maher, C.G.; Ferreira, M.L. Effectiveness of surgery for lumbar spinal stenosis: A systematic review and meta-analysis. *PLoS ONE* **2015**, *10*, e0122800. [CrossRef] [PubMed]
3. Martínez, C.R.; Lewandrowski, K.U.; Ortíz, J.G.; Cuéllar, G.O.; León, J.F. Transforaminal Endoscopic Discectomy Combined with an Interspinous Process Distraction System for Spinal Stenosis. *Int. J. Spine Surg.* **2020**, *14*, S4–S12. [CrossRef] [PubMed]
4. Tang, S.; Mok, T.N.; He, Q.; Li, L.; Lai, X.; Sin, T.H.; Deng, J.; Yu, S.; Li, J.; Wu, H. Comparison of clinical and radiological outcomes of full-endoscopic versus microscopic lumbar decompression laminectomy for the treatment of lumbar spinal stenosis: A systematic review and meta-analysis. *Ann. Palliat. Med.* **2021**, *10*, 10130–10146. [CrossRef] [PubMed]
5. Caspar, W.; Campbell, B.; Barbier, D.D.; Kretschmmer, R.; Gotfried, Y. The Caspar microsurgical discectomy and comparison with a conventional standard lumbar disc procedure. *Neurosurgery* **1991**, *28*, 78–86, discussion 86–87. [CrossRef]
6. Gibson, J.N.; Waddell, G. Surgical interventions for lumbar disc prolapse: Updated Cochrane Review. *Spine* **2007**, *32*, 1735–1747. [CrossRef]
7. Bono, C.M.; Vaccaro, A.R. Interspinous process devices in the lumbar spine. *J. Spinal Disord. Tech.* **2007**, *20*, 255–261. [CrossRef]
8. Benzel, E.C.; Mroz, T. Interlaminar spacers: Looks good, smells bad. *World Neurosurg.* **2010**, *74*, 576–578. [CrossRef]
9. Palmer, S.; Mahar, A.; Oka, R. Biomechanical and radiographic analysis of a novel, minimally invasive, extension-limiting device for the lumbar spine. *Neurosurg. Focus.* **2007**, *22*, E4. [CrossRef]
10. Andersson, G.B. Epidemiological features of chronic low-back pain. *Lancet* **1999**, *354*, 581–585. [CrossRef]
11. Ruetten, S.; Komp, M.; Merk, H.; Godolias, G. Use of newly developed instruments and endoscopes: Full-endoscopic resection of lumbar disc herniations via the interlaminar and lateral transforaminal approach. *J. Neurosurg. Spine* **2007**, *6*, 521–530. [CrossRef] [PubMed]
12. Ruetten, S.; Komp, M.; Godolias, G. An extreme lateral access for the surgery of lumbar disc herniations inside the spinal canal using the full-endoscopic uniportal transforaminal approach-technique and prospective results of 463 patients. *Spine* **2005**, *30*, 2570–2578. [CrossRef] [PubMed]
13. Hoogland, T.; van den Brekel-Dijkstra, K.; Schubert, M.; Miklitz, B. Endoscopic transforaminal discectomy for recurrent lumbar disc herniation: A prospective, cohort evaluation of 262 consecutive cases. *Spine* **2008**, *33*, 973–978. [CrossRef]
14. Ruetten, S.; Komp, M.; Merk, H.; Godolias, G. Full-endoscopic interlaminar and transforaminal lumbar discectomy versus conventional microsurgical technique: A prospective, randomized, controlled study. *Spine* **2008**, *33*, 931–939. [CrossRef] [PubMed]
15. Hua, W.; Zhang, Y.; Wu, X.; Gao, Y.; Li, S.; Wang, K.; Yang, S.; Yang, C. Full-Endoscopic Visualized Foraminoplasty and Discectomy Under General Anesthesia in the Treatment of L4-L5 and L5-S1 Disc Herniation. *Spine* **2019**, *44*, E984–E991. [CrossRef]
16. Choi, K.C.; Kim, J.S.; Park, C.K. Percutaneous Endoscopic Lumbar Discectomy as an Alternative to Open Lumbar Microdiscectomy for Large Lumbar Disc Herniation. *Pain Physician* **2016**, *19*, E291–E300.
17. Gibson, J.N.A.; Subramanian, A.S.; Scott, C.E.H. A randomised controlled trial of transforaminal endoscopic discectomy vs microdiscectomy. *Eur. Spine J.* **2017**, *26*, 847–856. [CrossRef]
18. Christie, S.D.; Song, J.K.; Fessler, R.G. Dynamic interspinous process technology. *Spine* **2005**, *30*, S73–S78. [CrossRef]
19. Zucherman, J.F.; Hsu, K.Y.; Hartjen, C.A.; Mehalic, T.F.; Implicito, D.A.; Martin, M.J.; Johnson, D.R.; Skidmore, G.A.; Vessa, P.P.; Dwyer, J.W.; et al. A prospective randomized multi-center study for the treatment of lumbar spinal stenosis with the X STOP interspinous implant: 1-year results. *Eur. Spine J.* **2004**, *13*, 22–31. [CrossRef]
20. Mariottini, A.; Pieri, S.; Giachi, S.; Carangelo, B.; Zalaffi, A.L.; Muzii, F.V.; Palma, L. Preliminary results of a soft novel lumbar intervertebral prothesis (DIAM) in the degenerative spinal pathology. *Acta Neurochir. Suppl.* **2005**, *92*, 129–131.

21. Kim, K.A.; McDonald, M.; Pik, J.H.; Khoueir, P.; Wang, M.Y. Dynamic intraspinous spacer technology for posterior stabilization: Case-control study on the safety, sagittal angulation, and pain outcome at 1-year follow-up evaluation. *Neurosurg. Focus.* **2007**, *22*, E7. [CrossRef]
22. Galarza, M.; Fabrizi, A.P.; Maina, R.; Gazzeri, R.; Martínez-Lage, J.F. Degenerative lumbar spinal stenosis with neurogenic intermittent claudication and treatment with the Aperius PercLID System: A preliminary report. *Neurosurg. Focus.* **2010**, *28*, E3. [CrossRef] [PubMed]
23. Sénégas, J.; Vital, J.M.; Pointillart, V.; Mangione, P. Long-term actuarial survivorship analysis of an interspinous stabilization system. *Eur. Spine J.* **2007**, *16*, 1279–1287. [CrossRef] [PubMed]
24. Galarza, M.; Gazzeri, R.; De la Rosa, P.; Martínez-Lage, J.F. Microdiscectomy with and without insertion of interspinous device for herniated disc at the L5-S1 level. *J. Clin. Neurosci.* **2014**, *21*, 1934–1939. [CrossRef] [PubMed]
25. Tsai, K.J.; Murakami, H.; Lowery, G.L.; Hutton, W.C. A biomechanical evaluation of an interspinous device (Coflex) used to stabilize the lumbar spine. *J. Surg. Orthop. Adv.* **2006**, *15*, 167–172.
26. Minns, R.J.; Walsh, W.K. Preliminary design and experimental studies of a novel soft implant for correcting sagittal plane instability in the lumbar spine. *Spine* **1997**, *22*, 1819–1825, discussion 1826–1827. [CrossRef]
27. Kim, D.H.; Albert, T.J. Interspinous process spacers. *J. Am. Acad. Orthop. Surg.* **2007**, *15*, 200–207. [CrossRef]
28. Jang, J.S.; An, S.H.; Lee, S.H. Transforaminal percutaneous endoscopic discectomy in the treatment of foraminal and extraforaminal lumbar disc herniations. *J. Spinal Disord. Tech.* **2006**, *19*, 338–343. [CrossRef]
29. Kapetanakis, S.; Gkantsinikoudis, N.; Charitoudis, G. Implementation of Percutaneous Transforaminal Endoscopic Discectomy in Competitive Elite Athletes with Lumbar Disc Herniation: Original Study and Review of the Literature. *Am. J. Sports Med.* **2021**, *49*, 3234–3241. [CrossRef]
30. Eum, J.H.; Heo, D.H.; Son, S.K.; Park, C.K. Percutaneous biportal endoscopic decompression for lumbar spinal stenosis: A technical note and preliminary clinical results. *J. Neurosurg. Spine* **2016**, *24*, 602–607. [CrossRef]
31. Kwon, O.; Yoo, S.J.; Park, J.Y. Comparison of Unilateral Biportal Endoscopic Discectomy with Other Surgical Technics: A Systemic Review of Indications and Outcomes of Unilateral Biportal Endoscopic Discectomy from the Current Literature. *World Neurosurg.* **2022**, *168*, 349–358. [CrossRef] [PubMed]
32. Ahn, Y.; Lee, S.G.; Son, S.; Keum, H.J. Transforaminal Endoscopic Lumbar Discectomy Versus Open Lumbar Microdiscectomy: A Comparative Cohort Study with a 5-Year Follow-Up. *Pain Physician* **2019**, *22*, 295–304. [CrossRef]
33. Choi, K.C.; Shim, H.K.; Kim, J.S.; Cha, K.H.; Lee, D.C.; Kim, E.R.; Kim, M.J.; Park, C.-K. Cost-effectiveness of microdiscectomy versus endoscopic discectomy for lumbar disc herniation. *Spine J.* **2019**, *19*, 1162–1169. [CrossRef] [PubMed]
34. Dabbs, V.M.; Dabbs, L.G. Correlation between disc height narrowing and low-back pain. *Spine* **1990**, *15*, 1366–1369. [CrossRef]
35. Hentenaar, B.; Spoor, A.B.; Malefijt, J.; Diekerhof, C.H.; den Oudsten, B.L. Clinical and radiological outcome of minimally invasive posterior lumbar interbody fusion in primary versus revision surgery. *J. Orthop. Surg. Res.* **2016**, *11*, 2. [CrossRef]
36. Narain, A.S.; Hijji, F.Y.; Duhancioglu, G.; Haws, B.E.; Khechen, B.; Manning, B.T.; Colman, M.W.; Singh, K. Patient Perceptions of Minimally Invasive Versus Open Spine Surgery. *Clin. Spine Surg.* **2018**, *31*, E184–E192. [CrossRef] [PubMed]
37. White, C.A.M.; Patel, A.V.B.; Butler, L.R.B.; Amakiri, U.O.B.; Yeshoua, B.J.M.; Steinberger, J.M.; Cho, S.K.; Kim, J.S. Comparison of Patient Preference, Understanding, and Sentiment for Minimally Invasive Versus Open Spine Surgery. *Spine* **2022**, *47*, 309–316. [CrossRef]
38. Chang, H.; Xu, J.; Yang, D.; Sun, J.; Gao, X.; Ding, W. Comparison of full-endoscopic foraminoplasty and lumbar discectomy (FEFLD), unilateral biportal endoscopic (UBE) discectomy, and microdiscectomy (MD) for symptomatic lumbar disc herniation. *Eur. Spine J.* **2023**, *32*, 542–554. [CrossRef] [PubMed]
39. Arriba, M.Á.P.; Maestre, C.; Martín-Gorroño, F.; Plasencia, P. Analysis of Long-Term Results of Lumbar Discectomy with and Without an Interspinous Device. *Int. J. Spine Surg.* **2022**, *16*, 681–689. [CrossRef]
40. Cai, H.; Liu, C.; Lin, H.; Wu, Z.; Chen, X.; Zhang, H. Full-endoscopic foraminoplasty for highly down-migrated lumbar disc herniation. *BMC Musculoskelet. Disord.* **2022**, *23*, 303. [CrossRef]
41. Kim, S.K.; Kang, S.S.; Hong, Y.H.; Park, S.W.; Lee, S.C. Clinical comparison of unilateral biportal endoscopic technique versus open microdiscectomy for single-level lumbar discectomy: A multicenter, retrospective analysis. *J. Orthop. Surg. Res.* **2018**, *13*, 22. [CrossRef] [PubMed]
42. Chen, C.-M.; Lin, G.-X.; Sharma, S.; Kim, H.-S.; Sun, L.-W.; Wu, H.-H.; Chang, K.-S.; Chen, Y.-C. Suprapedicular Retrocorporeal Technique of Transforaminal Full-Endoscopic Lumbar Discectomy for Highly Downward-Migrated Disc Herniation. *World Neurosurg.* **2020**, *143*, e631–e639. [CrossRef] [PubMed]
43. Eseonu, K.; Oduoza, U.; Monem, M.; Tahir, M. Systematic Review of Cost-Effectiveness Analyses Comparing Open and Minimally Invasive Lumbar Spinal Surgery. *Int. J. Spine Surg.* **2022**, *16*, 612–624. [CrossRef] [PubMed]
44. Jiang, H.W.; Chen, C.D.; Zhan, B.S.; Wang, Y.L.; Tang, P.; Jiang, X.S. Unilateral biportal endoscopic discectomy versus percutaneous endoscopic lumbar discectomy in the treatment of lumbar disc herniation: A retrospective study. *J. Orthop. Surg. Res.* **2022**, *17*, 30. [CrossRef] [PubMed]

45. Soliman, H.M. Irrigation endoscopic discectomy: A novel percutaneous approach for lumbar disc prolapse. *Eur. Spine J.* **2013**, *22*, 1037–1044. [CrossRef]
46. Cheng, X.; Bao, B.; Wu, Y.; Cheng, Y.; Xu, C.; Ye, Y.; Dou, C.; Chen, B.; Yan, H.; Tang, J. Clinical comparison of percutaneous transforaminal endoscopic discectomy and unilateral biportal endoscopic discectomy for single-level lumbar disc herniation. *Front. Surg.* **2022**, *9*, 1107883. [CrossRef]
47. Liu, Z.; Zhang, S.; Li, J.; Tang, H. Biomechanical comparison of different interspinous process devices in the treatment of lumbar spinal stenosis: A finite element analysis. *BMC Musculoskelet. Disord.* **2022**, *23*, 585. [CrossRef]
48. Gazzeri, R.; Galarza, M.; Neroni, M.; Fiore, C.; Faiola, A.; Puzzilli, F.; Callovini, G.; Alfieri, A. Failure rates and complications of interspinous process decompression devices: A European multicenter study. *Neurosurg. Focus.* **2015**, *39*, E14. [CrossRef]
49. Jansson, K.Å.; Németh, G.; Granath, F.; Blomqvist, P. Surgery for herniation of a lumbar disc in Sweden between 1987 and 1999. An analysis of 27,576 operations. *J. Bone Jt. Surg. Br.* **2004**, *86*, 841–847. [CrossRef]
50. Wiesel, S.W. The multiply operated lumbar spine. *Instr. Course Lect.* **1985**, *34*, 68–77.
51. Norton, W.L. Chemonucleolysis versus surgical discectomy. Comparison of costs and results in workers' compensation claimants. *Spine* **1986**, *11*, 440–443. [CrossRef] [PubMed]
52. Schaller, B. Failed back surgery syndrome: The role of symptomatic segmental single-level instability after lumbar microdiscectomy. *Eur. Spine J.* **2004**, *13*, 193–198. [CrossRef] [PubMed]
53. Erbulut, D.U.; Zafarparandeh, I.; Ozer, A.F.; Goel, V.K. Biomechanics of posterior dynamic stabilization systems. *Adv. Orthop.* **2013**, *2013*, 451956. [CrossRef] [PubMed]

Journal of
Clinical Medicine

MDPI

Article

Enhanced Recovery After Surgery Protocols in One- or Two-Level Posterior Lumbar Fusion: Improving Postoperative Outcomes

Ji Uk Choi, Tae-Hong Kee, Dong-Ho Lee, Chang Ju Hwang, Sehan Park and Jae Hwan Cho *

Department of Orthopedic Surgery, Asan Medical Center, University of Ulsan College of Medicine 88, Olympic-ro 43-gil, Songpa-gu, Seoul 05505, Republic of Korea; fairytales2@naver.com (J.U.C.); taehongkee@gmail.com (T.-H.K.); osdlee@gmail.com (D.-H.L.); baski47@gmail.com (C.J.H.); birdone86@gmail.com (S.P.)

* Correspondence: spinecjh@gmail.com

Abstract: Background/Objectives: Enhanced recovery after surgery (ERAS) protocols optimize perioperative care and improve recovery. This study evaluated the effectiveness of ERAS in one- or two-level posterior lumbar fusion surgeries, focusing on perioperative medication use, pain management, and functional outcomes. **Methods:** Eighty-eight patients undergoing lumbar fusion surgery between March 2021 and February 2022 were allocated into pre-ERAS ($n = 41$) and post-ERAS ($n = 47$) groups. Outcomes included opioid and antiemetic consumption, pain scores (numerical rating scale (NRS)), functional recovery (Oswestry Disability Index (ODI) and EuroQol 5 Dimension (EQ-5D)), and complication rates. Pain was assessed daily for the first four postoperative days and at 6 months. Linear Mixed Effects Model analysis evaluated pain trajectories. **Results:** The post-ERAS group showed significantly lower opioid ($p = 0.005$) and antiemetic ($p < 0.001$) use. No significant differences were observed in NRS pain scores in the first 4 postoperative days. At 6 months, the post-ERAS group reported significantly lower leg pain ($p = 0.002$). The time:group interaction was not significant for back ($p = 0.848$) or leg ($p = 0.503$) pain. Functional outcomes at 6 months, particularly ODI and EQ-5D scores, showed significant improvement in the post-ERAS group. Complication rates were lower in the post-ERAS group (4.3% vs. 19.5%, $p = 0.024$), while hospital stay and fusion rates remained similar. **Conclusions:** The ERAS protocol significantly reduced opioid and antiemetic use, improved long-term pain management and functional recovery, and lowered complication rates in lumbar fusion patients. These findings support the implementation of ERAS protocols in spinal surgery, emphasizing their role in enhancing postoperative care.

Keywords: enhanced recovery after surgery; ERAS; lumbar spinal fusion; opioid reduction; antiemetic use; multimodal analgesia; postoperative outcomes; postoperative pain management; functional recovery

1. Introduction

Enhanced Recovery After Surgery (ERAS) protocols are widely accepted across various surgical specialties as a method to optimize postoperative outcomes, reduce complication rates, and shorten the length of hospital stay [1]. This multimodal approach, initially introduced as "Fast-Track Surgery" by Henrik Kehlet in the 1990s to perioperative care, has evolved significantly [2]. Since its introduction in 2010, the ERAS Society has developed evidence-based guidelines tailored to numerous surgical procedures, with an emphasis on the importance of pre-operative education, early mobilization, multimodal analgesia, and enhanced nutritional support, which improve surgical outcomes and enhance patient experiences (http://www.erassociety.org, accessed on 1 March 2024) [1,3–5].

The integration of ERAS protocols into spine surgery, particularly lumbar fusion procedures, is a recent development [2]. Lumbar fusion remains a painful and complex surgical procedure despite significant advancements in spinal surgery techniques and a deeper understanding of spinal biomechanics [6,7]. Furthermore, it is frequently associated with considerable postoperative complications and a prolonged recovery period [8,9]. The increasing complexity of these procedures, combined with an aging population and the increasing demand for surgical interventions, underscores the critical need to implement standardized, evidence-based perioperative care protocols to improve recovery outcomes and reduce healthcare costs [2,10,11].

ERAS protocols can effectively reduce postoperative pain, decrease opioid consumption, and shorten the length of hospital stays following lumbar fusion surgery [2,12]. However, most previous studies have focused on broad patient populations or varied surgical procedures. Thus, the specific application of ERAS protocols in more narrowly defined contexts, such as one- or two-level posterior lumbar spinal fusion surgeries (which are commonly performed in Korea), remains unclear [13,14]. This gap in the literature underscores the necessity for conducting more focused investigations to determine the efficacy and safety of ERAS protocols in these specific surgical settings.

Therefore, this study aims to provide a detailed evaluation of the clinical effectiveness of ERAS protocols specifically in one- or two-level posterior lumbar spinal fusion surgery. This study strives to generate valuable data that contributes to the existing body of literature on ERAS by examining the postoperative outcomes. These findings will support the integration of ERAS protocols in spinal fusion surgery with a more targeted and evidence-based approach.

2. Materials and Methods

2.1. Study Design and Patient Selection

This retrospective cohort study, conducted at the Asan Medical Center, focused on 98 patients with lumbar degenerative disease who had undergone one- or two-level posterior lumbar spinal fusion between March 2021 and February 2022. Only patients who had undergone primary surgery were included. Individuals with degenerative or isthmic spondylolisthesis, as well as those with spinal stenosis or neural foraminal stenosis requiring fusion surgery, were eligible for inclusion in this study. Patients who had undergone concomitant procedures such as anterior lumbar interbody fusion (ALIF) or oblique lumbar interbody fusion (OLIF) were excluded. Thus, 88 patients were included in the final analysis after the exclusion of 10 cases. The ERAS protocol was implemented in September 2021. The patients were allocated into two groups: those who had undergone surgery before the implementation of the ERAS protocol (pre-ERAS group, $n = 41$) and those who had undergone surgery after its implementation (post-ERAS group, $n = 47$) (Figure 1).

This study was approved by the Institutional Review Board (IRB) of our institution. All procedures were conducted in accordance with ethical standards (2022-1632). The ERAS protocol used for lumbar spinal fusion surgery at our institution is outlined in Table 1. This protocol follows the general principles of ERAS guidelines, with minor adjustments to align with our institutional practices [1,3–5,15].

Table 1. Comparison of Pre-ERAS and ERAS protocols in lumbar spinal fusion surgery.

Stage	Pre-ERAS Protocol	ERAS Protocol
Pre-operative Management	• Fasting from midnight. • No routine administration of dexamethasone, pregabalin, or celecoxib. • Limited education and expectation management.	• Fasting from midnight. • Just before surgery: - IV administration of dexamethasone. - Oral administration of celecoxib and pregabalin. • Comprehensive education.
Intraoperative Management	• Less standardized pain management. • No routine use of long-acting local anesthetics. • Focus on general anesthesia and basic pain control.	• Long-acting local anesthetics (bupivacaine) at surgical site. • Tranexamic acid infusion (10 min pre-incision to wound closure). • Maintain normothermia.

Table 1. *Cont.*

Stage	Pre-ERAS Protocol	ERAS Protocol
Postoperative Management	• Opioid-based pain control (tramadol, hydromorphone, pethidine) as needed. • Antiemetics and PPI administration. • Delayed Foley catheter removal and ambulation. • Reliance on opioids, with lesser emphasis on multimodal analgesia.	• Multimodal analgesia. • Scheduled medications: • Acetaminophen 1 g IV post-surgery. • Antiemetics. • PPI. • PRN medications: • Tramadol, Hydromorphone, Pethidine. • POD 1~: Extended-release acetaminophen, pregabalin, celecoxib, magnesium oxide, antiemetics, prokinetics. • Early Foley removal. • Early mobilization. • Opioids as PRN.

ERAS, Enhanced Recovery After Surgery; PPI, proton pump inhibitor; PRN, Pro Re Nata (as needed); POD, postoperative day.

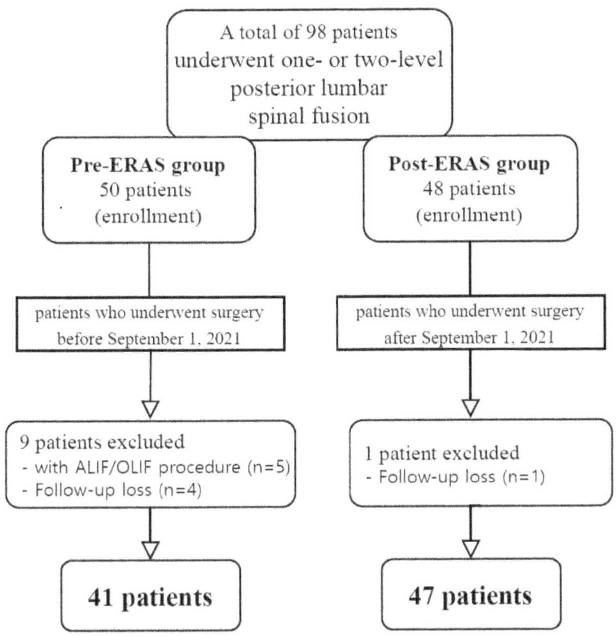

Figure 1. Flow diagram for the study sample selection. ERAS, Enhanced Recovery After Surgery; ALIF, anterior lumbar interbody fusion; OLIF, oblique lumbar interbody fusion.

2.2. Outcome Measures

The primary outcome measure of this study was pain management, as assessed using the numerical reporting scale (NRS) scores at multiple postoperative time points. The pain levels were assessed daily over the first four postoperative days (POD 1, 2, 3, and 4) using the average NRS score for each day to capture daily fluctuations in pain and provide a comprehensive evaluation of pain control during the critical early recovery period. The secondary outcome measure included the analysis of pain and functional outcomes at the 6-month postoperative time point. The NRS scores were recorded at 6 months to assess long-term pain management. The functional outcomes were evaluated using the Oswestry Disability Index (ODI) and EuroQol 5 Dimension (EQ-5D) scores recorded at 6 months postoperatively. Additional outcomes included the doses of antiemetics and opioids required, length of hospital days (HD), POD, complication rates, readmission rates within 30 days postoperatively, and fusion rates of the operated segments. The fusion rates were assessed using computed tomography (CT) at 1 year postoperatively, with fusion being defined as trabecular bridging within the cage in contact with the upper and lower endplates and the absence of a radiographic cleft [16].

2.3. Statistical Analysis

Descriptive statistics summarized patient demographics and baseline characteristics. Continuous variables were expressed as mean and standard deviation and categorical variables as frequencies and percentages. For the primary outcome of NRS pain scores, we used a Linear Mixed Effects Model to account for repeated measures and examine time and group effects. Separate models were fitted for back and leg pain NRS. Post hoc analyses compared group differences at each time point. Tukey-adjusted p-values for post hoc pairwise group comparisons at each timepoint in the Linear Mixed Effects Model were calculated to account for multiple comparisons. Secondary outcomes were analyzed using paired and independent t-tests for continuous variables, and Chi-square or Fisher's exact tests for categorical variables. These tests were also used to compare antiemetic and opioid doses, hospital stay, postoperative days, complication rates, readmission rates, and fusion rates between groups. A p-value less than 0.05 was considered statistically significant. All analyses were performed using SPSS version 21 (IBM, Armonk, NY, USA).

3. Results

3.1. Demographics

Table 1 presents the demographic data and preoperative characteristics. No significant differences were observed between the pre-ERAS and post-ERAS groups in terms of age (p = 0.201); sex (p = 0.666) or other comorbidities, such as hypertension, diabetes, heart disease, and smoking status (Table 2).

Table 2. Demographics.

	Pre-ERAS (n = 41)	Post-ERAS (n = 47)	p-Value
Male	14 (34.1)	14 (29.8)	0.666
Age	65.2 (±11.1)	67.8 (±8.0)	0.201
Height	158.67 (±8.06)	157.52 (±7.80)	0.501
Weight	63.98 (±12.66)	62.96 (±10.21)	0.678
BMI	25.30 (±3.81)	25.32 (±3.44)	0.980
HTN	22 (53.7)	25 (53.2)	0.966
DM	6 (14.6)	14 (29.8)	0.087
Heart disease	2 (4.9)	4 (8.5)	0.506
Liver disease	1 (2.4)	1 (2.1)	0.353
Pulmonary disease	1 (2.4)	3 (6.4)	0.381
Cancer	4 (9.8)	4 (8.5)	0.842
MDD	2 (4.9)	2 (4.3)	0.890
Smoking	5 (12.2)	5 (10.6)	0.678

ERAS, Enhanced Recovery After Surgery; HTN, hypertension; DM, diabetes mellitus; BMI, body mass index; MDD, major depressor disorder. Values are presented as number (%) of patients or mean (± SD) unless otherwise indicated.

3.2. Primary Outcomes

Analysis of the pain scores, measured using NRS, revealed consistent trends of lower pain scores in the post-ERAS group compared with that in the pre-ERAS group at most time points. No significant difference was observed between the two groups in terms of the pre-operative back pain scores (p = 0.056). The back pain scores on days 1, 2, 3, 4, and at 6 months were lower in the post-ERAS group, but these differences did not reach statistical significance (all $p > 0.05$). The most notable difference was observed on the third postoperative day (2.59 ± 0.21 vs. 2.35 ± 0.20, p = 0.060).

The pre-operative NRS scores for leg pain were comparable between the groups (p = 0.256). The postoperative leg pain scores in the post-ERAS group were consistently lower, but these differences were not statistically significant on days 1, 2, 3, or 4 postoperatively (all $p > 0.05$). However, a significant difference was observed at 6 months postoperatively, with the post-ERAS group reporting significantly lower leg pain (3.60 ± 0.40 vs. 2.64 ± 0.36, $p = 0.002$) (Table 3 and Figure 2).

Table 3. NRS in the pre-ERAS and post-ERAS groups.

		Pre-ERAS	Post-ERAS	*p* Value
NRS Back pain	Preop	7.20 (±0.22)	6.63 (±0.20)	0.056
	Postop#1D	3.20 (±0.21)	2.93 (±0.20)	0.358
	Postop#2D	2.87 (±0.21)	2.25 (±0.20)	0.266
	Postop#3D	2.59 (±0.21)	2.35 (±0.20)	0.060
	Postop#4D	2.57 (±0.21)	2.36 (±0.20)	0.446
	Postop#6M	2.70 (±0.30)	2.06 (±0.28)	0.119
NRS Leg pain	Preop	6.68 (±0.27)	6.88 (±0.26)	0.256
	Postop#1D	2.19 (±0.31)	2.33 (±0.30)	0.661
	Postop#2D	2.29 (±0.31)	2.03 (±0.31)	0.301
	Postop#3D	2.31 (±0.30)	2.14 (±0.30)	0.496
	Postop#4D	2.22 (±0.30)	1.77 (±0.30)	0.404
	Postop#6M	3.60 (±0.40) *	2.64 (±0.36) *	0.002

NRS, numerical reporting scale; Preop, Preoperative; Postop, Postoperative. Values are presented as mean (95% CI) unless otherwise indicated. * $p < 0.005$.

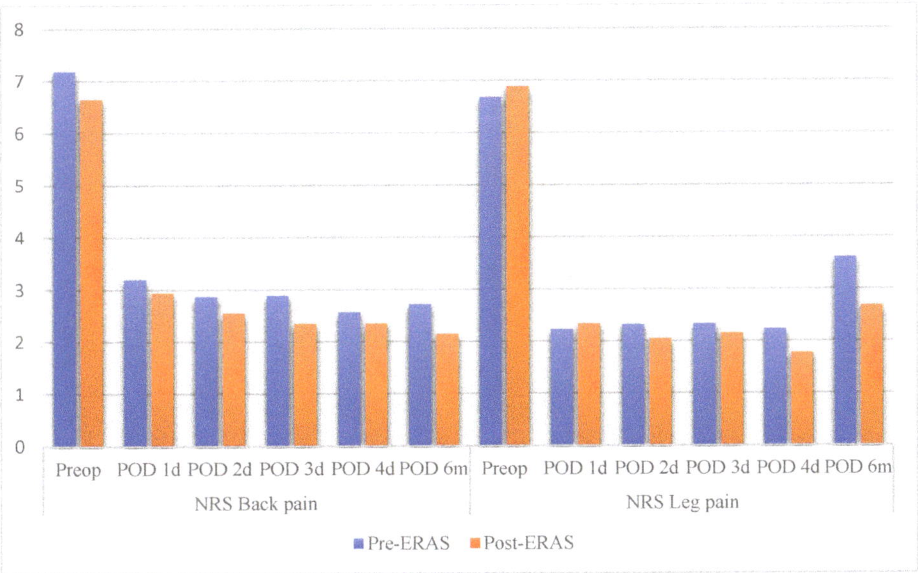

Figure 2. Comparison between the pre- and postoperative scores.

Further analysis using the Linear Mixed Effects Model showed that the time:group interaction was not statistically significant for either back pain NRS ($p = 0.848$) and leg pain NRS ($p = 0.503$), indicating that the pattern of pain scores over time did not differ significantly between the pre-ERAS and post-ERAS groups.

3.3. Secondary Outcomes

Significant improvements were observed in the pre-ERAS and post-ERAS groups at 6 months postoperatively in terms of functional outcomes, as summarized in Tables 4 and 5.

Table 4. ODI and EQ-5D scores in the pre-ERAS group.

ODI	Pre-Operative	Postoperative 6 m	*p*-Value
Pain	3.25 (±0.775)	2.38 (±1.746)	0.084
Personal care	2.00 (±0.632) *	0.69 (±0.793) *	0.000
Lifting	3.25 (±1.065)	3.44 (±1.209)	0.676
Walking	2.57 (±1.284) *	1.07 (±1.439) *	0.016
Sitting	2.50 (±1.095)	1.69 (±1.352)	0.055
Standing	3.56 (±1.153) *	2.06 (±1.526) *	0.005
Sleeping	2.50 (±1.414) *	0.63 (±1.025) *	0.001
Social life	2.94 (±0.854) *	1.50 (±1.211) *	0.000
Traveling	3.00 (±1.195) *	1.07 (±1.223) *	0.001
Sex life	-	-	
Total	27.00 (±7.598) *	14.50 (±7.755) *	0.000
EQ-5D			
Mobility	3.44 (±0.814) *	1.81 (±0.834) *	0.000
Self-care	2.19 (±0.750) *	1.38 (±0.619) *	0.001
Usual activity	3.19 (±0.911) *	1.69 (±0.704) *	0.000
Pain discomfort	3.88 (±0.719) *	3.00 (±1.265) *	0.039
Anxiety depression	2.25 (±1.000) *	1.38 (±0.619) *	0.001

ODI, Oswestry Disability Index; EQ-5D, EuroQol 5 Dimension (EQ-5D) questionnaire. Values are presented as mean (± SD) unless otherwise indicated. * $p < 0.005$.

Table 5. ODI and EQ-5D scores in the post-ERAS group.

ODI	Pre-Operative	Postoperative 6 m	*p*-Value
Pain	3.35 (±1.115) *	1.41 (±1.004) *	0.000
Personal care	2.35 (±1.412) *	0.47 (±0.624) *	0.000
Lifting	3.35 (±1.272)	3.00 (±1.803)	0.524
Walking	2.59 (±1.417) *	1.47 (±1.663) *	0.025
Sitting	2.65 (±1.057) *	1.29 (±1.404) *	0.001
Standing	3.35 (±1.367) *	1.29 (±1.448) *	0.000
Sleeping	1.65 (±1.169) *	0.76 (±0.903) *	0.020
Social life	2.82 (±1.185) *	1.41 (±1.661) *	0.008
Traveling	2.35 (±1.539)	2.12 (±2.118)	0.660
Sex life	4.00 (±0.000)	4.00 (±0.000)	1.000
Total	27.33 (±7.898) *	15.27 (±9.098) *	0.003
EQ-5D			
Mobility	3.44 (±1.094) *	1.94 (±0.854) *	0.000
Self-care	2.38 (±1.025) *	1.19 (±0.403) *	0.001
Usual activity	2.63 (±0.806) *	1.75 (±0.683) *	0.002
Pain discomfort	3.75 (±0.931) *	2.13 (±0.719) *	0.000
Anxiety depression	2.44 (±1.153) *	1.75 (±1.000) *	0.036

ODI, Oswestry Disability Index; EQ-5D, EuroQol 5 Dimension (EQ-5D) questionnaire. Values are presented as mean (± SD) unless otherwise indicated. * $p < 0.005$.

Notable improvements were observed in the following ODI domains in the pre-ERAS group: personal care ($p < 0.001$), walking ($p = 0.016$), standing ($p = 0.005$), sleeping ($p = 0.001$), social life ($p < 0.001$), and traveling ($p = 0.001$). A significant reduction in the total ODI score was observed ($p < 0.001$). Furthermore, significant improvements were observed in the following EQ-5D domains: mobility ($p < 0.001$), self-care ($p = 0.001$), usual activity ($p < 0.001$), pain/discomfort ($p = 0.039$), and anxiety/depression ($p = 0.001$).

Significant improvements were observed in the following domains in the post-ERAS group: pain ($p < 0.001$), personal care ($p < 0.001$), walking ($p = 0.025$), sitting ($p = 0.001$), standing ($p < 0.001$), sleeping ($p = 0.020$), and social life ($p = 0.008$). The total ODI score also exhibited a significant decrease ($p = 0.003$). The EQ-5D domains exhibiting significant improvements included mobility ($p < 0.001$), self-care ($p = 0.001$), usual activity ($p = 0.002$), pain/discomfort ($p < 0.001$), and anxiety/depression ($p = 0.036$).

Substantial functional recovery was observed postoperatively in both groups, with slightly greater improvements being observed in the post-ERAS group in key domains such as pain and standing, indicating the positive impact of the ERAS protocol.

3.4. Perioperative Medication

Analysis of perioperative medication usage revealed significant differences between the pre-ERAS and post-ERAS groups, particularly in terms of the total consumption of antiemetics and opioids.

The total usage of antiemetics in the post-ERAS group (1.41 amps) was significantly lower than that in the pre-ERAS group (2.73 amps, $p < 0.001$). No statistically significant differences were observed between the post-ERAS and pre-ERAS groups in terms of the use of individual antiemetics, such as ramosetron and palonosetron ($p = 0.074$ and $p = 0.151$, respectively); however, the overall reduction in antiemetic use in the post-ERAS group was notable.

Opioid consumption was also significantly reduced in the post-ERAS group. The mean number of amps of hydromorphone and pethidine administered in the post-ERAS and pre-ERAS groups were 1.64 and 3.13, respectively, indicating a statistically significant difference ($p = 0.005$) (Table 6).

Table 6. Perioperative medication.

Antiemetic Drug	**Pre-ERAS**		**Post-ERAS**		***p*-Value**
	Patient Number	**Ampule**	**Patient Number**	**Ampule**	
1. Ramosetron	41	2.32 (±0.82)	8	1.75 (±0.71)	0.074
2. Palonosetron	10	1.50 (±0.71)	37	1.14 (±0.48)	0.151
3. Macperan	2	1.00 (±0.00)	2	2.50 (±0.71)	0.095
4. Onseran	0	.	1	1.00 (±0.00)	
Total	41	2.73 (±1.34) *	44	1.41 (±1.15) *	<0.001
Opioid	**Pre-ERAS**		**Post-ERAS**		***p*-value**
	Patient number	**Ampule**	**Patient number**	**Ampule**	
Hydromorphone and Pethidine	23	3.13 * (±2.32)	14	1.64 * (±0.93)	0.005

ERAS, Enhanced Recovery After Surgery. Values are presented as mean (± SD) unless otherwise indicated. * $p < 0.005$.

3.5. Postoperative Outcomes

The comparison of postoperative outcomes between the pre-ERAS and post-ERAS groups revealed significant improvements in several key metrics following the implementation of the ERAS protocol.

3.5.1. Hospital Stay and Postoperative Days

No significant differences were observed between the pre-ERAS and post-ERAS groups in terms of the average HD (9.49 days vs. 9.43 days, respectively; $p = 0.814$). Similarly, the number of POD until discharge exhibited a trend toward shorter stays in the post-ERAS group (5.23 days) compared with that in the pre-ERAS group (5.59 days); however, this difference was not statistically significant ($p = 0.098$) (Table 7).

Table 7. Comparison between the postoperative data.

	Pre-ERAS	Post-ERAS	p-Value
HD	9.49 (±1.33)	9.43 (±1.16)	0.814
POD	5.59 (±1.07)	5.23 (±0.87)	0.098
Re-admission rate	7.3%	4.3%	0.549
Complication rate	19.5% *	4.3% *	0.024
Fusion rate	91.7%	94.7%	0.607

ERAS, Enhanced Recovery After Surgery; HD, Hospital day; POD, Postoperative day. Values are presented as mean (95% CI) unless otherwise indicated. * $p < 0.005$.

3.5.2. Complication and Re-Admission Rates

The complication rate in the post-ERAS group exhibited a significant reduction, with 4.3% (two patients) experiencing complications compared with 19.5% (eight patients) in the pre-ERAS group ($p = 0.024$). The complications observed in the pre-ERAS group included delirium (two cases), dural tear (one case), metal failure (one case), sciatica (two cases), seroma (one case), and urticaria (one case). In contrast, only one case of acute hepatitis and one case of sciatica were observed in the post-ERAS group, indicating a substantial reduction in postoperative complications following the implementation of the ERAS protocol. The re-admission rate did not differ significantly between the two groups (7.3% in pre-ERAS vs. 4.3% in post-ERAS, $p = 0.549$) (Table 7).

3.5.3. Fusion Rates

The spinal fusion rates were similar in the pre-ERAS and post-ERAS groups, with fusion rates of 91.7% and 94.7%, respectively ($p = 0.607$). This finding suggests that the ERAS protocol had no adverse effect on the technical success of the spinal fusion surgery (Table 6).

4. Discussion

The implementation of the ERAS protocol in one- or two-level posterior lumbar spinal fusion surgeries resulted in significant improvements in postoperative outcomes, with the substantial reduction in the use of antiemetics and opioids being one of the most important findings. This reduction highlights the effectiveness of the ERAS protocol in managing postoperative symptoms; furthermore, the role of ERAS in minimizing the risks associated with opioid use and medication-related side effects is demonstrated.

The use of antiemetics in the post-ERAS group was significantly lower ($p < 0.001$), with fewer patients requiring multiple doses. To validate these findings, we conducted post hoc power analyses for our main outcomes. Our post hoc analysis revealed 99.773% power to detect the observed mean difference in antiemetic use, strongly supporting the reliability of this finding. This reduction is particularly meaningful in the context of spine surgery, wherein the incidence of postoperative nausea and vomiting (PONV) can severely delay key recovery milestones, such as early mobilization and resumption of oral intake (which are critical for enhancing surgical recovery) [17]. The incidence of PONV prolongs the recovery period and increases the likelihood of unexpected hospital admissions, contributing to higher healthcare costs and patient discomfort [18,19]. The ERAS protocol effectively minimized the requirement for the administration of antiemetics by optimizing multimodal analgesia and reducing reliance on opioids, major contributors to PONV. This facilitated faster recovery and reduced the incidence of medication-related side effects. This outcome aligns with the ERAS goals of enhancing recovery by reducing complications such as PONV and promoting early ambulation [3–5,12].

The reduction in opioid use is equally crucial. The opioid consumption in the post-ERAS group was significantly lower ($p = 0.005$), with our post hoc analysis showing 96.432% power to detect this difference. This finding is consistent with the core objective of ERAS, which aims to limit opioid use by incorporating the use of non-opioid analgesics such as NSAIDs, acetaminophen, and pregabalin. Effective pain control using fewer opioids decreases the risk of opioid-related complications, such as respiratory depression and gastrointestinal dysfunction. Furthermore, it also mitigates the risk of long-term opioid dependence [20]. Pain is the predominant symptom reported by adult patients undergoing ambulatory surgery and the primary cause of unplanned healthcare visits [21]. Pain levels at 48 h postoperatively are a significant predictor of the ability of a patient to resume normal activities by day 7 [22]. The patients in the post-ERAS group in this present study possibly experienced smoother recovery owing to better pain control, which contributed to earlier mobilization and fewer side effects. Moreover, the effective management of acute pain plays a crucial role in preventing the transition to chronic pain, which is typically associated with functional decline, anxiety, and depression [15,23].

No significant differences were observed between the two groups in terms of the immediate postoperative pain scores (NRS) despite these benefits. This may be attributed to the fact that a comprehensive multimodal analgesic approach was already in place before the implementation of ERAS [24,25]. The patients in the pre-ERAS group received NSAIDs, acetaminophen, pregabalin, short-term narcotics, and patient-controlled analgesia (PCA) with fentanyl and ketorolac [26]. This may have led to effective pain control in both groups, making it difficult to detect significant differences in the NRS scores. Furthermore, variability in pain assessment during the immediate postoperative period owing to patient discomfort and the fluctuation in physical conditions may have contributed to fluctuating pain reports. Measures have been taken to address this issue by calculating the daily average NRS in this present study; however, discrepancies between the pain measured at the level requiring medication after surgery and NRS measured at periodic measurement time points may have also contributed to these results.

Interestingly, while immediate postoperative pain scores showed no significant differences, our analysis revealed a significant improvement in long-term pain management, particularly for leg pain. At 6 months postoperatively, the post-ERAS group reported significantly lower leg pain scores compared to the pre-ERAS group (3.60 ± 0.40 vs. 2.64 ± 0.36, $p = 0.002$). However, our post hoc analysis showed only 25.520% power for this outcome, indicating that these results should be interpreted cautiously and larger studies are needed to confirm this finding.

To further understand the pain trajectory over time, we conducted a Linear Mixed Effects Model analysis. This analysis showed no significant time:group interaction for both back pain NRS ($p = 0.848$) and leg pain NRS ($p = 0.503$). These results indicate that the effect of the ERAS protocol remained relatively consistent over time, suggesting a sustained benefit throughout the recovery period that culminated in significantly lower leg pain at 6 months.

The discrepancy between short-term and long-term pain outcomes observed in our study is intriguing and warrants further investigation. It is possible that the cumulative effects of various ERAS components, such as early mobilization, optimized nutrition, and patient education, contribute more significantly to improved long-term pain management than to immediate postoperative pain control. This finding suggests that the ERAS protocol may have a more pronounced effect on long-term pain management rather than immediate postoperative pain control. Future studies should focus on identifying which specific elements of the ERAS protocol are most influential in promoting long-term pain reduction, while also exploring ways to enhance its impact on immediate postoperative pain management. These studies should also aim to increase statistical power, particularly for long-term pain outcomes, to provide more definitive conclusions. The postoperative pain scores remained comparable; however, the functional outcomes exhibited significant improvements in the post-ERAS group. The post-ERAS group demonstrated better scores in terms of the ODI and EQ-5D scores, particularly in domains such as pain, standing, and quality of life, at 6 months postoperatively. Significant improvements were observed in ODI domains, such as pain ($p < 0.001$), personal care ($p < 0.001$), walking ($p = 0.025$), and standing ($p < 0.001$). Consistent with the findings of earlier studies, these results indicate that the ERAS protocol can enhance therapeutic outcomes more effectively and contribute to long-term functional recovery [27].

The implementation of the ERAS protocol in our study showed promising results in terms of postoperative outcomes, including a notable reduction in complication rates from 19.5% in the pre-ERAS group to 4.3% in the post-ERAS group ($p = 0.024$). However, it is important to interpret these findings with caution due to the retrospective nature of our study and potential confounding factors.

In this retrospective study, we took several measures to minimize potential selection bias between the pre- and post-ERAS groups. We implemented strict inclusion and exclusion criteria, with all patients undergoing one- or two-level posterior lumbar fusion at a single institution. To reduce potential bias from the surgeon's skill improvement over time, we kept the study period relatively short, from March 2021 to February 2022. We used consecutive sampling and compared baseline demographic and clinical characteristics to ensure no significant differences between groups.

Despite these efforts, the retrospective design and relatively small sample size limit our ability to draw definitive conclusions about the direct impact of ERAS on complication rates. The observed lower complication rate in the post-ERAS group might have been influenced by factors unrelated to the ERAS protocol itself, such as inherent patient variability or unaccounted perioperative care improvements. For instance, the reduced incidence of dural tears and metal failures, which are less likely to be directly influenced by ERAS protocols, suggests that the difference in complication rates may not be solely attributed to the protocol's implementation.

Nevertheless, the significance of our findings lies in demonstrating that the adoption of ERAS protocols, which emphasize early recovery and reduced length of hospital stay, did not lead to an increase in complication rates in the post-ERAS cohort. This is a noteworthy outcome, considering that early mobilization and accelerated recovery pathways have traditionally been associated with concerns regarding increased complications. The fact that the complication rates remained low, despite the implementation of a more aggressive postoperative recovery strategy, suggests that ERAS protocols can safely enhance recovery without compromising patient safety.

These results are consistent with previous studies showing that ERAS protocols can improve recovery and minimize the need for interventions associated with adverse effects [2,12]. Our findings support the notion that ERAS protocols can be safely implemented in lumbar fusion surgeries, potentially offering the benefits of faster recovery and shorter hospital stays without increasing the risk of complications.

No significant differences in length of stay (LOS) or readmission rates were observed between the two groups in this present study. This outcome may have been influenced by institutional policies and administrative factors during hospitalization. Our institution, a tertiary hospital, had already established a target for discharge on the third postoperative day, even before the implementation of the ERAS protocol. The patients were transferred to a rehabilitation facility or discharged home depending on their condition. Nevertheless, the similar re-admission rates confirm that the ERAS protocol did not increase the risk of postoperative complications after discharge, thereby reinforcing its safety and effectiveness. Early mobilization after spinal surgery and other major procedures is associated with a shorter LOS [28,29]. Thus, encouraging earlier and more consistent ambulation in the future could further reduce the duration of hospital stay.

The fusion rates in the pre-ERAS and post-ERAS groups were also similar ($p = 0.607$), indicating that the implementation of the ERAS protocol had no negative effect on the technical success of spinal fusion surgery. This finding supports the implementation of ERAS protocols, as they enhance perioperative care without compromising the surgical outcomes.

Future studies will focus on the implementation and evaluation of the Second Generation ERAS Protocol, which incorporates several novel components designed to further enhance patient recovery, at our institution. The key features include pre-operative anemia management, reduced preoperative fasting, administration of dexamethasone on the day of the surgery and the first postoperative day, early sitting and mobilization, and early initiation of oral nutrition. These studies are underway, and the outcomes will be reported in subsequent publications.

Certain limitations of this present study must be considered. First, causality cannot be established, and unmeasured factors may have influenced the results as this was a retrospective cohort study. Furthermore, the single-institution, single-surgeon design limits the generalizability of the findings to other settings or practices. Larger multi-center studies must be conducted to enhance external validity. The sample size, although sufficient for analysis, may also limit the broader applicability of the findings. Variability in the pain scores assessed using the NRS, which relies on patient-reported outcomes, may have affected the accuracy of pain measurements, particularly during the early postoperative period [24]. Lastly, the hospital policy of discharging patients on day 3, regardless of recovery status, may have restricted the observation of potential reductions in the LOS.

Nevertheless, this present study has several strengths. The effects of the ERAS protocol could be evaluated within a well-defined surgical context by focusing on a homogeneous patient population, specifically patients undergoing one- or two-level posterior lumbar spinal fusion surgeries. This homogeneity reduced the potential effects of confounding variables, which are often observed in studies involving more complex procedures, thereby improving the internal validity of our findings. In addition, unlike those of previous studies, the objective comparison of opioid and antiemetic drug usage performed in this present study provided quantifiable metrics, adding a layer of objectivity to the analysis. A more reliable evaluation of the impact of the ERAS protocol on perioperative care could be achieved by measuring the precise dosages of these medications.

The single-surgeon and retrospective design impose some limitations; however, the focus of this present study on a specific patient group and its objective data on drug use provides valuable insights into the effectiveness of the ERAS protocols in spine surgery.

5. Conclusions

The implementation of the ERAS protocol in one- or two-level posterior lumbar spinal fusion surgeries demonstrated several benefits. Our study shows that this protocol significantly reduces antiemetic and opioid use while potentially improving long-term pain management and functional recovery. Importantly, these benefits were achieved without increasing complication rates, underscoring the safety of the ERAS protocol in this surgical context.

These findings contribute to the growing body of evidence supporting the effectiveness and safety of ERAS protocols in spinal surgery, while also highlighting areas for potential optimization. Our results underscore the importance of considering both short-term and long-term outcomes in evaluating these protocols, supporting their wider implementation to enhance postoperative care and patient outcomes in spinal procedures.

Author Contributions: Conceptualization, J.U.C., T.-H.K. and J.H.C.; methodology, J.U.C. and T.-H.K.; software, not applicable; validation, J.U.C., D.-H.L., C.J.H. and J.H.C.; formal analysis, J.U.C.; investigation, J.U.C.; resources, J.U.C. and T.-H.K.; data curation, J.U.C. and T.-H.K.; writing—original draft preparation, J.U.C.; writing—review and editing, J.U.C., S.P. and J.H.C.; visualization, J.U.C.; supervision, D.-H.L. and J.H.C.; project administration, J.U.C. All authors have read and agreed to the published version of the manuscript.

Funding: This research received no external funding.

Institutional Review Board Statement: This study was approved by the Institutional Review Board (IRB) of Asan Medical Center, ensuring that all procedures were conducted in accordance with ethical standards (2022-1632, approved on 1 February 2022).

Informed Consent Statement: Patient consent was waived due to the retrospective nature of this study and the fact that it only involved medical records. This type of study posed a minimal risk to the participants, making individual informed consent unnecessary.

Data Availability Statement: The data supporting the findings of this study are not publicly available due to privacy and ethical restrictions. However, de-identified datasets are available from the corresponding author upon reasonable request, subject to approval by the Institutional Review Board of Asan Medical Center. The data will be shared in accordance with the principles of FAIR (Findable, Accessible, Interoperable, and Reusable) data practices while ensuring compliance with ethical guidelines and participant confidentiality.

Acknowledgments: The authors express their gratitude to Seonohk Ji for her support in data collection and to Seunghee Baek, for providing valuable statistical consultation.

Conflicts of Interest: The authors declare no conflicts of interest.

References

1. Kehlet, H. Multimodal approach to control postoperative pathophysiology and rehabilitation. *Br. J. Anaesth.* **1997**, *78*, 606–617. [CrossRef] [PubMed]
2. Debono, B.; Wainwright, T.W.; Wang, M.Y.; Sigmundsson, F.G.; Yang, M.M.H.; Smid-Nanninga, H.; Bonnal, A.; Le Huec, J.C.; Fawcett, W.J.; Ljungqvist, O.; et al. Consensus statement for perioperative care in lumbar spinal fusion: Enhanced Recovery After Surgery (ERAS(R)) Society recommendations. *Spine J.* **2021**, *21*, 729–752. [CrossRef] [PubMed]
3. Ljungqvist, O.; Scott, M.; Fearon, K.C. Enhanced Recovery After Surgery: A Review. *JAMA Surg.* **2017**, *152*, 292–298. [CrossRef] [PubMed]
4. Kim, H.J.; Steinhaus, M.; Punyala, A.; Shah, S.; Elysee, J.C.; Lafage, R.; Riviera, T.; Mendez, G.; Ojadi, A.; Tuohy, S.; et al. Enhanced recovery pathway in adult patients undergoing thoracolumbar deformity surgery. *Spine J.* **2021**, *21*, 753–764. [CrossRef]
5. Porche, K.; Yan, S.; Mohamed, B.; Garvan, C.; Samra, R.; Melnick, K.; Vaziri, S.; Seubert, C.; Decker, M.; Polifka, A.; et al. Enhanced recovery after surgery (ERAS) improves return of physiological function in frail patients undergoing one- to two-level TLIFs: An observational retrospective cohort study. *Spine J.* **2022**, *22*, 1513–1522. [CrossRef]
6. Devin, C.J.; McGirt, M.J. Best evidence in multimodal pain management in spine surgery and means of assessing postoperative pain and functional outcomes. *J. Clin. Neurosci.* **2015**, *22*, 930–938. [CrossRef]
7. Gerbershagen, H.J.; Aduckathil, S.; van Wijck, A.J.; Peelen, L.M.; Kalkman, C.J.; Meissner, W. Pain intensity on the first day after surgery: A prospective cohort study comparing 179 surgical procedures. *Anesthesiology* **2013**, *118*, 934–944. [CrossRef]
8. Sethi, R.K.; Pong, R.P.; Leveque, J.C.; Dean, T.C.; Olivar, S.J.; Rupp, S.M. The Seattle Spine Team Approach to Adult Deformity Surgery: A Systems-Based Approach to Perioperative Care and Subsequent Reduction in Perioperative Complication Rates. *Spine Deform.* **2014**, *2*, 95–103. [CrossRef]
9. Carli, F. Physiologic considerations of Enhanced Recovery After Surgery (ERAS) programs: Implications of the stress response. *Can. J. Anaesth.* **2015**, *62*, 110–119. [CrossRef]
10. Mendivil, A.A.; Busch, J.R.; Richards, D.C.; Vittori, H.; Goldstein, B.H. The Impact of an Enhanced Recovery After Surgery Program on Patients Treated for Gynecologic Cancer in the Community Hospital Setting. *Int. J. Gynecol. Cancer* **2018**, *28*, 581–585. [CrossRef]
11. Adamina, M.; Kehlet, H.; Tomlinson, G.A.; Senagore, A.J.; Delaney, C.P. Enhanced recovery pathways optimize health outcomes and resource utilization: A meta-analysis of randomized controlled trials in colorectal surgery. *Surgery* **2011**, *149*, 830–840. [CrossRef] [PubMed]
12. Wainwright, T.W.; Immins, T.; Middleton, R.G. Enhanced recovery after surgery (ERAS) and its applicability for major spine surgery. *Best. Pract. Res. Clin. Anaesthesiol.* **2016**, *30*, 91–102. [CrossRef] [PubMed]
13. Kim, Y.H.; Ha, K.Y.; Kim, Y.S.; Kim, K.W.; Rhyu, K.W.; Park, J.B.; Shin, J.H.; Kim, Y.Y.; Lee, J.S.; Park, H.Y.; et al. Lumbar Interbody Fusion and Osteobiologics for Lumbar Fusion. *Asian Spine J.* **2022**, *16*, 1022–1033. [CrossRef] [PubMed]
14. Lewis, D.; Marya, S.; Carrasco, R.; Sabou, S.; Leach, J. Comparative Outcome Data Using Different Techniques for Posterior Lumbar Fusion: A Large Single-Center Study. *Asian Spine J.* **2023**, *17*, 807–817. [CrossRef]
15. Thomas, D.A.; Chang, D.; Zhu, R.; Rayaz, H.; Vadivelu, N. Concept of the Ambulatory Pain Physician. *Curr. Pain. Headache Rep.* **2017**, *21*, 7. [CrossRef]
16. Lee, J.H.; Lee, J.H.; Park, J.W.; Lee, H.S. Fusion rates of a morselized local bone graft in polyetheretherketone cages in posterior lumbar interbody fusion by quantitative analysis using consecutive three-dimensional computed tomography scans. *Spine J.* **2011**, *11*, 647–653. [CrossRef]
17. Joshi, G.P.; Kehlet, H. Enhanced Recovery Pathways: Looking into the Future. *Anesth. Analg.* **2019**, *128*, 5–7. [CrossRef]
18. Gan, T.J.; Diemunsch, P.; Habib, A.S.; Kovac, A.; Kranke, P.; Meyer, T.A.; Watcha, M.; Chung, F.; Angus, S.; Apfel, C.C.; et al. Consensus guidelines for the management of postoperative nausea and vomiting. *Anesth. Analg.* **2014**, *118*, 85–113. [CrossRef] [PubMed]
19. Rajan, N.; Joshi, G.P. Management of postoperative nausea and vomiting in adults: Current controversies. *Curr. Opin. Anaesthesiol.* **2021**, *34*, 695–702. [CrossRef]
20. Soffin, E.M.; Waldman, S.A.; Stack, R.J.; Liguori, G.A. An Evidence-Based Approach to the Prescription Opioid Epidemic in Orthopedic Surgery. *Anesth. Analg.* **2017**, *125*, 1704–1713. [CrossRef]

21. Odom-Forren, J.; Rayens, M.K.; Gokun, Y.; Jalota, L.; Radke, O.; Hooper, V.; Wiggins, A.T.; Apfel, C.C. The Relationship of Pain and Nausea in Postoperative Patients for 1 Week After Ambulatory Surgery. *Clin. J. Pain.* **2015**, *31*, 845–851. [CrossRef] [PubMed]
22. Rosén, H.I.; Bergh, I.H.; Odén, A.; Mårtensson, L.B. Patients' experiences of pain following day surgery—At 48 hours, seven days, and three months. *Open Nurs. J.* **2011**, *5*, 52–59. [CrossRef] [PubMed]
23. Apfel, C.; Jahr, J.R.; Kelly, C.L.; Ang, R.Y.; Oderda, G.M. Effect of i.v. acetaminophen on total hip or knee replacement surgery: A case-matched evaluation of a national patient database. *Am. J. Health Syst. Pharm.* **2015**, *72*, 1961–1968. [CrossRef]
24. American Society of Anesthesiologists Task Force on Acute Pain Management. Practice guidelines for acute pain management in the perioperative setting: An updated report by the American Society of Anesthesiologists Task Force on Acute Pain Management. *Anesthesiology* **2012**, *116*, 248–273. [CrossRef]
25. Chalermkitpanit, P.; Yingsakmongkol, W.; Limthongkul, W.; Tanasansomboon, T.; Pannangpetch, P.; Tangchitcharoen, N.; Singhatanadgige, W. Perioperative Intravenous Nefopam on Pain Management and Ambulation after Open Spine Surgery: A Randomized Double-Blind Controlled Study. *Asian Spine J.* **2023**, *17*, 632–638. [CrossRef]
26. Jeong, Y.B.; Lee, M.S.; Choi, B.M.; Chin, J.H.; Noh, G.J. A Clinical Study to Evaluate the Safety and Efficacy of a Patient-Controlled Analgesia Pump in Post-Surgical Patients. *Korean J. Anesthesiol.* **2007**, *52*, 161–165. [CrossRef]
27. Jin, X.; Xu, Y. Differences in postoperative knee joint function and prognostic quality of life in patients undergoing posterior cruciate ligament reconstruction at different surgical timing under enhanced recovery after surgery. *Medicine* **2023**, *102*, e34345. [CrossRef]
28. Burgess, L.C.; Wainwright, T.W. What Is the Evidence for Early Mobilisation in Elective Spine Surgery? A Narrative Review. *Healthcare* **2019**, *7*, 92. [CrossRef]
29. Epstein, N.E. A review article on the benefits of early mobilization following spinal surgery and other medical/surgical procedures. *Surg. Neurol. Int.* **2014**, *5*, S66–S73. [CrossRef]

Journal of
Clinical Medicine

MDPI

Review

The Future of Motion Preservation and Arthroplasty in the Degenerative Lumbar Spine

Michael S. Pheasant [1], Matthew W. Parry [1], Mina Girgis [1], Alex Tang [1] and Tan Chen [2,*]

[1] Geisinger Musculoskeletal Institute, Danville, PA 17822, USA
[2] Division of Orthopedic Spine Surgery, Geisinger Musculoskeletal Institute, Danville, PA 17822, USA
* Correspondence: tchen1@geisinger.edu

Abstract: The lumbar degenerative cascade is a pathological process that affects most of the aging adult population and has significant negative economic consequences. Lumbar fusion surgery remains a mainstay of treatment for refractory degenerative disease but carries significant long-term consequences. More recently, lumbar arthroplasty and motion-sparing technology has become an increasingly popular alternative surgical option in carefully indicated patients. Arthroplasty technology carries the theoretical benefits of spinal segment motion preservation and decreased degeneration of adjacent segments as compared to traditional fusion procedures. This article will review the lumbar degenerative cascade and its related anatomic considerations, current management strategies and the challenges surrounding lumbar spinal fusion, including adjacent segment disease. This article will also review the theoretical benefits of lumbar arthroplasty and motion preservation. Furthermore, this paper will highlight the current state of lumbar arthroplasty, including current concepts of implant design, limitations, outcomes and ongoing development. It will review the development and current state of artificial disk arthroplasty, total joint arthroplasty and posterior column motion-preserving implants, including flexible rods and facet joint replacement.

Keywords: lumbar spine degeneration; lumbar arthroplasty; motion-preserving surgery

1. Introduction

Degeneration of the lumbar spine is a significant contributor to disability throughout the world, with an incidence of 3.63% worldwide [1]. Lumbar degeneration is a complex process which encompasses disk degeneration, lumbar spinal stenosis, facet arthropathy and deformity [2]. The degenerative process involves the complex interplay between the anterior and posterior column and presents a challenge for management as there may be numerous pain generators involved. The resultant low back pain can have a major impact on function and quality of life [3].

To date, the most common surgical strategy for lumbar degeneration is lumbar fusion, which has long been considered the gold standard [4]. Despite the segmental loss of motion that occurs with fusion, the lumbar spine, unlike the appendicular skeleton, can compensate for loss of motion with a compensatory increase in the adjacent segments, reducing the functional burden of arthrodesis in the short term and leading to an acceptable clinical result. Furthermore, rapid advances in spinal fusion technologies have in part driven the use of fusion in practice [5]. Despite its widespread use, spinal fusion has drawn scrutiny over its multiple drawbacks, including pseudoarthrosis, adjacent segment pathology, hardware failure and additional surgery. Given these factors, there has been long-standing interest in motion-preserving surgery [6,7].

The concept of motion preservation in lumbar spine surgery has made several technological and clinical advances and has shown promising results in the literature, but widespread adoption remains limited. This has been due to several factors, mainly concerns over the longevity of arthroplasty implants and potential need for revision. Furthermore, the triad of joints that make up a single spinal level complicates the prospect of resurfacing and motion preservation from an implant development standpoint and from the perspective of patient selection. For example, concomitant facet arthropathy in the setting of disk degeneration would contraindicate isolated disk arthroplasty which would not address the degeneration of the posterior column. These considerations make patient selection and surgical indications challenging. Despite these hurdles, there have been several significant advances and milestones reached in lumbar arthroplasty, which will likely accelerate the use of arthroplasty implants in the coming years [5]. This article will provide a narrative review of the historical and current concepts along with the future direction of lumbar arthroplasty.

2. Materials and Methods

In this narrative review, the historical background, current concepts and future direction of lumbar arthroplasty will be described and discussed. To this end, current data, along with case reports and articles of historical significance, will be utilized to illustrate the historical context, current concepts and clinical experience thus far.

This article will discuss the current concepts of the lumbar degenerative cascade and the anatomical effects on the disc, ligaments and facet joints; the theoretical benefits of lumbar arthroplasty and motion preservation; and the disadvantages of spinal fusion.

Furthermore, the review will address specific implant categories, including artificial lumbar disc arthroplasty, facet joint replacement, dynamic stabilization and total joint arthroplasty. We will discuss implant designs, along with the respective advantages and disadvantages of each.

3. Current Concepts on the Lumbar Degenerative Cascade and the Anatomical Effects on the Disc, Ligaments and Facet Joints

Spine degeneration is a complex process which occurs with aging but can also occur independently in the setting of early degeneration [2]. The lumbar spine is a three-joint complex with intervertebral discs and two facet joints which biomechanically collaborate to distribute physiologic loads and stresses [8]. In the lumbar spine, the facet joints are designed to prevent rotational instability while providing flexibility in the sagittal plane. The interplay between the anterior and posterior columns is complex and has been well studied throughout the past decades.

The degenerative cascade was described by Kirkaldy-Willis in the 1970s and predicably follows a three-phase process. In phase one, trauma in the form of torsional stress causes damage to the anulus fibrosus, which weakens the circumferential structure of the annulus. This leads to instability in the disk in phase two, at which point the nucleus pulposus can migrate, leading to a loss of disk height, or the nucleus migrates through the anulus, which occurs in the setting of a herniation. In either case, the compensatory re-stabilization process leads to increased bony hypertrophy in the form of osteophytosis [9].

In comparison, during normal aging, disk degeneration can occur following a three-phase molecular pattern. In phase one, there is an accumulation of molecular damage to protein and DNA structures the intervertebral disk over time. Subsequently, in phase two, there is a resultant change in the ECM of the disk, which in phase three, leads to a loss of biologic structure and function of the disk, with compensatory bone changes and increased stresses placed on the facet joints. The compensatory changes that then occur in the facet joints include facet degeneration and arthropathy [2].

More recently, the interplay between the intervertebral disk and facet joints has been better elucidated. Studies involving MRI review of the lumbar spine over time have demonstrated the interplay between disc degeneration and facet tropism. In many cases, disk degeneration appears to precede facet degeneration, with facet arthropathy occurring as a result of microinstability at the intervertebral disk [8]. Instability at the intervertebral disk and the subsequent imbalance in kinematic forces places increased strain on the facet joints. The facet joint undergoes synovitis, cartilage destruction, capsular laxity and, ultimately, instability. This cascade of changes leads to degenerative rotational and translational deformities, such as degenerative spondylolisthesis and degenerative scoliosis [9,10]. In other cases, a posterior-to-anterior cascade of degeneration has been observed. MRI studies have shown that variations of facet morphology appear to correlate with early disk degeneration and concomitant facet degeneration, suggesting that variations in facet morphology may alter the stress distribution on the intervertebral disk and play a role in accelerating disk degeneration [8]. Regardless of the degenerative pathway, lumbar degeneration may involve either the anterior column, the posterior elements or both, and treatment strategies need to be tailored to best address the pathology involved.

4. Disadvantages of Spinal Fusion

In the orthopedic treatment of degenerative joints of the appendicular skeleton, arthrodesis has been largely abandoned in favor of arthroplasty. Management of spine degeneration has been an exception, with fusion of the diseased spinal level remaining the gold standard for surgical management. Fusion of the lumbar spine is accepted as a reasonable treatment of spine degeneration, since adjacent levels can compensate for the fused level, reducing the impact of arthrodesis on functional motion and resulting in a clinically acceptable outcome [11]. Despite being the standard of care, lumbar spinal fusion has several well-established complications, including pseudoarthrosis, hardware failure and adjacent level degeneration [3,12]. These post-operative complications lead to poor and often dreaded outcomes that commonly lead to a need for revision surgery.

Adjacent segment degeneration occurs in response to the loss of motion above and/or below a fused level. The increased stresses placed on the adjacent levels in compensation for loss of motion at the fused level lead to accelerated degeneration at the adjacent levels. This is a significant concern following lumbar fusion and is a common cause of revision surgery [11]. Adjacent segment degeneration (ASDe) is defined as the radiographic changes that occur at the levels adjacent to a fused level, including disk height collapse of >20% and disk wedging > 5 degrees [13]. Adjacent segment disease (ASDi), by comparison, is defined as radiographic degeneration with concomitant symptomatic worsening. ASDi has been defined as the radiographic findings of ASDe in the setting of an Oswestry disability index score with a >20 increase from baseline and VAS score > 5 for back or leg pain at follow-up [14].

Pseudoarthrosis, another feared complication of spinal fusion, occurs when bony fusion fails to occur and pseudoarthrosis forms. Incidence of pseudoarthrosis has decreased over time as fusion techniques have improved; however, this remains a common complication of lumbar fusion with an incidence of 5–15% [15]. Similarly, hardware failure rates have also decreased over time with advances in implant technology but also remain a risk following lumbar fusion. Irmola et al. found a revision rate of 12.5% in a cohort of 433 consecutive lumbar fusion patients [16].

Given the significant complications which plague spinal fusion, it is not surprising that clinical success at 5 years is only 51% [3]. Concerns regarding these outcomes have driven an increased interest in motion-preserving treatments which has parallelled the rapid development in fusion technologies and surgical techniques.

5. Theoretical Benefits of Lumbar Arthroplasty and Motion Preservation

Many of the complications of spinal fusion center around the loss of motion at the fused level, adding to the appeal of motion-sparing surgery. Treatment of the degenerate joint while maintaining motion would, in theory, reduce the stresses placed at the adjacent levels at a minimum, and at best, restore native biomechanical strain. Furthermore, a motion-preserving construct eliminates the need to achieve bony fusion and the concern of pseudoarthrosis. In practice, these once-theoretical goals have been demonstrated in practice over the past decades as arthroplasty technologies have advanced; however, the literature has been limited thus far.

Successful motion preservation with lumbar arthroplasty as a proof of concept was demonstrated in several studies [11,17]. In a prospective cohort study by Rasouli et al. [17], 159 patients underwent adjacent two-level (n = 114), three-level (n = 41) or four-level (n = 4) lumbar total disk replacement (TDR). Patients were followed, and VAS-S, VAS-P, Oswestry disability index and sagittal motion on pre- and post-op radiographs at both the operative segments and adjacent segments were recorded. Patients were followed at 6 weeks, 3 months and annually from 2 to 6 years. At pre-operative radiograph, across motion segments for both groups, the mean ROM was 10.15 ± 2.71 degrees pre-operatively versus 12.30 ± 2.25 degrees post-operatively. Motion was improved at all segments except for L5-S1, where the mean pre-operative motion was 7.60 ± 3.90 versus 5.81 ± 3.1 post-operatively. Importantly, in the segment adjacent to the TDR, the mean pre-operative ROM was 8.20 ± 2.88 degrees compared with the ROM at the latest follow-up, which was 8.40 ± 2.4 degrees. Thus, there was no loss of motion demonstrated in the motion of adjacent segments in TDR patients at the 6-year follow-up [17]. These findings helped to propel lumbar arthroplasty beyond proof of concept to a viable motion-preserving alternative to lumbar fusion. Despite these promising findings, the body of evidence is limited, and additional long-term radiographic and outcome studies are needed to support the concept of motion preservation and the overall long-term efficacy of lumbar arthroplasty.

6. Artificial Lumbar Disc Arthroplasty

Lumbar disc replacement has become increasingly popular in the past decades as an alternative to spinal fusion and has been the leading construct in motion-preserving lumbar spine surgery. Disk replacement only addresses degeneration at the intervertebral disk; therefore, patients with concomitant facet degeneration are contraindicated, as they will have continued pain and poor outcomes following an otherwise successful disk replacement. In addition to facet degeneration, adequate bone quality, (t score > −1.0) and an absence of significant deformity are all imperative in candidates for disk arthroplasty [18]. In properly indicated patients, disk arthroplasty has shown success at both short-term and long-term follow-up [11]. Despite these promising studies, there has been concern regarding the durability and safety of disk arthroplasty. Concerns largely centered around the risk of implant stability and durability and the risk associated with revision surgery. Since most implants require an anterior approach, revision could risk damage to ureter and anterior vascular structures. A retrospective review by Schwender et al. found that revision anterior lumbar spine surgery carried a three to five times increased rate of complication when compared with primary cases [19]. Therefore, the risks of revision surgery have made durability and stability paramount factors in implant development. As the field cautiously advances, there are several implants that have been widely used and have paved the way for motion-preserving lumbar spine surgery.

The lumbar disc replacement was first developed in 1982 in Germany with the Charité artificial disc. The device consisted of an ultra-high-molecular-weight polyethylene (UHMWPE) core positioned between two polished metal end plates. The endplates featured 11 teeth used to anchor the device to the native vertebral endplate [20]. The second generation of the device featured two lateral wings with five anchoring teeth. The second-generation device experienced fractures in the end plate and was ultimately abandoned for a third-generation device developed in conjunction with Waldemar Link Gmbh & Co, (Hamburg, Germany). The Charité implant was later FDA approved in the US in 2004 and gained popularity following a prospective multicenter randomized controlled trial under FDA IDE status, which examined the Charité implant against a posterior fusion cohort. In the study, 304 patients from 14 centers were randomized into an arthroplasty group or control instrumented ALIF group at a 2:1 ratio. The outcome measures, including back pain, the Oswestry disability index and SF36 health surveys, were assessed at 6 weeks and 3, 6, 12 and 24 months post-operation. At each time point, the arthroplasty group had lower levels of disability and pain, with the exception of 24 months, which resulted in equal scores for pain. The arthroplasty group had a 1 day shorter hospital stay and expressed higher satisfaction and willingness to have the same procedure again compared to the ALIF group [21]. These results propelled disk arthroplasty forward in the spine community as a reasonable alternative to fusion in the appropriate patient.

Currently, there are two disk implants which are FDA approved for use in the US, the ProDisc-L (Centinel Spine, West Chester, PA, USA) and the activeL (Aesculap/B. Braun, Center Valley, PA, USA), approved for two and one levels, respectively, with five other implants on the global market CE marks for use in Europe: the Baguera® L (SpineArt, Geneva, Switzerland), M6-L Artificial disk (Orthofix, Lewisville, TX, USA) Freedom® Lumbar disk (Axiomed, Malden, MA, USA), LP-ESP® Lumbar disk prosthesis (Spine Innovations, Ecully, France), Orbit™ Anterior Lumbar disk (Globus Medical, Audubon, PA, USA) Aditus Lumbar Disk Prosthesis (Aditus Medical, Berlin, Germany) and Mobidisk® L Lumbar disk prosthesis (HighRidge medical, Westminster, CO, USA).

The ProDisc-L, (Centinel Spine, West Chester, PA, USA) (Figure 1) is a semi-constrained ball-and-socket design currently FDA approved for one-level or two-consecutive-level arthroplasty L3-S1. The device features a midline keel on both the superior and inferior cobalt chrome alloy endplates which house the ultra-high-molecular-weight polyethylene inlay. Both the implant footprint and lordotic angle are offered in variable sizes. The devices performed well with an FDA investigational device exemption study which compared single-level (between L3 and S1) and 360-degree spinal fusion. Single-level TDR patients treated with the ProDisc-L experienced 0% major complications, significantly higher SF36 scores, neurologic success and VAS pain scores, along with higher improvement in ODI for pain and disability scores than the fusion cohort [22]. In terms of adverse events, the device demonstrated a favorable safety profile, with persistent back pain being a leading complication but at lower rates than in their fusion counterparts. The early successful outcomes of the implant led to its FDA approval for use in two contiguous levels in 2020 [5]. The longevity of the device and lumbar disk arthroplasty at large were recently validated in a 7–21-year follow-up by Marnay et al. In this study, 1187 patients were reviewed who had undergone one-level (n = 772) and two-level (n = 415) TDRs. Notably, of the entire group, 373 patients had undergone prior surgery at the index level. All groups demonstrated marked improvements in ODI at 3 months and sustained the improvement over time, with no difference in pain scores in patients who had undergone prior surgery. Rates of revision surgery and adjacent level surgery were also low at 7 (0.67%) and 21 (1.85%) years, demonstrating the long-term clinical efficacy and durability of the ProDisk-L for TDR [11].

This study confirmed, in the long term, a low revision rate with TDR which had been seen in earlier short-term studies.

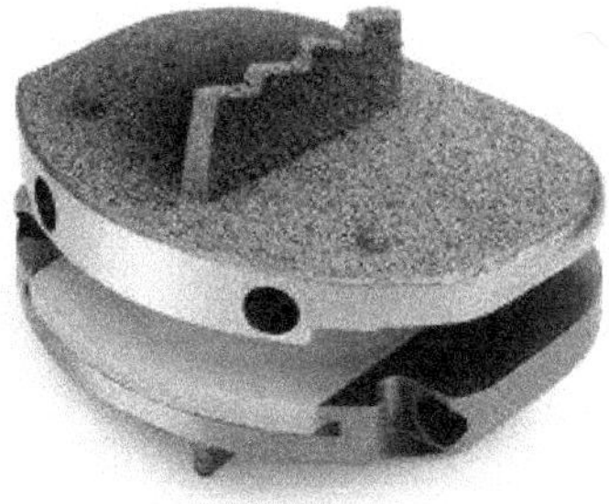

Figure 1. Prodisc® L (courtesy of FDA SSED: https://www.accessdata.fda.gov/cdrh_docs/pdf5/P050010S020B.pdf (accessed on 24 March 2025)).

Additionally, a retrospective review of 2141 patients over a 20-year period found a 1.26% revision/removal rate. Twenty-five patients (0.99%) had implants removed (twelve patients for loosening or implant migration, three following trauma, two for ongoing pain, two for lymphocytic reaction, one for implant sizing, one for vertebral body fracture, one for implant subsidence with facet arthrosis, one for a lytic lesion and one for infection); three patients (0.12%) underwent revision to a second arthroplasty (one for core repositioning, one for core replacement due to wear and one for implant repositioning). A subset of 258 patients with a minimum 15-year follow-up were surveyed and only 1 patient underwent revision/removal after 15 years post-implant [23]. Overall, the study reiterated the longevity of these implants despite initial concerns regarding reoperation. A 2024 meta-analysis reviewing complications and clinical outcomes in lumbar disk replacement and interbody fusion was also promising in terms of reoperation risk and overall noninferiority to fusion. The 2024 retrospective study involving 1720 patients revealed no difference in EBL, length of stay, OR time, ODI leg pain, complications and reoperations between total disk replacement and lumbar fusion groups. However, the total disk replacement group had lower back pain scores [3].

Currently, in the US, FDA approval has been limited to two-level TDR. However, there has been some conflicting evidence on two-level TDR success. A 2007 study placed 99 patients into 3 groups, one-level TDR at L4-5, (n = 22), one-level TDR at L5-S1 (n = 57) and two-level TDR at L4-5 and L5-S1 (n = 20), and followed them to 24 months. The two-level fusion group had a significantly higher complication rate than the single-level group. Also of note is that this study confirmed, via fluoroscopic guided spine infiltrations, that the incidence of post-operative back pain from posterior joint structures was 9.1% (n = 2) for L4-5 TDR, 28.1% (n = 16) for L5-S1 TDR and 60.0% (n = 12) for two-level TDR (L4-5 + L5-S1) [24]. Findings such as these demonstrate a possible limitation of expanding TDR to multiple levels and also serve as a reminder of the innate inability of isolated TDR to address the posterior column. Despite these findings, recent multi-level studies have not redemonstrated a difference in one- vs multi-level TDR. In the above-mentioned trial by Rasouli et al., multi-level TDR patients uniformly demonstrated improved clinical outcome scores. Furthermore, the study also included 41 three-level TDR cases and 4 four-level cases, all of which demonstrated similar improvements in satisfaction and VAS pain scores at 24–72 months. These results are promising for the expansion of FDA approval to three levels; however, FDA trials have not yet addressed three-level implantation [5].

7. Facet Joint Replacement

While there were early patent applications for facet arthroplasty in the 1980s, the Graf ligament device was one of the earliest attempts at posterior dynamic stabilization and was implanted via the tension band construction of braided polypropylene against titanium pedicle screws of adjacent levels [25]. The goal was to control rotary movement in young patients with axial back pain. Grevitt et al. reported improved ODI scores (59% to 31%) in a retrospective cohort of 50 patients at 2 years [26]. Similarly, Markwalder et al. found improvement in subjective pain perception in (37/41) 90% of patients. However, the design is plagued by resultant lateral canal stenosis, segmental lordosis and early failure in 72% of patients by 2 years, likely due to altered biomechanical strain of the posterior column [27,28]. While this design may be appropriate for patients with spondylolisthesis, it should not be employed in settings of scoliosis or lateral listhesis.

The Total Facet Arthroplasty System (TFAS) (Archus Orthopaedics, Redmond, WA, USA) was designed as an anatomic facet joint arthroplasty system. The design included cement-augmented pedicle screw insertion to anchor the device, which utilizes high-carbon-content cobalt chromium bearings articulating with cobalt chromium spheres to replicate the motion and stability of the facet joints [29] (Palmer et al., 2011). Unfortunately, the system experienced two cases of rod fracture in early clinical trials. The design was ultimately discontinued during phase III clinical trials in light of the hardware failures and following the financial acquisition of Archus in 2009 [30].

Similar to TFAS, however, the Anatomic Facet Replacement System (AFRS) (Facet Solutions Inc., Logan, UT, USA) was an anatomically designed facet prosthesis also utilizing pedicle screw fixation to affix wear-resistant alloy cobalt–chromium molybdenum-articulating surfaces. A finite element analysis (FEA) and parallel in vitro biomechanical study from 2007 demonstrated that the AFRS can predictably restore native facets and intradiscal pressures throughout the spinal range of motion [31]. This datum suggested that the device may be able to restore native biomechanics and therefore restore native adjacent segmental motion, theoretically reducing abnormal contact stress and lowering the risk of adjacent segment disease. Sjovold et al. produced a second FEA and parallel biomechanical study to evaluate the pull-out strength of the implant compared to a rigid posterior fusion construct [32]. The group found that rigid fixation devices were subjected to greater implant loads in extension and lateral bending. They also confirmed a normal intradiscal pressure through the range of motion [32].

The ACADIA device (GLOBUS Medical, Audubon, PA, USA) is a non-anatomic facet joint replacement system available outside the United States. Dryer et al. conducted an IDE and performed a prospective randomized trial with 158 patients randomized to either standard PLIF or the ACADIA trial group [33]. Outcomes demonstrated 52% follow-up at 2 years and found no significant difference between groups with regards to VAS, ZCQ and ODI scores from pre-operation to post-operation at 2 years [33]. The group therefore concluded that the ACADIA implant was a reasonable alternative to PLIF. The ACADIA implant has not been granted FDA approval in the United States but is available for elective intervention outside the United States. Notably, a recent case series of five patients demonstrated a metal-on-metal (MOM)-associated reaction in two (40%) patients necessitating subsequent explanation with PLIF at less than 2 years post-operation [34]. The occurrence of metal-on-metal crevice corrosion is a well-documented danger in orthopedic implant design and may signal a critical design flaw of the ACADIA implant precluding further utilization and FDA approval [35].

The Total Posterior Spine (TOPS) system (Premia Spine Ltd., Nowalk, CT, USA) (Figure 2) is a non-anatomic facet arthroplasty system that received FDA approval for use in the United States for patients between 35 and 80 years of age with grade 1 spondylolisthesis of L3–L5 in June, 2023, but has been on the global market since 2012. The device consists of four pedicle screws placed at adjacent levels with metal plates and a central internal motion device surrounded by a polycarbonate boot.

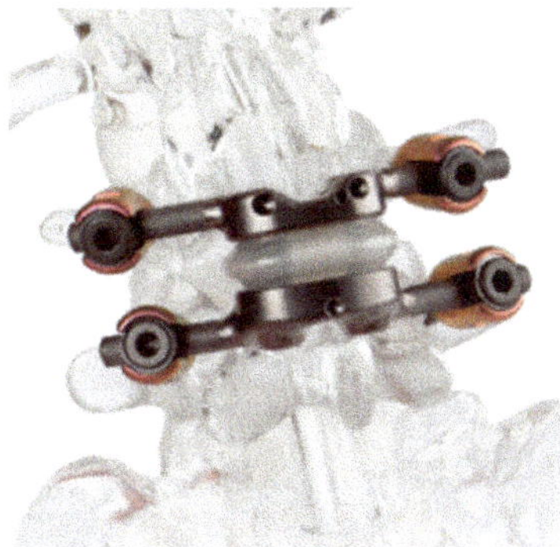

Figure 2. TOPS system (courtesy of FDA: https://www.fda.gov/medical-devices/recently-approved-devices/tops-system-p220002 (accessed on 1 April 2025)).

Smorgick et al. reported 11-year post-operative outcomes for 10 patients who underwent isolated total facet arthroplasty with the TOPS system for neurogenic claudication and single-level spondylolisthesis of L4–L5 [36]. The group reported sustained improvements in VAS (5.6 to 1.4), ODI (49.1 to 17) and SF-36 (43.2 to 70.9) at 11 years compared to their pre-operative states. Four (36%) patients experienced adjacent segment disc degeneration by 11 years, without requiring surgery. One early device failure occurred and required revision at 6 weeks. Results were similar in a separate group of ten patients at 5 years of follow-up [37].

A multi-staged prospective randomized trial group has demonstrated promising findings over the past several years [38–40]. Patients were randomized to either decompression and fusion or decompression and total facet arthroplasty. A total of 321 patients were enrolled and randomized in a 2:1 fashion with 113 arthroplasty (51.6%) and 47 (46.1%) fusion patients with 2 years of completed follow-up or early failure [40]. The arthroplasty cohort demonstrated improved VAS (back pain), ODI and ZCQ and lower higher rates of adjacent segment disease [40]. There was no significant difference in complications or revision rates (11.5% vs. 10.6%). Of note is that there were no statistical comparisons of the time points in which complications occurred. Furthermore, 6.8% (14/206) of the patients in the arthroplasty group suffered a dural tear compared to only 2.2% (2/93) in the fusion group ($p = 0.16$). Notably, the rate of adjacent segment disease in the arthroplasty group was 0% compared to 5% in the fusion group, demonstrating successful proof of concept despite the concerns surrounding dural tear events [40]. Currently, there is active monitoring and continued data collection with multiple clinical trials ongoing [38–40].

Future directions for total facet arthroplasty will need to include considerations of long-term safety; specifically, the TOPS device mechanism will require continued observation. Based on the present data, there may be a paradoxical increase in adjacent segment disease within arthroplasty cohorts compared to fusion; however, larger groups and longer follow-ups will be required. Minimally invasive strategies may also be advantageous for patient recovery. Similarly, patient-specific implantation and device design that respects the native facet joint architecture with thoughtful design criteria could also provide improved patient outcomes.

8. Dynamic Stabilization

Posterior dynamic stabilization (PDS), as discussed previously, was first described in the 1980s, with early attempts including the Graf ligament device [25]. The primary goal of PDS is to allow micromotion for better fusion, decrease rigidity and allow improved load sharing, which has been associated with decreased risk of ASDi and ASDe. Broadly, PDS is achieved via 1. altered rod shape, 2. elastic rod materials, 3. polyaxial pedicle screws, 4. semi-dynamic plating devices and 5. unique mechanical constructs, or some combination of the above. There has been a myriad of devices released to achieve PDS; however, there are several examples worthy of discussion, notable for both clinical successes and failures, many of which warrant further investigation.

The Dynamic Neutralization System (Dynesys) was developed in 1994 by Gilles Dubois (Centerpulse Orthopaedics Ltd., Winterthur, Switzerland), with the first results formally published in 2002 [41]. This original device was designed to connect standard pedicle screws with hollow rods made of PCU with PET cords inside the hollow shell, allowing for flexible multidirectional control [41]. Early indications included spinal stenosis and DJD. Importantly, this design differed from the Graf ligament because it theoretically prevented foraminal collapse with spinal extension. The Dynesys received 510 k approval in 2004; however, it has failed to obtain FDA standalone approval for dynamic stabilization, largely due to inconclusive data on its efficacy and long-term outcomes.

A recent literature review outlined the short-term, mid-term and long-term results of the Dynesys device over the past 20 years [42]. Short-term results at 2 years have shown no significant differences in ODI, VAS, range of motion of adjacent segments or risk of adjacent segment disease [42,43]. A more recent meta-analysis of mid-term and long-term time points evaluated 17 studies with 1296 patients which found that the Dynesys patients experienced more natural index and adjacent level motion associated with improved back pain compared to the instrumented fusion cohort's levels [44]. The longest time point included was 93.6 months, with 58 patients (33 in the Dynesys group), in a study conducted by Bredin et al. [45]. This retrospective comparative cohort study found significantly better VAS (1.8 vs. 3.6), ODI (14.6 vs. 19.4) and decreased rates of adjacent segment disease (12.1% vs. 36%) at final follow-up compared to the rigid instrumented fusion cohort [45].

One prospective randomized controlled trial exists on the product and was completed in China [46]. Results at 2 years demonstrated significantly greater ROM of the operated segment without significant differences in VAS and ODI when compared to the fusion cohort [46]. While the Dynesys device may protect normal spinal motion, large, long-term level I studies will be critical to elucidate the validity of these preliminary findings.

Although there have been some promising data with the Dynesys, other flexible rod systems have demonstrated poor outcomes or a need for further monitoring. The Accuflex Rod System produced by Globus Medical (no longer on the market) was a standard 6.5 mm titanium rod with a variable circumferential helical cut to allow customized flexibility [47]. Mandigo et al. reported results from 170 patients (54 in the Accuflex cohort) who underwent posterior instrumented fusion and found similar fusion rates without a difference in clinical outcomes [47]. However, a report of 20 patients demonstrated fatigue failure at a rate of 22.22%, requiring revision surgery [48]. The Accuflex Rod System might be prone to catastrophic mechanical fracture due to cyclic failure and is no longer offered on the US market and should not be implemented.

The Isobar TTL System (Scient'x) is a titanium rod with a damper component in the longitudinal axis and first received FDA clearance in 1999. The damper provides 2.25 degrees of angular range of motion in flexion–extension and lateral bending without axial rotation restriction [49]. Guan et al. recently published a systematic review of current results for the Isobar system [49]. When evaluating fusion surgery and hybrid fusion surgery, the group found greater than 88.5% fusion at final follow-up [49]. Barrey et al. found a fusion rate of 89% by ten years with stable symptomatic improvement after fusion with the Isobar system [50]. Importantly, there is a paucity of literature evaluating the rate of ASD; however, the small cohort in the study conducted by Barrey et al. does report a low rate of only 44.4% by ten years. Notably, the largest series of patients treated with the Isobar system was published by Perrin et al., with a collection of 800 patients who underwent dynamic stabilization, dynamic fusion and hybrid fusion, with an overall fusion rate of 98% without any mechanical complications [51]. In another cohort series by Li et al., the incidence of adjacent segment disease was 15% (6/40) at 79 months [52]. Unfortunately, this was a retrospective case series, and there was no direct comparison between PDS instrumentation and standard rigid fusion instrumentation. Thus, limited data have been reported on ASD after PDS with flexible rods, particularly Isobar. In short, the Isobar system may be indicated for young patients with single-level pathology, including spinal stenosis and spondylolisthesis, and may be better suited for hybrid, non-fusion techniques. Further high-quality investigations are warranted.

Compared to standard pedicle screws in rigid fixation, dynamic pedicle screws allow varying degrees of freedom and motion between the fixation (threaded) and rod fixation (tulip). Hayati et al. reported on a retrospective cohort series of 101 patients treated with standard pedicle screw fusion or dynamic pedicle screw fixation and found a non-significant decreased rate of radiographic adjacent segment disease at 79 months post-operation in those with dynamic screws [53]. Furthermore, these results did not correlate to any significant clinical benefit, including VAS, ODI or complication profiles. A prospective randomized double-blinded multicenter study by Meyer et al. evaluated standard instrumented fusion with posterior stabilized and pedicle-based dynamic stabilization without fusion [54]. The dynamic group received the Cosmic MIA system, which has a hinged joint between the screw head and the threaded screw, allowing sagittal motion [54]. The group found that non-instrumented dynamic stabilization was non-inferior to standard instrumented fusion, with no significant differences between the groups with regard to VAS and ODI at 24 months. This study may suggest that posterior or posterolateral dynamic fixation without fusion is a sufficient treatment for DJD of the lumbar spine compared to standard instrumented fusion [54].

Classic titanium rods have a high modulus of elasticity (110 GPa), which can lead to immediate segmental stability; however, they may be related to stress shielding and pseudoarthrosis. Polyetheretherketone (PEEK) is a material with a modulus of elasticity of only 3.6 GPa, which allows for a more flexible construct, increased load sharing to the anterior column, improved stress-shielding and, overall, a more natural physiologic loading of the spinal column [55].

Several meta-analyses exist on the topic of PEEK rod implementation for lumbar fusion [56,57]. Li et al.'s was the most recent and evaluated eight prospective and seven retrospective studies comparing rigid titanium rods and PEEK rod stabilization with intervertebral bone grafting at a minimum of 6 months from surgery [57]. Based on the random effects model, Li et al. concluded that the PEEK flexible rod group had superior improvement in VAS, ODI and JOA scores and fusion rates by 12 weeks from surgery sustained to final follow-up. Critically, while Li et al. (2023) included eight prospective studies, the level of evidence was limited by retrospective data inclusion and limited follow-up length. Furthermore, the group was unable to compare the incidence of adjacent segment disease—the primary theoretical benefit of flexible posterior instrumentation. Overall, the evidence for PEEK rod implementation remains low quality and should be improved over time.

The DSS-HPS® System (Paradigm Spine, Germany) is a unique modular system with an internal coupler designed to limit spinal range of motion to 50% of the physiologic motion with an allowed 2 mm of displacement (1.33 mm in tension and 0.66 mm in compression), maintaining a fixed center of rotation [58]. Paradigm Spine implemented an internal registry of patient information for the long-term tracking of clinical outcomes; however, the data remain unpublished and accessible only to Paradigm Spine internal use. Few studies have been published on clinical outcomes; however, Angelini et al. reported results of 27 consecutive patients treated with hybrid stabilization [59]. The group found that 40.7% of the patients experienced disc space degeneration at both the instrumented levels and adjacent levels at one year after surgery [59]. They concluded that the device may not function as well as other systems such as the Dynesys with regards to ASD. The DSS system remains unavailable in the USA.

The landscape of posterior dynamic stabilization is tenuous. While multiple products are currently available for implementation in lumbar spine surgery, all products with FDA approval are approved for only single-level instrumentation in grade 1 spondylolisthesis. Off-label utilization is a common occurrence across many fields in medicine and allows further investigation and understanding of the use criteria; however, it can cause patient harm. Future directions for posterior dynamic stabilization systems include attaining a higher quality of evidence with prospectively designed studies, investigating multi-segment disease and combination treatment with multi-column fixation and arthroplasty, among other focused investigational study strategies. From an engineering perspective, flexible rods present a design challenge in a construct innately at risk for cyclic load failure. With regard to future development, currently, many companies are creating their own version of a PEEK rod or other dynamic rod due to its documented success and hope to gain market share. This competition will ideally lower the cost of implants over time. Future development of technology such as microsensors for stress/strain evaluation in vivo, microprocessor dynamic control and patient-specific implants could provide helpful insight and improve patient outcomes.

9. Total Joint Arthroplasty

Total joint spinal arthroplasty (TJR) involves the replacement of both the anterior and posterior columns simultaneously from a single approach, including the degenerative intervertebral disc and facet joints, to relieve pain or neural compression while preserving motion and spinal alignment. TJR in theory fills the gap left off by isolated disk replacement as a treatment for patients that have not only disk degeneration but also concomitant facet degeneration as well. Currently, TJR is indicated for grade 1 spondylolisthesis, recurrent disc herniation with severe disc degeneration, severe foraminal or central stenosis requiring extensive facet or pars removal and degenerative disc disease with concurrent facet arthrosis [60]. Contraindications include trauma, tumors, infections, severe deformity and osteoporosis, with pre-operative bone density assessment recommended to ensure adequate implant fixation [60]. The only currently available implant for total spinal arthroplasty in the US is the MOTUS (3Spine, Chattanooga, TN, USA) (Figure 3), which is used at levels L1-L2 to L5-S1. The TJR implant is designed to replace both the intervertebral disc and facet joints while allowing for wide neural decompression. The surgical approach involves a posterior bilateral transforaminal technique, incorporating laminectomy, bilateral facetectomy and partial discectomy to achieve decompression, followed by implantation of the MOTUS device to reconstruct the motion segment.

A key consideration in the long-term success of TJR of the spine is implant durability, particularly wear resistance, which directly impacts device longevity and clinical outcomes. Siskey et al. evaluated the wear performance of a vitamin-E-stabilized highly crosslinked polyethylene (VE-HXLPE) lumbar TJR, designed to replace both the intervertebral disc and facet joints via a posterior approach [61]. Standard wear testing demonstrated a low mean wear rate of 1.2 ± 0.5 mg per million cycles (MC), significantly lower than traditional anterior disc replacement designs, which range from 2.7 mg/MC to 13.8 mg/MC. Abrasive wear testing resulted in a similar wear rate (1.1 ± 0.6 mg/MC), indicating resistance to third-body wear. Impingement testing showed slightly increased wear rates, ranging from 1.7 ± 1.1 mg/MC (smallest implant size) to 3.9 ± 1.1 mg/MC (largest size). Importantly, no mechanical failures were observed, and the VE-HXLPE implant outperformed traditional ultra-high-molecular-weight polyethylene under similar conditions. These findings support the FDA-regulated clinical trial of VE-HXLPE TJR and highlight its potential as a durable, motion-preserving alternative to both fusion and conventional ADRs. The material's superior wear resistance and stability suggests it may reduce long-term complications such as osteolysis and implant failure, which are common concerns with traditional polyethylene designs.

Polyethylene wear is not the only area where TJR shows promise; early clinical outcomes suggest it may offer comparable or improved symptom relief and functional recovery compared to traditional fusion procedures. A recent study by Sielatycki et al. compared posterior-based lumbar TJR to transforaminal lumbar interbody fusion (TLIF) for degenerative lumbar conditions requiring surgical intervention [60]. The TJR implant was evaluated for its ability to provide motion preservation while allowing for wide neural decompression. The study conducted a retrospective analysis of 208 propensity-matched patients, with 52 undergoing TJR and 156 undergoing TLIF. Patient-reported outcomes at 3 and 12 months post-operation were measured using the Oswestry disability index (ODI) and Numeric Rating Scale (NRS) for back and leg pain. Both groups showed significant improvements at 3 months, but at 1 year, LTJR continued to show improvements in ODI and NRS scores, whereas the TLIF group plateaued. Specifically, the LTJR group had a significantly lower ODI at 12 months (12.4 ± 12.8) compared to TLIF (23.8 ± 17.3, $p < 0.001$), and lower NRS back pain scores (2.1 ± 2.3 vs. 3.4 ± 2.8, $p = 0.006$). Further analysis demonstrated that LTJR patients had 3.3 times greater odds of achieving a minimal clinical symptom state (MSS) ($p = 0.001$), 2.4 times greater odds of achieving a substantial clinical benefit (SCB) ($p = 0.028$) and 4.1 times greater odds of achieving a minimal clinically important difference (MCID) ($p = 0.006$) compared to TLIF patients. Furthermore, a recent case report by Nel et al. provided the first valuable long-term data on TJR of the lumbar spine, a novel motion-preserving alternative to spinal fusion for degenerative lumbar disease [62]. In this case study, the authors presented the first two patients to undergo lumbar TJR, both of whom had severe degenerative lumbar disease with chronic, refractory back and leg pain. Sixteen years post-operation, both patients reported complete and sustained symptom resolution, with full functional recovery and unrestricted participation in daily and occupational activities. Importantly, long-term imaging demonstrated no evidence of adjacent segment degeneration, implant failure, or progressive arthropathy. These findings suggest that lumbar TJR may provide durable pain relief and functional benefits in both the short term and the long term while mitigating the adverse effects of fusion. Furthermore, the lumbar TJR implant has demonstrated favorable wear properties and the potential for long-term durability. While further research and long-term trials are needed, these findings support the continued exploration of TJR as a viable option for select patients with lumbar spine degeneration.

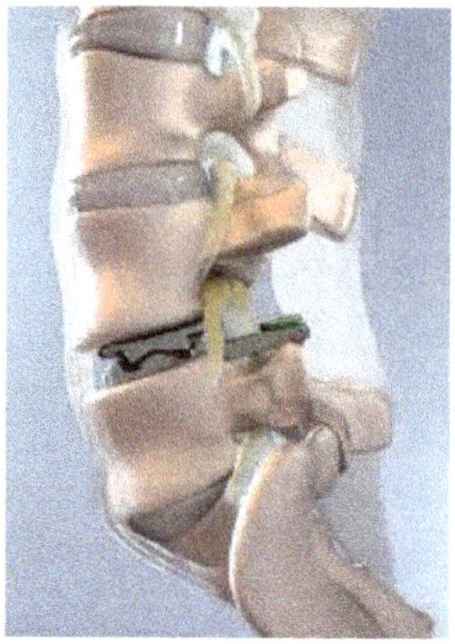

Figure 3. MOTUS 3Spine (courtesy of Nel et al. [62]).

10. Discussion

The gold standard for surgical management of lumbar spine degeneration has been spinal fusion, despite the known complications and associated risk of additional surgery. Lumbar arthroplasty is a motion-preserving alternative to spinal fusion for surgical treatment of lumbar degeneration. (Table 1) Arthroplasty has not been widely accepted due to concerns regarding implant survival, revision risk and a lack of long-term follow-up data. The lack of long-term data has often been cited as the reason for apprehension toward lumbar arthroplasty. The three-joint complex of a single lumbar spine segment adds complexity to the prospect of lumbar arthroplasty. Therefore, patient selection and selection of surgical treatment are critical for clinical success. Total disk replacement for isolated disk degeneration has led the way in the field, with recent promising results in 21-year follow-up data from a large cohort [11]. With these recent favorable results from the long-term experience of Thierry and Guyer, the durability and long-term efficacy of lumbar arthroplasty has been further validated as a favorable and reliable alternative to fusion in patients without facet arthropathy [11,23]. Furthermore, success in lumbar disk arthroplasty at one and two levels has demonstrated that TDR is a reasonable multilevel treatment as well. Indications for lumbar arthroplasty have been generally limited to early disk degeneration; as the field progresses, the clinical pathway for arthroplasty will need to be critically evaluated as indications expand. Pitfalls such as the misdiagnosis of spinal epidural lipomatosis upon MRI could lead to inappropriate surgery and should be considered during patient evaluation [63]. Also, as mentioned previously, concomitant facet arthropathy should be identified as a contraindication to isolated disk arthroplasty.

Addressing lumbar facet pathology has been a challenging hurdle to overcome to expand the indication of lumbar arthroplasty. While devices such as TOPS have shown some early success, other implants, such as some dynamic rods, have demonstrated notable clinical failures, highlighting the need for further observation, monitoring and implant development [40,48]. Total joint arthroplasty (TJR), which addresses the degenerative disk as well as the facets from the same posterior approach, has shown good results in both short- and long-term studies. These are exciting advances for motion-preserving treatment of posterior column degeneration. Although limited, current data point to the possible expansion of lumbar arthroplasty as an option for lumbar degeneration beyond isolated disk disease. While lumbar fusion will likely remain the workhorse salvage procedure for advanced lumbar degeneration, the progress in lumbar arthroplasty is a promising alternative for early degeneration across all three joints of a lumbar spinal level.

When coupled with advances in navigated technology and minimally invasive techniques, arthroplasty has the potential to provide customized treatment options to address the challenge of lumbar degeneration. In totality, these findings indicate a cautious optimism toward the future of lumbar spine arthroplasty and motion-preserving surgery.

Table 1. Summary table comparing advantages and disadvantages of different spinal implants.

Implant Type	Advantages	Disadvantages
Lumbar Interbody Fusion (LIF)	- Widely practiced and understood surgery with multiple approaches and techniques to address the degenerative lumbar spine and deformity correction - Current standard of care - Minimally invasive surgery is an option - Able to extend to multiple levels (useful in complex or revision settings) - Acceptable short-term clinical outcomes	- Pseudoarthrosis - Hardware failure - Loss of motion at the fused level accelerates adjacent segment degeneration
Artificial Lumbar Disc Arthroplasty	- Leading alternative construct in preserving motion at the index lumbar level - Low adjacent segment stress forces with lower rates of adjacent segment degeneration - Lower levels of early disability scores, higher patient satisfaction and shorter length of hospital stay compared to LIF	- Only addresses degenerative intervertebral disc; unable to address posterior column pathology - Contraindicated in facet degeneration, poor bone quality and significant deformity - Anterior approach risks (vascular/ureter injury) - Concerns with implant stability and durability may increase risk of revision surgery - Currently only two FDA-approved implants that can be used for one to two contiguous levels
Facet Joint Replacement	- Addresses posterior column - Offers patient-specific instrumentation and device design that respects the native facet joint architecture - Restores native biomechanics while preserving motion - Minimally invasive surgery is an option	- Limited FDA-approved options due to mixed results and high complication rates among different implant options - Latest devices are limited to single-level spondylolisthesis of L3–L5 - Some early evidence of paradoxical increases in adjacent segment disease, although larger long-term studies are needed
Flexible Rods	- Allow micromotion, decrease rigidity and improve load sharing with a theoretical decreased risk of adjacent segment disease - Multiple implant options for posterior dynamic stabilization	- Despite multiple options, the data are largely inconclusive on the efficacy and long-term outcomes due to low-level evidence - All FDA-approved products are only approved for single-level instrumentation in grade 1 spondylolisthesis - Off-label use is common - Implant design and construct is innately at risk for cyclic load failure
Total Joint Arthroplasty (TJR)	- Addresses both anterior column and posterior column pathology while preserving motion and spinal alignment - Single posterior approach utilizing bilateral transforaminal technique to replace both the intervertebral disc and facet joints, providing wide neural decompression - Improved implant durability and long-term success secondary to superior wear resistance rates from using vitamin-E-stabilized highly crosslinked polyethylene (VE-HXLPE)	- Currently only one implant available for implementation - Limited use at L1–L2 and L5-S1, highlighting the importance of appropriate patient selection - Current data are promising but remain limited due to low-level evidence

11. Conclusions

Lumbar arthroplasty has the theoretical potential to provide a motion-preserving alternative to lumbar fusion for patients with lumbar spine degeneration. Although substantial long-term outcome studies are still needed, there have been promising data thus far indicating a cautious optimism toward the future of motion preservation in degenerative lumbar spine surgery.

Author Contributions: Conceptualization, T.C.; writing—original draft preparation, M.S.P., M.W.P. and M.G.; writing—review and editing, M.S.P.; supervision, A.T. and T.C. All authors have read and agreed to the published version of the manuscript.

Funding: This research received no external funding.

Acknowledgments: Steven D. Pheasant PT, for insight and resources on biomechanics of lumbar degeneration.

Conflicts of Interest: The authors declare no conflicts of interest.

Abbreviations

The following abbreviations are used in this manuscript:

TDR	total disk replacement
TJR	total joint replacement
ASDe	adjacent segment degeneration
ASDi	adjacent segment disease

References

1. Ravindra, V.M.; Senglaub, S.S.; Rattani, A.; Dewan, M.C.; Härtl, R.; Bisson, E.; Park, K.B.; Shrime, M.G. Degenerative Lumbar Spine Disease: Estimating Global Incidence and Worldwide Volume. *Glob. Spine J.* **2018**, *8*, 784–794. [CrossRef]
2. Vo, N.V.; Hartman, R.A.; Patil, P.R.; Risbud, M.V.; Kletsas, D.; Iatridis, J.C.; Hoyland, J.A.; Le Maitre, C.L.; Sowa, G.A.; Kang, J.D. Molecular mechanisms of biological aging in intervertebral discs. *J. Orthop. Res.* **2016**, *34*, 1289–1306. [CrossRef]
3. Daher, M.; Nassar, J.; Balmaceno-Criss, M.; Diebo, B.G.; Daniels, A.H. Lumbar Disc Replacement Versus Interbody Fusion: Meta-analysis of Complications and Clinical Outcomes. *Orthop. Rev.* **2024**, *16*, 116900. [CrossRef]
4. Fujiya, M.; Saita, M.; Kaneda, K.; Abumi, K. Clinical study on stability of combined distraction and compression rod instrumentation with posterolateral fusion for unstable degenerative spondylolisthesis. *Spine* **1990**, *15*, 1216–1222. [CrossRef] [PubMed]
5. Fiani, B.; Nanney, J.M.; Villait, A.; Sekhon, M.; Doan, T. Investigational Research: Timeline, Trials, and Future Directions of Spinal Disc Arthroplasty. *Cureus* **2021**, *13*, e16739. [CrossRef] [PubMed]
6. Freeman, B.J.C.; Davenport, J. Total disc replacement in the lumbar spine: A systematic review of the literature. *Eur. Spine J.* **2006**, *15* (Suppl. S3), 439–447. [CrossRef]
7. Humphreys, S.C.; Hodges, S.D.; Sielatycki, J.A.; Sivaganesan, A.; Block, J.E. Are We Finally Ready for Total Joint Replacement of the Spine? An Extension of Charnley's Vision. *Int. J. Spine Surg.* **2024**, *18*, 24–31. [CrossRef] [PubMed]
8. Putz, R. The functional morphology of the superior articular processes of the lumbar vertebrae. *J. Anat.* **1985**, *143*, 181–187. [PubMed]
9. Kirkaldy-Willis, W.H.M.; Wedge, J.H.M.; Yong-Hing, K.M.; Reilly, J.M. Pathology and pathogenesis of lumbar spondylosis and stenosis. *Spine* **1978**, *3*, 319–328. [CrossRef]
10. Botwin, K.P.; Gruber, R.D. Lumbar spinal stenosis: Anatomy and pathogenesis. *Phys. Med. Rehabil. Clin. N. Am.* **2003**, *14*, 1–15. [CrossRef]
11. Marnay, T.P.; Geneste, G.Y.; Edgard-Rosa, G.W.; Grau-Ortiz, M.M.; Hirsch, C.C.; Negre, G.G. Clinical Outcomes After 1 and 2-Level Lumbar Total Disc Arthroplasty. *J. Bone Jt. Surg.* **2025**, *107*, 53–65. [CrossRef]
12. Turner, J.A.; Ersek, M.; Herron, L.; Haselkorn, J.; Kent, D.; Ciol, M.A.; Deyo, R. Patient outcomes after lumbar spinal fusions. *J. Am. Med. Assoc.* **1992**, *268*, 907–911. [CrossRef]
13. Okuda, S.; Oda, T.; Miyauchi, A.; Tamura, S.; Hashimoto, Y.; Yamasaki, S.; Haku, T.; Kanematsu, F.; Ariga, K.; Ohwada, T.; et al. Lamina Horizontalization and Facet Tropism as the Risk Factors for Adjacent Segment Degeneration After PLIF. *Spine* **2008**, *33*, 2754–2758. [CrossRef] [PubMed]
14. Fuster, S.; Martínez-Anda, J.J.; Castillo-Rivera, S.A.; Vargas-Reverón, C.; Tornero, E. Dynamic Fixation Techniques for the Prevention of Adjacent Segment Disease: A Retrospective Controlled Study. *Asian Spine J.* **2022**, *16*, 401–410. [CrossRef] [PubMed]
15. Boonsirikamchai, W.; Wilartratsami, S.; Ruangchainikom, M.; Korwutthikulrangsri, E.; Tongsai, S.; Luksanapruksa, P. Pseudarthrosis risk factors in lumbar fusion: A systematic review and meta-analysis. *BMC Musculoskelet. Disord.* **2024**, *25*, 433. [CrossRef]

16. Irmola, T.M.; Häkkinen, A.; Järvenpää, S.; Marttinen, I.; Vihtonen, K.; Neva, M. Reoperation Rates Following Instrumented Lumbar Spine Fusion. *Spine* **2018**, *43*, 295–301. [CrossRef]
17. Rasouli, A.; Cuellar, J.M.; Kanim, L.; Delamarter, R. Multiple-Level Lumbar Total Disk Replacement: A Prospective Clinical and Radiographic Analysis of Motion Preserva-tion at 24–72 Months. *Clin. Spine Surg.* **2019**, *32*, 38–42. [CrossRef]
18. Büttner-Janz, K.; Guyer, R.D.; Ohnmeiss, D.D. Indications for lumbar total disc replacement: Selecting the right patient with the right indication for the right total disc. *Int. J. Spine Surg.* **2014**, *8*, 12. [CrossRef]
19. Schwender, J.D.; Casnellie, M.T.; Perra, J.H.; Transfeldt, E.E.; Pinto, M.R.; Denis, F.; Garvey, T.A.; Polly, D.W.; Mehbod, A.A.; Dykes, D.C.; et al. Perioperative Complications in Revision Anterior Lumbar Spine Surgery. *Spine* **2009**, *34*, 87–90. [CrossRef]
20. Link, H.D. History, design and biomechanics of the LINK SB Charité artificial disc. *Eur. Spine J.* **2002**, *11* (Suppl. S2), S98–S105. [CrossRef]
21. Blumenthal, S.; McAfee, P.C.; Guyer, R.D.; Hochschuler, S.H.; Geisler, F.H.; Holt, R.T.; Garcia, R.; Regan, J.J.; Ohnmeiss, D.D. A prospective, randomized, multicenter Food and Drug Administration investigational device exemptions study of lumbar total disc replacement with the CHARITE artificial disc versus lumbar fusion: Part I: Evaluation of clinical out-comes. *Spine* **2005**, *30*, 1565–1575. [CrossRef]
22. Zigler, J.; Delamarter, R.; Spivak, J.M.; Linovitz, R.J.; Danielson, G.O.; Haider, T.T.; Cammisa, F.; Zuchermann, J.; Balderston, R.; Kitchel, S.; et al. Results of the Prospective, Randomized, Multicenter Food and Drug Administration Investigational Device Exemption Study of the ProDisc®-L Total Disc Replacement Versus Circumferential Fusion for the Treatment of 1-Level Degenerative Disc Disease. *Spine* **2007**, *32*, 1155–1162. [CrossRef] [PubMed]
23. Guyer, R.D.; Blumenthal, S.L.; Shellock, J.L.; Zigler, J.E.; Ohnmeiss, D.D. Lumbar Total Disk Replacement Device Removals and Revisions Performed During a 20-Year Experience with 2141 Patients. *Spine* **2024**, *49*, 671–676. [CrossRef] [PubMed]
24. Siepe, C.J.; Mayer, H.M.; Heinz-Leisenheimer, M.; Korge, A. Total Lumbar Disc Replacement. *Spine* **2007**, *32*, 782–790. [CrossRef]
25. Graf, H. Evaluation of the therapeutic effect of the graf stabilization system. In Proceedings of the 2nd Annual Meeting of the European Spine Society, Rome, Italy, 17–19 October 1991.
26. Grevitt, M.P.; Gardner, A.D.H.; Spilsbury, J.; Shackleford, I.M.; Baskerville, R.; Pursell, L.M.; Hassaan, A.; Mulholland, R.C. The Graf stabilisation system: Early results in 50 patients. *Eur. Spine J.* **1995**, *4*, 169–175. [CrossRef]
27. Markwalder, T.-M.; Wenger, M. Dynamic stabilization of lumbar motion segments by use of Graf's ligaments: Results with an average follow-up of 7.4 years in 39 highly selected, consecutive patients. *Acta Neurochir.* **2003**, *145*, 209–214. [CrossRef]
28. Hadlow, S.V.; Fagan, A.B.; Hillier, T.M.; Fraser, R.D. The Graf ligamentoplasty procedure. Comparison with posterolateral fusion in the management of low back pain. *Spine* **1998**, *23*, 1172–1179. [CrossRef] [PubMed]
29. Palmer, D.K.; Inceoglu, S.; Cheng, W.K. Stem fracture after total facet replacement in the lumbar spine: A report of two cases and review of the literature. *Spine J.* **2011**, *11*, e15–e19. [CrossRef]
30. Archus Orthopedics, Inc. Spine Device Maker that Raised $60M, Shuts Down Amid Cash Crunch. 2009. Available online: https://www.biospace.com/archus-orthopedics-inc-spine-device-maker-that-raised-60m-shuts-down-amid-cash-crunch (accessed on 1 April 2025).
31. Goel, V.K.; Mehta, A.; Jangra, J.; Faizan, A.; Kiapour, A.; Hoy, R.W.; Fauth, A.R. Anatomic Facet Replacement System (AFRS) Restoration of Lumbar Segment Mechanics to Intact: A Finite Element Study and In Vitro Cadaver Investigation. *Int. J. Spine Surg.* **2007**, *1*, 46–54. [CrossRef]
32. Sjovold, S.G.; Zhu, Q.; Bowden, A.; Larson, C.R.; de Bakker, P.M.; Villarraga, M.L.; Ochoa, J.A.; Rosler, D.M.; Cripton, P.A. Biomechanical evaluation of the Total Facet Arthroplasty System® (TFAS®): Loading as compared to a rigid posterior instrumentation system. *Eur. Spine J.* **2012**, *21*, 1660–1673. [CrossRef]
33. Dryer, R.; Youssef, J.A.; Lorio, M.P.; DiRisio, D.J.; Myer, J.; Baker, K. ACADIA™ Facet Replacement System IDE Clinical Trial: Preliminary Two-Year Outcomes. *Spine J.* **2012**, *12*, S140–S141. [CrossRef]
34. Goodwin, M.L.; Spiker, W.R.; Brodke, D.S.; Lawrence, B.D. Failure of facet replacement system with metal-on-metal bearing surface and subsequent discovery of cobalt allergy: Report of 2 cases. *J. Neurosurg. Spine* **2018**, *29*, 81–84. [CrossRef]
35. Eliaz, N. Corrosion of Metallic Biomaterials: A Review. *Materials* **2019**, *12*, 407. [CrossRef]
36. Smorgick, Y.; Mirovsky, Y.; Floman, Y.; Rand, N.; Millgram, M.; Anekstein, Y. Long-term results for total lumbar facet joint replacement in the management of lumbar degenerative spondylolisthesis. *J. Neurosurg. Spine* **2020**, *32*, 36–41. [CrossRef] [PubMed]
37. Haleem, S.; Ahmed, A.; Ganesan, S.; McGillion, S.F.; Fowler, J.L. Mean 5-Year Follow-Up Results of a Facet Replacement Device in the Treatment of Lumbar Spinal Stenosis and Degenerative Spondylolisthesis. *World Neurosurg.* **2021**, *152*, e645–e651. [CrossRef] [PubMed]
38. Pinter, Z.W.; Freedman, B.A.; Nassr, A.; Sebastian, A.S.; Coric, D.; Welch, W.C.; Steinmetz, M.P.; Robbins, S.E.; Ament, J.; Anand, N.; et al. A Prospective Study of Lumbar Facet Arthroplasty in the Treatment of Degenerative Spondylolisthesis and Stenosis: Results from the Total Posterior Spine System (TOPS) IDE Study. *Clin. Spine Surg.* **2023**, *36*, E59–E69. [CrossRef]

39. Coric, D.; Nassr, A.; Kim, P.K.; Welch, W.C.; Robbins, S.; DeLuca, S.; Whiting, D.; Chahlavi, A.; Pirris, S.M.; Groff, M.W.; et al. Prospective, randomized controlled multicenter study of posterior lumbar facet arthroplasty for the treatment of spondylolisthesis. *J. Neurosurg. Spine* **2023**, *38*, 115–125. [CrossRef]
40. Nassr, A.; Coric, D.; Pinter, Z.W.; Sebastian, A.S.; Freedman, B.A.; Whiting, D.; Chahlavi, A.; Pirris, S.; Phan, N.; Meyer, S.A.; et al. Lumbar Facet Arthroplasty Versus Fusion for Grade-I Degenerative Spondylolisthesis with Stenosis. *J. Bone Jt. Surg.* **2024**, *106*, 1041–1053. [CrossRef]
41. Stoll, T.M.; Dubois, G.; Schwarzenbach, O. The dynamic neutralization system for the spine: A multi-center study of a novel non-fusion system. *Eur. Spine J.* **2002**, *11* (Suppl. S2), S170–S178. [CrossRef]
42. Peng, B.-G.; Gao, C.-H. Is Dynesys dynamic stabilization system superior to posterior lumbar fusion in the treatment of lumbar degenerative diseases? *World J. Clin. Cases* **2020**, *8*, 5496–5500. [CrossRef]
43. Kumar, A.; Beastall, J.; Hughes, J.; Karadimas, E.J.; Nicol, M.; Smith, F.; Wardlaw, D. Disc changes in the bridged and adjacent segments after Dynesys dynamic stabilization system after two years. *Spine* **2008**, *33*, 2909–2914. [CrossRef]
44. Zhou, L.-P.; Zhang, R.-J.; Wang, J.-Q.; Zhang, H.-Q.; Shang, J.; Gao, Y.; Jia, C.-Y.; Ding, J.-Y.; Zhang, L.; Shen, C.-L. Medium and long-term radiographic and clinical outcomes of Dynesys dynamic stabilization versus instrumented fusion for degenerative lumbar spine diseases. *BMC Surg.* **2023**, *23*, 46. [CrossRef]
45. Bredin, S.; Demay, O.; Mensa, C.; Madi, K.; Ohl, X. Posterolateral fusion versus Dynesys dynamic stabilization: Retrospective study at a minimum 5.5 years' follow-up. *Orthop. Traumatol. Surg. Res.* **2017**, *103*, 1241–1244. [CrossRef] [PubMed]
46. Yu, S.-W.; Yang, S.-C.; Ma, C.-H.; Wu, C.-H.; Yen, C.-Y.; Tu, Y.-K. Comparison of Dynesys posterior stabilization and posterior lumbar interbody fusion for spinal stenosis L4L5. *Acta Orthop. Belg.* **2012**, *78*, 230–239. [PubMed]
47. Mandigo, C.E.; Sampath, P.; Kaiser, M.G. Posterior dynamic stabilization of the lumbar spine: Pedicle-based stabilization with the AccuFlex rod system. *Neurosurg. Focus* **2007**, *22*, E9. [CrossRef]
48. Reyes-Sánchez, A.; Zárate-Kalfópulos, B.; Ramírez-Mora, I.; Rosales-Olivarez, L.M.; Alpizar-Aguirre, A.; Sánchez-Bringas, G. Posterior dynamic stabilization of the lumbar spine with the Accuflex rod system as a stand-alone device: Experience in 20 patients with 2-year follow-up. *Eur. Spine J.* **2010**, *19*, 2164–2170. [CrossRef]
49. Guan, J.; Liu, T.; Yu, X.; Li, W.; Feng, N.; Jiang, G.; Zhao, H.; Yang, Y. Biomechanical and clinical research of Isobar semi-rigid stabilization devices for lumbar degenerative diseases: A systematic review. *Biomed. Eng. Online* **2023**, *22*, 95. [CrossRef] [PubMed]
50. Barrey, C.; Perrin, G.; Champain, S. Pedicle-Screw-Based Dynamic Systems and Degenerative Lumbar Diseases: Biomechanical and Clinical Experiences of Dynamic Fusion with Isobar TTL. *ISRN Orthop.* **2013**, *2013*, 183702. [CrossRef]
51. Perrin, G.; Cristini, A. Prevention of adjacent level degeneration above a fused vertebral segment: Long term effect, after a mean follow-up of 8.27 years, of the semirigid intervertebral fixation as a protective technique for pathological adjacent disc. In Proceedings of the International Meeting for Advanced Spine Technologies, Rome, Italy, 10–12 July 2003.
52. Li, J.; Li, Q.; Deng, Z.; Wang, L.; Wang, L.; Song, Y. Long-term Outcome of Isobar TTL System for the Treatment of Lumbar Degenerative Disc Diseases. *Orthop. Surg.* **2024**, *16*, 912–920. [CrossRef]
53. Aygun, H.; Yaray, O.; Mutlu, M. Does the Addition of a Dynamic Pedicle Screw to a Fusion Segment Prevent Adjacent Segment Pathology in the Lumbar Spine? *Asian Spine J.* **2017**, *11*, 715–721. [CrossRef]
54. Meyer, B.; Thomé, C.; Vajkoczy, P.; Kehl, V.; Dodel, R.; Ringel, F.; Dynorfuse Study Group. Lumbar dynamic pedicle-based stabilization versus fusion in degenerative disease: A multicenter, double-blind, prospective, randomized controlled trial. *J. Neurosurg. Spine* **2022**, *37*, 515–524. [CrossRef] [PubMed]
55. Li, J.; Cao, S.; Zhao, B. Biomechanical comparison of polyetheretherketone rods and titanium alloy rods in transforaminal lumbar interbody fusion: A finite element analysis. *BMC Surg.* **2024**, *24*, 169. [CrossRef] [PubMed]
56. Li, C.; Liu, L.; Shi, J.-Y.; Yan, K.-Z.; Shen, W.-Z.; Yang, Z.-R. Clinical and biomechanical researches of polyetheretherketone (PEEK) rods for semi-rigid lumbar fusion: A systematic review. *Neurosurg. Rev.* **2018**, *41*, 375–389. [CrossRef]
57. Li, W.; Zhao, H.; Li, C.; Liu, T.; Guan, J.; Yang, Y.; Yu, X. Polyetheretherketone (PEEK) rods versus titanium rods for posterior lumbar fusion surgery: A systematic review and meta-analysis. *J. Orthop. Surg. Res.* **2023**, *18*, 348. [CrossRef] [PubMed]
58. Wilke, H.-J.; Heuer, F.; Schmidt, H. Prospective design delineation and subsequent in vitro evaluation of a new posterior dynamic stabilization system. *Spine* **2009**, *34*, 255–261. [CrossRef]
59. Angelini, A.; Baracco, R.; Procura, A.; Nena, U.; Ruggieri, P. Lumbar Stabilization with DSS-HPS® System: Radiological Outcomes and Correlation with Adjacent Segment Degeneration. *Diagnostics* **2021**, *11*, 1891. [CrossRef]
60. Sielatycki, J.A.; Devin, C.J.; Pennings, J.; Koscielski, M.; Metcalf, T.; Archer, K.R.; Dunn, R.; Humphreys, S.C.; Hodges, S. A novel lumbar total joint replacement may be an improvement over fusion for degenerative lumbar conditions: A comparative analysis of patient-reported outcomes at one year. *Spine J.* **2021**, *21*, 829–840. [CrossRef]
61. Siskey, R.L.; Yarbrough, R.V.; Spece, H.; Hodges, S.D.; Humphreys, S.C.; Kurtz, S.M. In Vitro Wear of a Novel Vitamin E Crosslinked Polyethylene Lumbar Total Joint Replacement. *Bioengineering* **2023**, *10*, 1198. [CrossRef]

62. Nel, L.J.; Humphreys, S.C.; Sielatycki, J.A.; Block, J.E.; Hodges, S.D. Total joint replacement of the lumbar spine: Report of the first two cases with 16 years of follow-up. *J. Spine Surg.* **2024**, *10*, 583–589. [CrossRef]
63. Malone, J.B.; Bevan, P.J.; Lewis, T.J.; Nelson, A.D.; Blaty, D.E.; Kahan, M.E. Incidence of spinal epidural lipomatosis in patients with spinal stenosis. *J. Orthop.* **2017**, *15*, 36–39. [CrossRef] [PubMed] [PubMed Central]

Journal of
Clinical Medicine

MDPI

Technical Note

Lumbopelvic Fixation: How to Be Less Invasive When You Cannot Be Minimally Invasive—A New Subcutaneous Supra-Fascial Approach to Minimize Open Iliac Screwing

Carlo Brembilla [1,*], Emanuele Stucchi [1,2], Mario De Robertis [1,2], Giorgio Cracchiolo [3], Ali Baram [1], Gabriele Capo [1], Zefferino Rossini [1], Andrea Franzini [1], Marco Riva [1,2], Federico Pessina [1,2] and Maurizio Fornari [1]

1 Department of Neurosurgery, IRCCS Humanitas Research Hospital, Via Alessandro Manzoni 56, 20089 Rozzano, MI, Italy; emanuele.stucchi@humanitas.it (E.S.); mario.derobertis@humanitas.it (M.D.R.); ali.baram@humanitas.it (A.B.); gabriele.capo@humanitas.it (G.C.); zefferino.rossini@humanitas.it (Z.R.); andrea.franzini@humanitas.it (A.F.); federico.pessina@hunimed.eu (F.P.); maurizio.fornari@humanitas.it (M.F.)

2 Department of Biomedical Sciences, Humanitas University, Via Rita Levi Montalcini 4, 20090 Pieve Emanuele, MI, Italy

3 School of Medicine and Surgery, University of Milano-Bicocca, 24127 Bergamo, BG, Italy; g.cracchiolo@campus.unimib.it

* Correspondence: carlo.brembilla@humanitas.it

Abstract: Background/Objectives: Lumbopelvic fixation (LPF) is essential for stabilizing the lumbosacral junction (LSJ) in cases of trauma, tumors, and other pathologies. While minimally invasive percutaneous techniques are preferred when feasible, open LPF remains necessary when direct sacral access is required. This study describes a modified open LPF technique designed to minimize invasiveness while maintaining effective stabilization. **Methods:** We present a case of sacral metastasis requiring LPF. The surgical technique involves a linear midline incision, meticulous subfascial dissection to preserve the Longissimus thoracis and Iliocostalis lumborum muscles, and a subcutaneous suprafascial approach for iliac screw placement guided by intraoperative CT navigation. A U-shaped cross-link is used for final construct stability. The case illustrates the application of this technique in a 56-year-old female patient with metastatic breast carcinoma involving the sacrum, complicated by nerve compression and urinary retention. **Results:** The patient underwent successful LPF with nerve root decompression and partial tumor resection. Postoperatively, she experienced no new neurological deficits and demonstrated progressive improvement in sphincter function. The described surgical approach minimized soft tissue disruption, blood loss, and potential complications associated with more extensive dissection. Six-month follow-up CT scans confirmed the stability of the LPF construct and the residual lesion. **Conclusions:** When open LPF is unavoidable, the described subcutaneous supra-fascial approach for iliac screw placement, combined with muscle preservation and a U-shaped cross-link, offers a less invasive alternative that minimizes soft tissue trauma, reduces potential complications, and facilitates faster patient recovery. This technique can be particularly beneficial in patients with sacral metastases requiring nerve decompression and tumor resection.

Keywords: lumbopelvic fixation; lumbosacral junction; iliac screw fixation; minimally invasive surgery (MIS); sacral metastasis; U-shaped cross-link

1. Introduction

Lumbopelvic fixation (LPF) is a crucial technique for achieving solid construct stability across the lumbosacral junction (LSJ). Indications for LPF include unstable sacral fractures, pseudarthrosis, infections, and tumors at the LSJ, particularly when associated with significant bone loss and/or neurological deficits [1,2]. Biomechanically, LPF is considered superior to other approaches due to its ability to directly transfer vertical loads from the lumbar spine to the iliac bones, effectively bypassing the sacrum. Optimal placement of pelvic screws is critical for LPF success. The ideal entry point for iliac screw placement is located close to the posterior inferior iliac spine, ensuring secure fixation within the dense cortical bone of the ilium [3,4].

Traditional open iliac screw placement techniques can have several drawbacks. Extensive soft tissue dissection for accurate screw placement can increase the risk of tissue devitalization, leading to potential complications such as increased blood loss, prolonged operative times, and a heightened risk of infection [5].

Percutaneous techniques offer a less invasive alternative, allowing for rapid fixation of posterior pelvic or sacral pathologies while minimizing soft tissue disruption. They are particularly well suited for conditions requiring stabilization of the LSJ, such as many traumatic and oncological fractures [6–8]. However, percutaneous approaches are limited in cases requiring direct access to the sacrum for procedures such as nerve decompression, tumor resection, open reduction in sacral fractures, or sacral reconstruction [9].

This paper presents a case of sacral metastases. We describe a refined surgical technique for open LPF, developed to minimize invasiveness while ensuring robust and reliable fixation.

2. Case Presentation

A 56-year-old woman with a history of infiltrating mucinous breast carcinoma and ductal carcinoma in situ (DCIS) underwent right quadrantectomy in 2020, followed by adjuvant radiotherapy and oral Tamoxifen. Subsequent follow-up examinations revealed no evidence of disease recurrence.

In June 2023, she presented with left-sided gluteal pain radiating along the posterior aspect of the ipsilateral thigh. The pain was described as burning, with an initial severity of 8/10 on the Numerical Rating Scale (NRS) [10]. Further investigation with pelvic CT in November 2023 revealed an expansive lesion completely replacing the first three sacral vertebrae, with associated spinal canal invasion. Subsequent sacral spine MRI confirmed a heterogeneous, vascularized lesion measuring approximately 80 × 50 mm. Concurrently, a similar lesion was identified in the right femoral neck. A whole-body 18F-FDG PET/CT scan did not reveal any other sites of significant metabolic activity. Biopsy of the sacral lesion confirmed metastatic involvement from her previous breast carcinoma. Immunohistochemical analysis demonstrated estrogen receptor (ER) positivity, progesterone receptor (PR) negativity, and a Ki67 proliferation index of less than 3%. In January 2024, the patient underwent hypofractionated radiotherapy targeting the sacral and right femoral lesions, delivering a total dose of 46 Gy in 12 daily fractions. Concurrent systemic therapy with Ribociclib and Fulvestrant was initiated. Following radiotherapy, the patient reported a partial reduction in pain intensity to 5/10 on the NRS.

In May 2024, the patient experienced a recurrence and worsening of symptoms. Right-sided gluteal pain, now radiating to the posterior thigh, calf, and lateral foot, emerged, accompanied by tingling paresthesia. Left-sided gluteal pain persisted at a moderate intensity (NRS 8/10). Over the following weeks, she developed urinary symptoms, including urgency, incontinence, and incomplete bladder emptying.

In June 2024, the patient presented to the Emergency Department with acute urinary retention, necessitating the placement of an indwelling urinary catheter. Subsequent MRI (Figure 1A–D) and CT scans confirmed progression of the sacral lesion with significant compression of sacral nerve roots. Based on the clinical and radiological findings, lumbopelvic fixation (LPF) was planned, including nerve root decompression and intralesional resection of the sacral lesion (Figure 1E). The surgical procedure had a total duration of 250 min, with intraoperative blood loss of 180 cc.

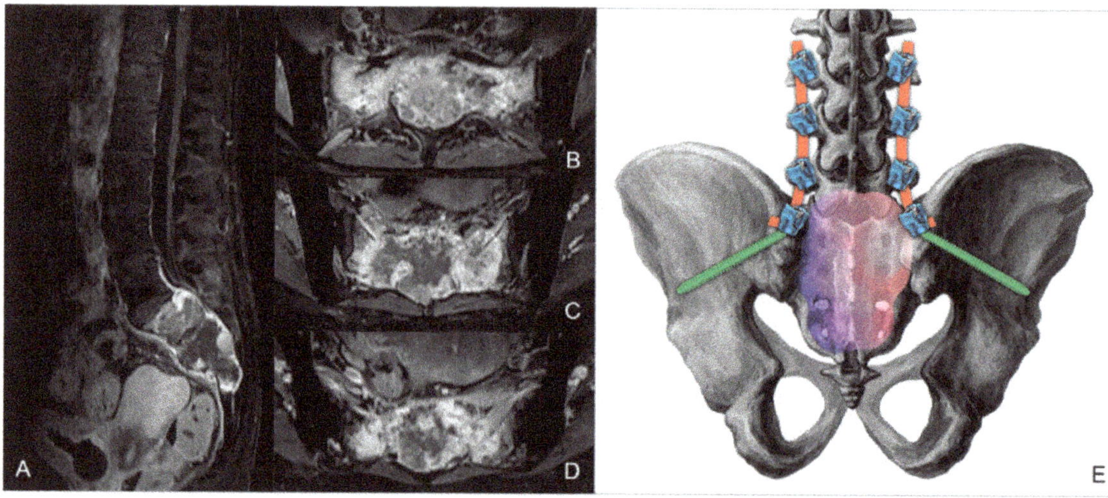

Figure 1. Preoperative MRI of the sacral metastatic lesion, in sagittal (**A**) and axial (**B–D**) planes. (**E**) Three-dimensional reconstruction of the planned LPF, including nerve root decompression and tumor resection.

The postoperative course was uneventful, with no new-onset neurological deficits and progressive restoration of sphincter function. The drains were removed on the second postoperative day, and the patient began ambulating with a lumbar elastic support. The patient was discharged home on the tenth postoperative day with a neurorehabilitation program. At discharge, she was able to perform all activities of daily living (ADL) and was free of urinary catheter, as no active urinary retention was observed at catheterization; her pain level had decreased from 8/10 to 2/10 on the NRS. Histomolecular analysis of the intraoperative tissue revealed metastatic involvement of breast carcinoma with a triple-negative phenotype (ER negative, PR negative, Ki67 1%, HER-2 low − score 1+). Given the systemic disease control achieved with the ongoing treatment despite the triple-negative profile of the lesion, therapy was modified to include Ribociclib and Fulvestrant in combination with Denosumab to manage lytic bone involvement. Six-month-follow-up CT scans demonstrated the stability of the residual lesion and the LPF construct.

3. Surgical Technique

The patient was positioned prone. Intraoperative CT imaging was performed using a Medtronic O-arm™ Navigation System (Littleton, MA, USA). A midline longitudinal skin incision was made from L3 to the sacrum. Subcutaneous dissection exposed the supraspinous ligament between L3 and the sacrum. The thoracolumbar fascia was then dissected bilaterally, extending to the level of the posterior superior iliac spine (PSIS) (Figures 2A,B and 3A). The subcutaneous dissection was extended sufficiently to allow comfortable access to the PSIS for screw placement and was wide enough to permit subsequent retraction of the skin and subcutaneous tissues for the tightening of fixation rods. Standard midline skeletonization was then performed to expose the vertebrae from L3 to the sacrum and identify the lumbar screw entry points. Medial portions of the Longissimus thoracis and Multifidus muscles were carefully disinserted to expose the vertebrae, while preserving the lateral muscle mass for optimal function and minimizing soft tissue trauma. Following frame placement for intraoperative CT navigation, polyaxial screws were inserted into the L3, L4, and L5 vertebral bodies (Figure 4A,B).

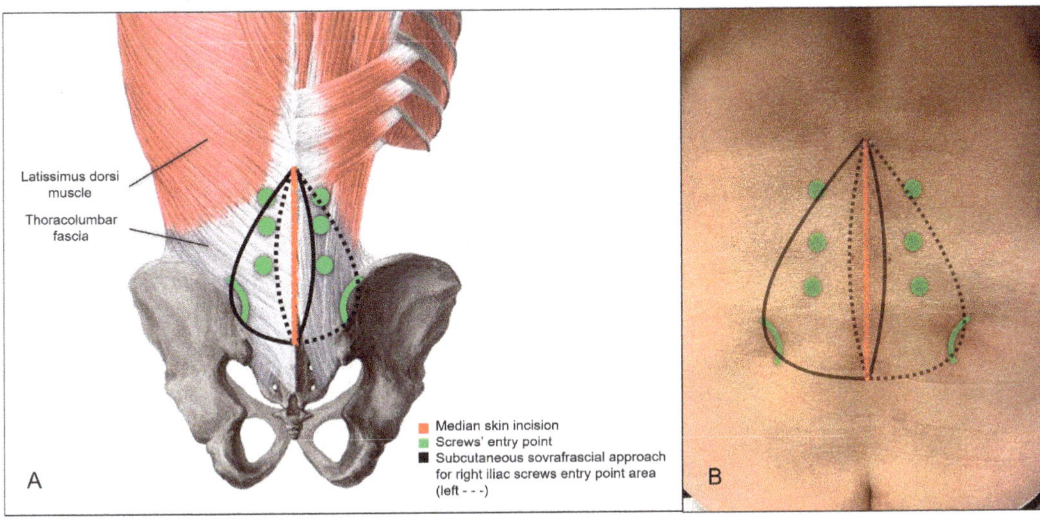

Figure 2. Surgical approach for LPF. (**A**) Illustration of the linear lumbosacral skin incision and the subcutaneous supra-fascial dissection to expose the PSIS. (**B**) Six-month postoperative view of the surgical field, demonstrating the well-healed incision.

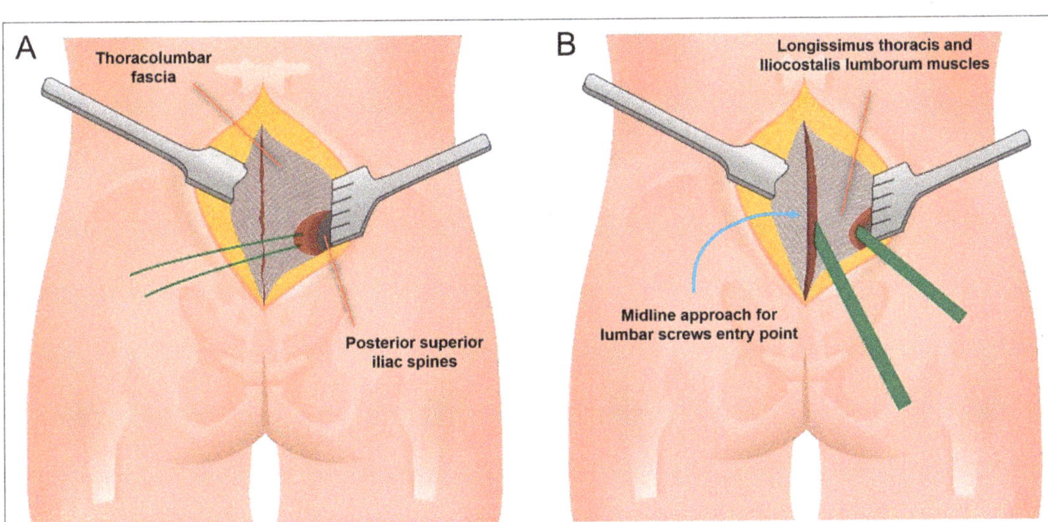

Figure 3. (**A**) Subcutaneous exposure of the thoracolumbar fascia and posterior superior iliac spine (PSIS). (**B**) Creation of the submuscular/subfascial tunnel via digital dissection (digitoclasia), preserving the distal attachments of the Longissimus thoracis, Iliocostalis lumborum, and Multifidus muscles.

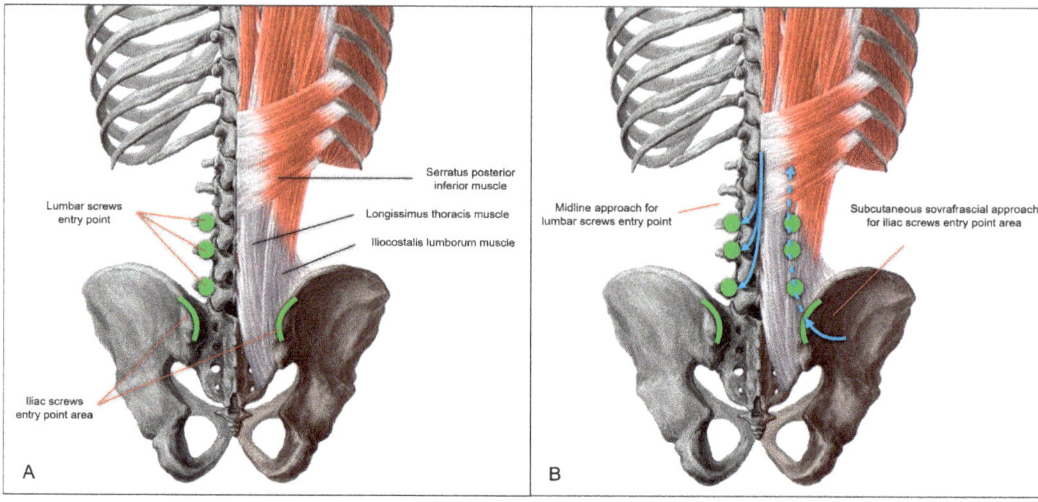

Figure 4. (**A**) Illustration of lumbar and iliac screw entry points. (**B**) Midline approach for lumbar screw entry points (left), and subcutaneous sovrafrascial approach (right) for iliac screw entry point area.

For iliac screw placement, the thoracolumbar fascia was incised along the medial margin of the PSIS bilaterally. A small portion of the Iliocostalis lumborum muscle was dissected to expose the medial margin of the PSIS, creating sufficient space for iliac screw insertion. Two iliac screws were placed per side using the subcutaneous supra-fascial approach (Figure 4A,B). A submuscular/subfascial channel was then created by blunt dissection, connecting the space obtained at the level of the iliac spines to the midline surgical cavity. With their fingers (digitoclasia: digital dissection), the surgeon gently dissected along the bony plane, following the course of the sacroiliac joint (Figures 3B and 5). This digital dissection technique, linking the medial and PSIS surgical fields, is crucial for maintaining the integrity of the distal attachments of the Longissimus thoracis and the majority of the Iliocostalis lumborum and the Multifidus muscles, thereby minimizing muscular trauma. Pre-contoured rods with appropriate lordosis were then inserted through the medial surgical cavity, passed beneath the previously created submuscular/subfascial tunnel, and positioned in the tulips of the iliac screws. In this case, the rods were connected to the iliac screw tulips using dedicated connector. The previous creation of adequate subcutaneous space is paramount for successful rod placement, as it allows for sufficient retraction of the superficial soft tissues and prevents compression or impingement. The rods were secondarily secured within the tulips of the lumbar screws, for easer manipulation through the median approach.

A sacral laminectomy was then performed. The spinal canal was found to be occupied by the tumor, compressing the cauda equina nerve roots. Careful debulking of the sacral tumor was performed to decompress the nerve roots (subtotal resection—STR). A U-shaped cross-link, crafted from a 5.5 mm diameter rod, was finally placed between the rods through the midline approach and secured with dedicated connectors. At the end of the procedure, the fixation system demonstrated stability, and the nerve roots were adequately decompressed (Figure 6A–D). Lumbopelvic fixation was achieved using polyaxial titanium alloy screws from the Cortical Fix Expedium Spinal System (DePuy Synthes, LLC, a Johnson & Johnson Company, New Brunswick, NJ, USA).

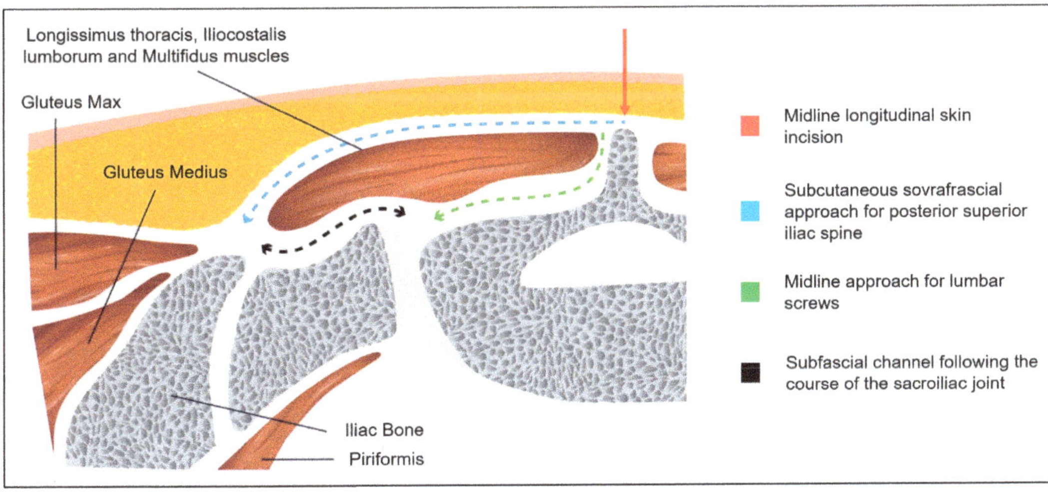

Figure 5. Cross-sectional view at the S1 level: (red) midline longitudinal skin incision; (blue) subcutaneous supra-fascial approach for PSIS; (green) midline approach for lumbar screws; (black) subfascial/submuscular channel for rod insertion.

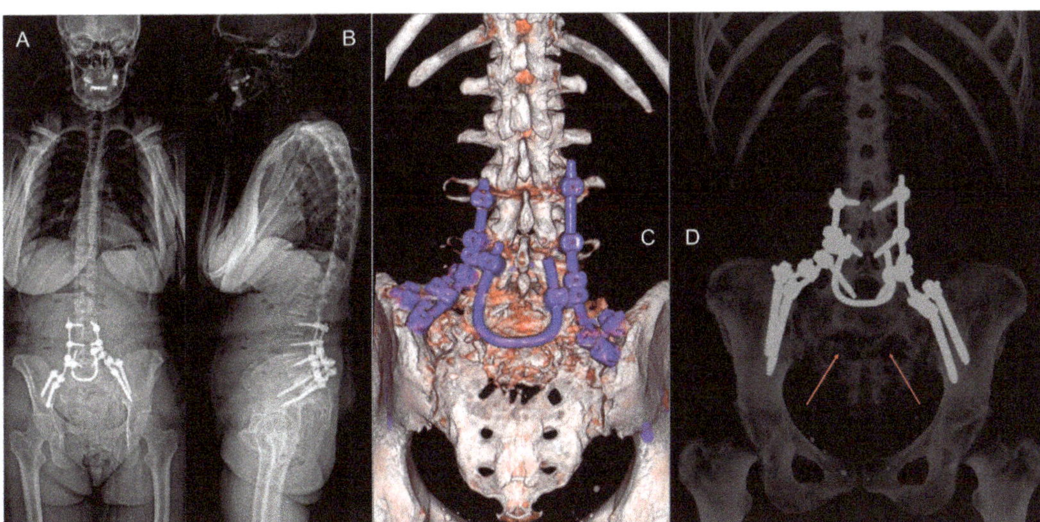

Figure 6. (**A**,**B**) Post-operative standing X-ray. (**C**,**D**) Six-month 3D CT scan reconstruction demonstrating the stability of the LPF and the residual sacral defect (red arrows).

During closure, the thoracolumbar fascia was meticulously sutured at the level of the PSIS, and the supraspinous ligament too. Two drains were placed: one in the midline subfascial surgical cavity and one in the subcutaneous layer.

4. Discussion

LSJ pathologies present a complex surgical challenge due to the unique anatomical and biomechanical characteristics of this transitional zone between the mobile spine and the relatively fixed pelvis. The inherent biomechanics of the LSJ, coupled with the destructive nature of pathological processes affecting the sacrum, create a significant challenge for spinal stabilization. LPF is a cornerstone of LSJ stabilization, leveraging the human pelvis as a stable anchor point. While various implants have been used over the years, iliac screw fixation has become increasingly prominent due to its demonstrated ability to prevent LPF failure and sacral fractures [3,11,12].

Open LPF is a major procedure. The extensive muscle and soft tissue dissection required for accurate iliac screw insertion can increase the risk of tissue devitalization, leading to increased blood loss, prolonged operative times, and infection. Percutaneous approaches, often guided by intraoperative CT navigation or robotic assistance, aim to mitigate these risks and allow for rapid LPF [8,12,13]. These minimally invasive techniques are limited when direct access to the sacrum is necessary for procedures such as nerve decompression, tumor resection, open reduction in sacral fractures, or sacral reconstruction.

The S2-alar-iliac (S2AI) screw has recently gained significant popularity as it provides similar biomechanical fixation without the extensive tissue dissection associated with traditional iliac screws [14]. Highly destructive lesions of the sacral spine, however, may preclude S2AI instrumentation [15].

In our experience, we have prioritized minimizing invasiveness even in open LPF procedures requiring sacral access. Linear skin incision is less problematic than U-shaped or inverted Y-shaped (Mercedes star) incisions. The sacral region is prone to pressure sores postoperatively, especially given that patients rest in the supine position. Extensive dissection can make early mobilization difficult. A single linear incision helps maintain better vascularization of the soft tissues, reducing the risk of necrosis and infection [16].

Maintaining a functionally intact muscle plane is crucial. Preserving the Longissimus thoracis and Iliocostalis lumborum muscles maintains the functionality and support of the posterior paravertebral muscle compartment. Dissection between the subcutaneous plane and the muscle fascia allows easy access to the PSIS. While the minimal detachment of the Longissimus thoracis muscle provides sufficient access for iliac screw placement, precise screw placement within this limited exposure is critically dependent on intraoperative CT navigation due to the lack of anatomical landmarks. Following screw placement, the supraperiosteal space needed for rod placement between the Longissimus muscle and the sacroiliac region can be easily created with smooth dissection.

In pathologies requiring open sacral access for partial or total sacrectomy and LSJ reconstruction, the resulting cavity from bone resection presents a challenge [9,17,18]. Preserving the Longissimus thoracis and Iliocostalis lumborum muscles helps maintain a separation between the cavity and the external surface, supporting the overlying subcutaneous tissues and skin. For final LPF construct torsional stability, the cross-link is essential. This additional stability is crucial for minimizing micromotion at the LSJ, promoting bone fusion, and reducing the risk of implant failure. The recent literature has highlighted the strength and resistance of U-shaped cross-links in LSJ constructs [19,20], among other solutions. Moreover, in our experience, the U-shaped cross-link also acts as a support for the overlying tissues (muscle, subcutaneous tissue, and skin), minimizing tissue depression above the surgical cavity.

These minimally invasive surgical techniques have, in our experience, resulted in reduced blood loss, less tissue necrosis, and lower risk of infection, facilitating faster patient mobilization and reducing the risk of pressure sores.

This surgical technique is the result of years of clinical expertise gained by our team in the treatment of traumatic sacral fractures. Starting from a traditional open approach, we have progressively developed a refined method that maintains the strength of fixation while significantly reducing invasiveness. This article presents a single clinical case, which inherently limits the generalizability of our findings and the ability to definitively assess the overall effectiveness and safety of the described technique. While the presented case demonstrates the successful application of the method in a specific clinical scenario, it cannot provide statistically significant evidence of efficacy or identify any potential complications that may arise in a larger patient population, including the risk of infection, implant loosening, and neurological complications. Specifically, this case report cannot establish the technique's applicability to other patient populations with varying comorbidities, disease severity, or anatomical variations. Furthermore, the absence of a control group limits our ability to compare the outcomes of this technique with those of traditional open or minimally invasive approaches. Finally, the short-term follow-up period in this case report precludes the assessment of long-term outcomes, such as implant stability, pain relief durability, and the potential for late complications.

5. Conclusions

LPF provides excellent stability for LSJ pathologies. Percutaneous or robotic-assisted methods offer the least invasive approach when feasible. However, these techniques are not always applicable, particularly in cases of traumatic and, especially, oncological pathologies requiring sacral access. In such cases, the described subcutaneous supra-fascial approach for iliac screw placement, combined with the use of a U-shaped cross-link, represents, in our experience, a surgical technique that minimizes the major drawbacks of open LPF, including hemorrhage, tissue necrosis, prolonged recovery, pressure sores, and infection.

Author Contributions: C.B. and E.S. conceived of the presented idea, and wrote the main manuscript text. M.D.R., G.C. (Giorgio Cracchiolo), A.B., G.C. (Gabriele Capo), Z.R. and A.F. collected the data, and prepared the figures. All authors discussed the design and contributed to the final manuscript. C.B., M.R., F.P. and M.F. supervised the project. All authors have read and agreed to the published version of the manuscript.

Funding: The publication fee for this work was covered by the Italian Ministry of Health's "Ricerca Corrente" funding to the IRCCS Humanitas Research Hospital. This research received no other external funding.

Institutional Review Board Statement: The ethical review and approval were waived for this study because it involves procedures considered standard clinical practice and routinely performed at our institution. These procedures are part of the established treatment protocols. The decision to use these techniques was made solely based on clinical judgement and patient needs, independent of study inclusion. No modifications to standard care were made for research purposes.

Informed Consent Statement: Informed consent was obtained from the subject involved in the study.

Data Availability Statement: We excluded the data availability section since our study did not report on any data present in public datasets.

Acknowledgments: The authors gratefully acknowledge Kenhub (Kenhub Image License Store) for providing the anatomical images that were adapted and modified for use in Figures 1, 2 and 4 of this manuscript. A scientific license was obtained for these images. I would also like to acknowledge Olena Kogrusheva for creating Figures 3 and 5 featured in this article.

Conflicts of Interest: The authors declare no conflicts of interest.

References

1. Jones, C.B.; Sietsema, D.L.; Hoffmann, M.F. Can lumbopelvic fixation salvage unstable complex sacral fractures? *Clin. Orthop. Relat. Res.* **2012**, *470*, 2132–2141. [CrossRef] [PubMed] [PubMed Central]
2. Suk, S.I.; Chung, E.R.; Lee, S.M.; Lee, J.H.; Kim, S.S.; Kim, J.H. Posterior vertebral column resection in fixed lumbosacral deformity. *Spine* **2005**, *30*, E703–E710. [CrossRef] [PubMed]
3. Jain, A.; Hassanzadeh, H.; Strike, S.A.; Menga, E.N.; Sponseller, P.D.; Kebaish, K.M. Pelvic Fixation in Adult and Pediatric Spine Surgery: Historical Perspective, Indications, and Techniques: AAOS Exhibit Selection. *J. Bone Jt. Surg. Am.* **2015**, *97*, 1521–1528. [CrossRef] [PubMed]

vertebral bodies, with further imaging with computed tomography (CT) and magnetic resonance imaging (MRI) recommended for preoperative planning [5].

Surgical treatment is the only definitive method to decompress the spinal canal and can be achieved via anterior or posterior approaches to the cervical spine. Anterior decompression often involves corpectomy followed by direct removal of the pathology or the floating technique, while the posterior approach typically involves indirect decompression through laminoplasty or laminectomy with fusion [6,7]. Open-door laminoplasty, an indirect decompression technique, expands the dimensions and area of the spinal canal by freeing the laminae on one side and securing them in a more posterior position. Numerous studies have reported sufficient decompression and neurological recovery following laminoplasty [8,9].

Additionally, some reports suggest the radiological effectiveness of surgical decompression and subsequent neurological recovery, as measured by the spinal canal dimensions and the percentage of occupancy after the procedure [10,11]. However, few studies have analyzed the relationships between increased spinal canal area and various clinical symptoms, including not only neurological recovery but also axial or radicular pain.

This study aimed to measure and compare the bony canal area, spinal canal area, and OPLL before and after multilevel open-door laminoplasty in patients with cervical OPLL and myelopathy and to determine the relationships between these radiologic measurements and clinical outcomes.

2. Materials and Methods

This retrospective study included 36 patients who underwent surgery for cervical myelopathy due to OPLL between 2009 and 2021. The inclusion criteria were as follows: myelopathy associated with multilevel OPLL (involving two or more cervical levels), absence of cervical kyphosis, absence of dynamic instability, and a minimum follow-up period of more than two years post-surgery. Myelopathy symptoms included hand numbness, loss of fine motor function, bilateral paresthesia, impaired gait, lower extremity weakness, and urinary or fecal urgency and incontinence [12]. Exclusion criteria included myelopathy caused by cervical disc herniation or spondylosis, cervical kyphosis, previous cervical surgery, spine trauma, tumor, infection, or incomplete medical and radiographic records. All patients underwent a single surgical procedure and received conservative postoperative treatment, including pain management medication. This study was ethically approved by the institutional review board (KC21RISI0093).

2.1. Surgical Procedure

After general anesthesia and prone positioning, a posterior cervical approach was performed. The paravertebral muscles were detached from the spinous processes on both sides of the affected level. Once the spinous process and laminae were exposed, a high-speed burr was used to cut through one side of the lamina on the opening side and partially through the other side, preserving one cortex on the hinge side as part of the open-door laminoplasty technique [9]. A Medtronic mini-plate (Centerpiece, Medtronic, Minneapolis, MN, USA) was then applied and secured with one screw on the medial lamina and two screws on the lateral mass. Plates ranging in length from 10 mm to 12 mm were used. Previous studies have demonstrated that C3 laminectomy, when combined with multilevel open-door laminoplasty for OPLL, can effectively reduce postoperative axial neck pain [13,14]. C3 laminectomy offers distinct advantages over C3 laminoplasty: prevention of C2–3 bone fusion and preservation of posterior cervical musculature attachments [15]. Based on this evidence, our institution has implemented C3 laminectomy in conjunction with multilevel open-door laminoplasty as a standard surgical protocol since 2018. Intraoperative neuromonitoring with transcranial motor-evoked and somatosensory-evoked potentials was utilized during the surgery.

2.2. Radiologic Parameters

Cervical spine anteroposterior and lateral views, along with CT scans obtained before and after surgery, were analyzed. Radiographic measurements of cervical lordosis (CL) and cervical sagittal vertical axis (CSVA) were performed on neutral lateral views. CL was measured using the inferior endplate of C2 as the superior reference and the inferior endplate of C7 as the inferior reference. CSVA was determined by measuring the distance between a plumb line dropped from the center of the C2 body and the posterior superior corner of C7 [16].

Radiographic measurements of cross-sectional areas of the bony canal and the spinal canal were performed by two independent observers, similar to the methodology used by Dong et al. [10]. The bony canal area (BCA) was delineated by the posterior border of the vertebral body, pedicles, and the union of both laminae. After surgery, the plate replaced the posterior border of the operated laminae. If one or both pedicles were not visible on the CT scan, the posterior margin of the nerve root was used as the border. The entire external border of the OPLL was delineated, and the area was measured. The spinal canal area (SCA) was defined anteriorly by the posterior margin of the PLL or OPLL and posteriorly by the inner margin of the ligamentum flavum (Figure 1). BCA, SCA, and the cross-sectional area of the OPLL were measured at all levels before surgery and two years after surgery.

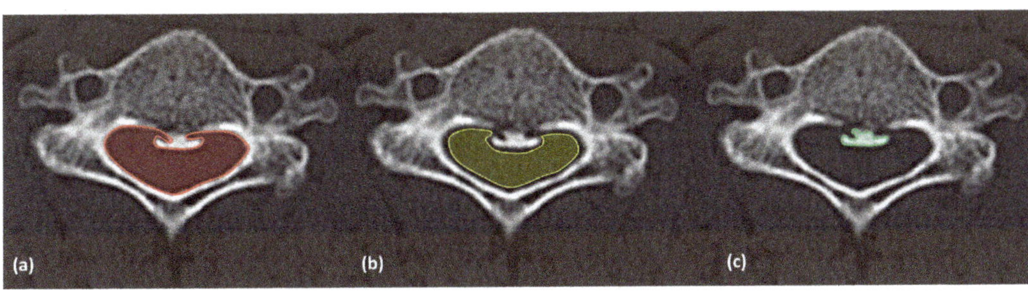

Figure 1. (**a**) Bony Canal Area (BCA) in red, defined by the posterior edge of the vertebral body, the pedicles, and the union of the laminae. (**b**) Spinal Canal Area (SCA) in yellow, bounded anteriorly by the posterior limit of the posterior longitudinal ligament (PLL) or ossification of the posterior longitudinal ligament (OPLL) and posteriorly by the inner edge of the ligamentum flavum. (**c**) OPLL in green, showing the outer boundary of the ossified posterior longitudinal ligament.

2.3. Clinical Parameters

Clinical outcomes were evaluated using the Numerical Rating Scale (NRS) for neck pain (NRS-neck) and radicular pain in the right and left arms (NRS-right arm [NRS-R] and NRS-left arm [NRS-L]), the Neck Disability Index (NDI), and the Japanese Orthopaedic Association (JOA) score. These parameters were assessed preoperatively and two years postoperatively [17,18]. Patients were stratified according to their JOA scores; those with scores ≤ 11 were categorized as severe myelopathy, whereas those with scores ≥ 12 were classified as mild to moderate myelopathy [19]. Because postoperative neck pain has been reported as the most significant difference between C3 laminectomy and laminoplasty, the NRS-neck scores were compared between the C3 laminectomy group and the laminoplasty group through subgroup analysis [15].

2.4. Statistical Analysis

Statistical analyses were conducted using SPSS software version 24.0.0 (SPSS Inc., Chicago, IL, USA). A p-value of less than 0.05 was considered statistically significant. For the comparison of paired data, either the paired t-test or the Wilcoxon signed-rank test was used, depending on the normality of the data distribution. Pearson's correlation analysis was performed to evaluate the relationships between clinical outcomes and radiologic measurements. To assess the intra-observer reproducibility and inter-observer reliability of BCA and SCA, an agreement was quantified using the intraclass correlation coefficient (ICC). Two independent researchers (an orthopedic spine surgeon with 1 year of experience and an orthopedic resident with 3 years of experience) performed two series of BCA and SCA measurements on the CT scans.

3. Results

Of the 36 patients, 11 were female and 25 were male, with an average age of 64.06 years (range: 41–81 years). No perioperative complications related to the surgery were reported. OPLL was observed in all 36 patients at the C5–6 level, followed by C4–5 (91.7%), C3–4 (69.4%), and C6–7 (58.3%) (Table 1). All patients underwent decompression surgery from C3 to C6, with 15 patients receiving laminoplasty at C3 and 21 patients undergoing C3 laminectomy. The surgeries were performed by two experienced surgeons using the same standardized technique, as described in the surgical technique section.

Table 1. Distribution of OPLL in included patients.

Segment	Number (Percentage)
C1–2	3 (8.3%)
C2–3	16 (44.4%)
C3–4	25 (69.4%)
C4–5	33 (91.7%)
C5–6	36 (100.0%)
C6–7	21 (58.3%)
C7-T1	8 (22.2%)

3.1. Radiologic Outcomes

In the analysis of cervical alignment before and after surgery, CL significantly decreased from 15.54 ± 8.99 degrees to 12.49 ± 6.93 degrees (p = 0.005). CSVA changed from 22.12 ± 11.11 mm to 23.89 ± 10.80 mm, although this change was not statistically significant (p = 0.341). The results of cross-sectional area measurements of the BCA, SCA, and OPLL are presented in Table 2. Both BCA and SCA showed significant increases after surgery at all levels (Figure 2). The average BCA across all levels increased from 239.12 ± 29.48 mm^2 to 351.19 ± 39.51 mm^2, representing a change of 112.07 mm^2 (46.87%). Similarly, the average SCA increased from 157.35 ± 32.13 mm^2 to 257.85 ± 44.19 mm^2, with a change of 100.50 mm^2 (63.87%).

Table 2. Radiologic parameters before and after open-door laminoplasty.

		Preoperative	Postoperative	Rate of Change	p-Value
CL (°)		15.54 ± 8.99	12.49 ± 6.93	−19.60%	**0.005**
CSVA (mm)		22.12 ± 11.11	23.89 ± 10.80	8.01%	0.341
C3 (mm^2) *	BCA	226.33 ± 24.40	317.80 ± 25.96	40.41%	**0.001**
	SCA	150.67 ± 39.47	225.00 ± 48.64	49.34%	**0.001**
	OPLL	29.47 ± 27.42	30.47 ± 28.39	3.39%	0.198
C4 (mm^2)	BCA	233.27 ± 34.72	341.58 ± 38.80	46.43%	**0.000**
	SCA	147.12 ± 36.92	248.79 ± 55.67	69.10%	**0.000**
	OPLL	31.82 ± 25.30	30.48 ± 23.72	−4.19%	**0.014**
C5 (mm^2)	BCA	241.77 ± 36.51	354.77 ± 49.50	46.74%	**0.000**
	SCA	161.66 ± 38.20	262.97 ± 46.18	62.67%	**0.000**
	OPLL	29.17 ± 17.76	29.17 ± 16.88	0.59%	0.827

Table 2. *Cont.*

		Preoperative	Postoperative	Rate of Change	*p*-Value
C6 (mm^2)	BCA	246.14 ± 33.90	367.89 ± 54.04	49.46%	**0.000**
	SCA	167.31 ± 42.02	276.31 ± 54.54	65.12%	**0.000**
	OPLL	27.26 ± 17.46	26.60 ± 17.00	−2.41%	0.190
Average (mm^2)	BCA	239.12 ± 29.48	351.19 ± 39.51	46.87%	**0.000**
	SCA	157.35 ± 32.13	257.85 ± 44.19	63.87%	**0.000**
	OPLL	29.95 ± 15.99	29.53 ± 15.73	−1.41%	0.246

Note: CL—cervical lordosis, CSVA—cervical sagittal vertical axis, BCA—bony canal area, SCA—spinal canal area, OPLL—ossified posterior longitudinal ligament. * 15 patients undergoing C3 laminoplasty except C3 laminectomy. Statistically significant values in bold.

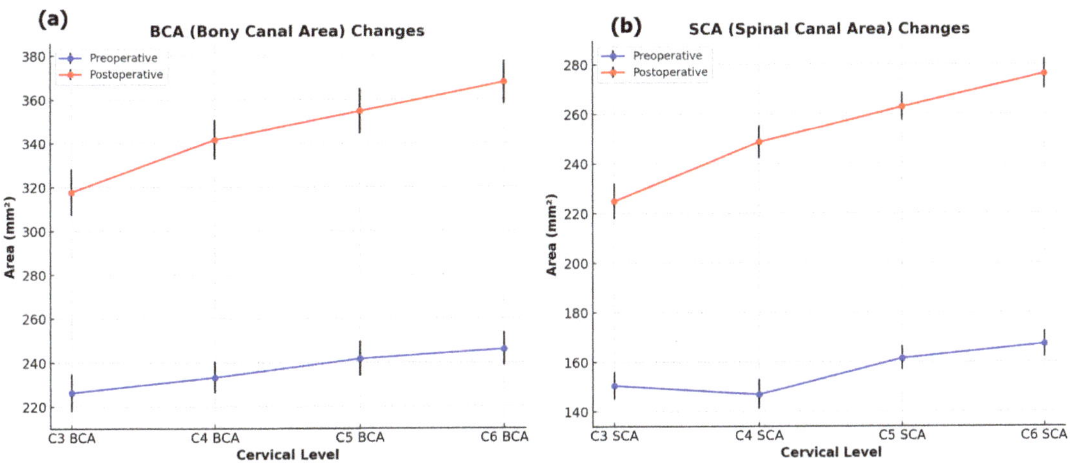

Figure 2. (**a**) Changes in the bony canal area (BCA) preoperatively and postoperatively. (**b**) Changes in the spinal canal area (SCA) preoperatively and postoperatively.

The inter-observer and intra-observer ICC for the measurement of BCA and SCA were above 0.9, ranging from 0.936 to 0.961, indicating excellent intra-observer reproducibility and inter-observer reliability (Table 3).

Table 3. Inter-class correlation coefficient for bony canal area and spinal canal area measurements.

	Inter-ICC	95%CI	Intra-ICC	95%CI
BCA	0.936	0.909–0.956	0.948	0.912–0.962
SCA	0.961	0.942–0.973	0.956	0.919–0.971

Note: BCA—bony canal area, SCA—spinal canal area, ICC—inter-class correlation coefficient.

3.2. Clinical Outcomes

In the analysis of clinical outcomes before and two years after surgery, the JOA score improved from 11.97 ± 3.54 to 12.30 ± 3.52, and the NDI improved from 28.63 ± 21.44 to 23.07 ± 20.39, although these improvements were not statistically significant (p = 0.587 and p = 0.179, respectively). NRS-neck, NRS-R, and NRS-L scores also showed improvements, although these improvements were not statistically significant (Table 4). According to the surgical method, the degree of NRS-neck improvement was compared between the C3 laminoplasty group (n = 15) and the C3 laminectomy group (n = 21). No significant difference was found between the two groups (0.52 ± 3.50 vs. 1.14 ± 3.25, p = 0.804).

Table 4. Clinical outcomes before and after open-door laminoplasty.

	Preoperative	Postoperative	*p*-Value
JOA	11.97 ± 3.54	12.30 ± 3.52	0.587
NDI	28.63 ± 21.44	23.07 ± 20.39	0.179
NRS-neck	3.94 ± 2.65	2.97 ± 2.91	0.051
NRS-R	3.97 ± 3.07	3.53 ± 3.58	0.493
NRS-L	3.38 ± 3.16	3.25 ± 3.57	0.852

Note: JOA—Japanese orthopedic association score, NDI—neck disability index, NRS-neck—numeric rating scale of neck pain, NRS-R—numeric rating scale of right arm pain, NRS-L—numeric rating scale of left arm pain.

Clinical outcomes were further analyzed by classifying patients according to the severity of myelopathy using the JOA score (JOA score of 11 or less = severe; JOA score of 12 or more = mild to moderate) (Table 5). In the severe group, the JOA score significantly improved from 8.33 ± 2.23 to 10.83 ± 3.69 after surgery ($p = 0.009$). In contrast, in the mild to moderate group, NDI ($p = 0.010$), NRS-neck ($p = 0.047$), and NRS-R ($p = 0.038$) scores showed significant improvements (Figure 3).

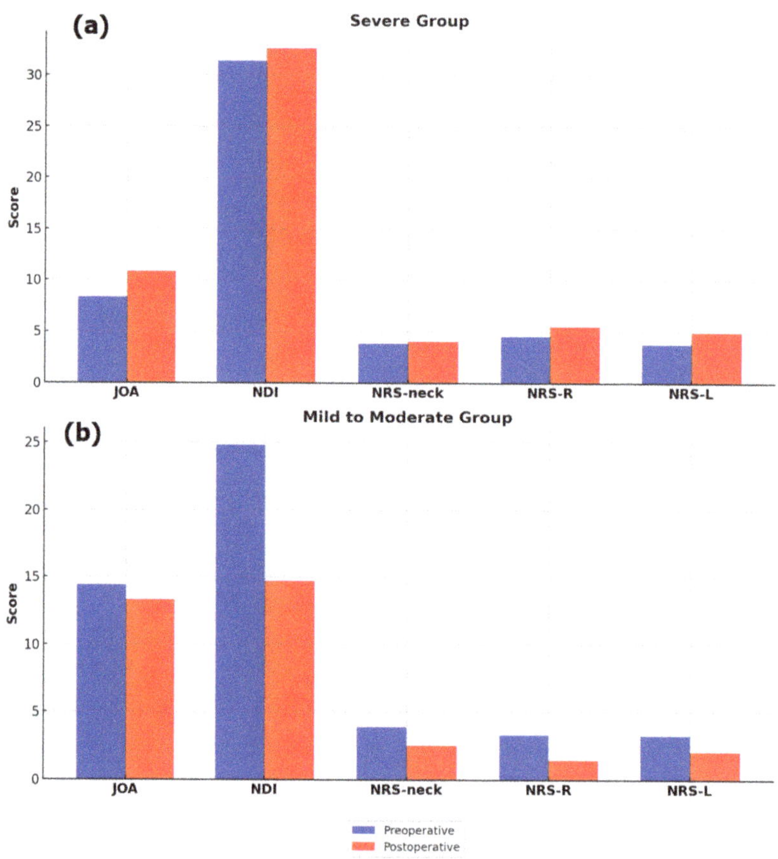

Figure 3. (**a**) Changes in clinical metrics, including JOA score, NDI, NRS-neck, NRS-R, and NRS-L, preoperatively and postoperatively in the severe group. (**b**) Changes in the same clinical metrics preoperatively and postoperatively in the mild to moderate group.

Table 5. Clinical outcomes before and after surgery according to severity of myelopathy.

	Severity *	Preoperative	Postoperative	p-Value
JOA	Severe (n = 14)	8.33 ± 2.23	10.83 ± 3.69	**0.009**
	mild to moderate (n = 22)	14.39 ± 1.61	13.28 ± 3.14	0.161
NDI	Severe (n = 14)	31.33 ± 20.50	32.55 ± 23.71	0.582
	mild to moderate (n = 22)	24.81 ± 20.32	14.65 ± 12.22	**0.010**
NRS-neck	Severe (n = 14)	3.83 ± 2.79	4.00 ± 3.54	0.693
	mild to moderate (n = 22)	3.89 ± 2.54	2.50 ± 2.56	**0.047**
NRS-R	Severe (n = 14)	4.50 ± 3.12	5.50 ± 3.80	0.248
	mild to moderate (n = 22)	3.31 ± 2.44	1.43 ± 1.97	**0.038**
NRS-L	Severe (n = 14)	3.75 ± 3.31	4.92 ± 4.36	0.421
	mild to moderate (n = 22)	3.25 ± 2.98	2.06 ± 2.62	0.211

Note: JOA—Japanese orthopedic association score, NDI—neck disability index, NRS-neck—numeric rating scale of neck pain, NRS-R—numeric rating scale of right arm pain, NRS-L—numeric rating scale of left arm pain. * A JOA score of 11 or less was classified as severe, and a score of 12 or more was classified as mild to moderate. Statistically significant values in bold.

3.3. Correlations Between Radiologic and Clinical Outcomes

The correlation between radiological canal expansions and clinical outcomes is presented in Table 6. Improvement of NRS-neck showed significant correlations with expansions of both BCA (r = 0.533, p = 0.001) and SCA (r = 0.537, p = 0.001). Improvement in NDI also showed a significant correlation with BCA expansion (r = 0.351, p = 0.045). However, improvement in JOA scores showed no significant correlation with the expansion of BCA or SCA (p = 0.265 and 0.292, respectively). Similarly, NRS-R and NRS-L were not associated with canal expansion (all p-values > 0.05).

Table 6. Correlations between radiologic changes and clinical outcomes.

	Variables	Pearson's Correlation Coefficient	p-Value
ΔJOA	ΔBCA	−0.210	0.265
	ΔSCA	−0.199	0.292
	Preoperative OPLL	0.038	0.842
	ΔCL	0.254	0.176
	ΔCSVA	−0.003	0.989
ΔNDI	ΔBCA	0.351	**0.045**
	ΔSCA	0.279	0.116
	Preoperative OPLL	−0.089	0.623
	ΔCL	−0.018	0.921
	ΔCSVA	0.009	0.962
ΔNRS-neck	ΔBCA	0.533	**0.001**
	ΔSCA	0.537	**0.001**
	Preoperative OPLL	−0.077	0.667
	ΔCL	−0.074	0.677
	ΔCSVA	−0.089	0.617

Table 6. *Cont.*

	Variables	Pearson's Correlation Coefficient	*p*-Value
ΔNRS-R	ΔBCA	−0.002	0.990
	ΔSCA	−0.070	0.699
	Preoperative OPLL	−0.048	0.789
	ΔCL	0.058	0.748
	ΔCSVA	0.170	0.344
ΔNRS-L	ΔBCA	−0.114	0.526
	ΔSCA	−0.187	0.297
	Preoperative OPLL	0.055	0.761
	ΔCL	0.267	0.133
	ΔCSVA	0.186	0.301

Note: JOA—Japanese orthopedic association score, NDI—neck disability index, NRS-neck—numeric rating scale of neck pain, NRS-R—numeric rating scale of right arm pain, NRS-L—numeric rating scale of left arm pain, BCA—bony canal area, SCA—spinal canal area, OPLL—ossification of posterior longitudinal ligament, CL—cervical lordosis, CSVA—cervical sagittal vertical axis. Statistically significant values in bold.

4. Discussion

Management strategies for OPLL vary according to symptom severity; asymptomatic or mildly symptomatic patients can be managed conservatively, whereas patients with neurological manifestations typically require surgical decompression through anterior, posterior, or combined approaches [1,20]. Among the various surgical options, open-door laminoplasty has demonstrated efficacy in treating OPLL-associated cervical myelopathy when appropriate patient selection criteria are met [21–23]. Recent advances have introduced minimally invasive open-door laminoplasty techniques, which have shown superior outcomes in reducing postoperative axial symptoms compared to conventional expansive open-door laminoplasty [24]. The present study validates these findings while investigating the correlations between clinical symptom recovery (including axial neck pain, radiculopathy, and myelopathy), the extent of spinal canal decompression, and alterations in cervical sagittal alignment.

In the analysis of radiologic outcomes, cervical lordosis was reduced before and after surgery. This reduction in lordosis has also been observed in previous studies [21,25,26]. It is thought to be related to the detachment of cervical extensor muscles attached to the spinous process and resection of the interspinous ligament during surgery [27]. A recent study reported that risk factors for decreased cervical lordosis after laminoplasty differ between cervical spondylotic myelopathy and OPLL. Preoperative CSVA was identified as an independent risk factor in OPLL patients, suggesting that greater preoperative CSVA should be carefully considered in these cases [28].

Studies on the size and compression of the cervical spinal canal have been conducted. Lee et al. [29] measured the spinal canal diameter from C3 to C7 in 469 cadavers and reported a range of 9 to 20.9 mm, with a median diameter of 14.4 mm. The Torg–Pavlov ratio, one of the most common methods, compared the sagittal diameter of the spinal canal with the width of the vertebral body [30]. More recently, direct measurements of bony and spinal canal areas using CT scans have been reported by Dong et al. [10]. They described the volume-occupying rate of the spinal canal by obtaining the area through direct measurement and then used an integration formula to calculate the volume-occupying rate. They concluded that the volume-occupying rate had a significantly higher correlation with JOA scores than the sagittal diameter of the secondary cervical spinal canal and the effective cervical spinal canal ratio.

However, specific studies focused on the relationship between the spinal canal and OPLL are lacking [11,31]. Wang et al. [31] measured the amount of SCA expansion in 82 patients with cervical myelopathy after open-door laminoplasty and found an increase of 123.01 ± 17.06 mm^2. Park et al. [11] have described a bony spinal canal dimension that increased from 204.3 to 331.7 mm^2 after a single open-door laminoplasty. Similarly, in our study, the average BCA increased from 239.12 mm^2 to 351.19 mm^2 (46.9%), and the average SCA increased from 157.35 mm^2 to 257.85 mm^2 (63.9%).

Neurologically, conservative management is generally indicated for patients maintaining JOA scores ≥ 15, with most spine surgeons considering JOA scores of 12–13 as the surgical intervention threshold [32]. While overall cohort analysis revealed no significant differences in pre- and postoperative JOA scores, stratified analysis by myelopathy severity demonstrated significant postoperative improvement in the severe group (8.33 vs. 10.83, $p < 0.05$) but not in the mild-to-moderate group. Similarly, initial analysis of the entire cohort showed no significant differences in NDI, NRS-neck, NRS-R, and NRS-L scores between pre- and postoperative states. However, subgroup analysis revealed significant improvements in NDI (31.33 vs. 32.55, $p < 0.05$) and NRS-neck scores (3.89 vs. 2.50, $p < 0.05$) within the mild-to-moderate group. These findings suggest two important clinical implications. First, clinical outcomes following surgical intervention for OPLL appear to be dependent on preoperative myelopathy severity. Second, contrary to previous reports suggesting axial neck pain as a potential complication of open-door laminoplasty in cervical myelopathy [33,34], our findings demonstrate improvements in both NDI and NRS-neck scores postoperatively.

Although OPLL patients may initially present as asymptomatic, they frequently experience axial neck pain or radicular symptoms prior to developing myelopathic manifestations [35]. During early-stage myelopathy, clinical deterioration may be more readily detected through NRS or NDI scores rather than JOA scores, which are more specific to myelopathy. Meanwhile, neurological recovery has been identified as an independent factor significantly associated with the reduction in postoperative neck pain in patients with cervical myelopathy due to OPLL who underwent cervical spine surgery [36]. Additionally, recent studies suggest that axial neck pain does not necessarily worsen after laminoplasty when appropriate patient selection and surgical techniques are applied [37,38].

These results were consistent with the observed relationship between radiologic and clinical outcomes. The degree of BCA expansion was found to be related to improvements in neck pain, as reflected by NDI and NRS-neck scores. In contrast, myelopathy symptoms, as represented by JOA scores, did not show a significant correlation with canal expansion. Consequently, canal expansion appears to be more closely associated with neck pain than with neurological symptoms.

Previous studies investigating French-door laminoplasty in degenerative cervical myelopathy have reported that insufficient spinal cord expansion following adequate decompression may predict suboptimal neurological recovery [39]. However, evidence explaining the relationship between spinal canal expansion and the improvement of clinical outcomes remains limited. Our findings suggest that alleviation of spinal canal compression may primarily contribute to the improvement of early myelopathic symptoms, particularly neck pain and functional disability. The lack of significant correlation between JOA scores and canal expansion in our study may be attributed to the disproportionate distribution of myelopathy severity in our cohort (mild-moderate: $n = 22$; severe: $n = 14$). Based on these observations, laminoplasty may be indicated not only for spinal canal decompression in severe myelopathy but also for the amelioration of neck pain and functional disability in patients with OPLL-associated myelopathy.

This study has several limitations. First, the sample size was relatively small, with only 36 patients, due to the strict inclusion criteria. In addition, the severity of myelopathy in the included patients varied according to JOA scores. Further studies with larger cohorts are needed to validate these results, as clinical outcomes may vary significantly depending on the severity of myelopathy and the number of patients in this study was limited. Second, not all patients underwent the same surgical technique. C3 laminectomy was performed in 21 patients, while laminoplasty was performed on C3 in 15 patients. Some authors have reported that C3 laminoplasty can affect axial neck pain postoperatively [13,14,37].

However, in our subgroup analysis, there was no significant difference in neck pain between the C3 laminoplasty group and the laminectomy group. Third, long-term follow-up results were not analyzed. This study evaluated clinical scores two years after surgery, while previous studies have reported that recovery in patients with cervical myelopathy typically reaches a plateau between 6 months and 1 year after surgery [40,41].

Despite these limitations, this study is meaningful in that it analyzed the relationships between radiologic measurements and clinical outcomes. In addition to improving myelopathy symptoms in severe cases, cervical open-door laminoplasty could be effective in improving neck pain and NDI through spinal canal expansion.

5. Conclusions

Cervical open-door laminoplasty is an effective surgical technique for increasing the bony canal and spinal canal area in patients with OPLL. This study demonstrated that spinal canal expansion improved myelopathy symptoms in severe cases and was significantly correlated with improvements in neck pain and disability. While laminoplasty is typically considered for relieving myelopathy, it may also improve quality of life through the alleviation of neck pain and disability. Further research is needed to validate the long-term clinical benefits and to better understand the relationship between spinal canal expansion and clinical outcomes in OPLL patients.

Author Contributions: Conceptualization, Y.-H.K. and H.-Y.P.; methodology, J.B. and S.-I.K.; validation, M.-S.K. and B.J.H.; formal analysis, Y.-I.K. and C.B.; investigation, Y.-I.K. and S.-I.K.; data curation, J.B. and B.J.H.; writing—original draft preparation, Y.-I.K. and H.-Y.P.; writing—review and editing, Y.-H.K. and H.-Y.P.; supervision, Y.-H.K. and S.-I.K.; project administration, H.-Y.P.; funding acquisition, Y.-H.K. All authors have read and agreed to the published version of the manuscript.

Funding: This work was supported by a grant (No.NRF-2019R1F1A1063013) of the National Research Foundation (NRF) funded by the Ministry of Science and ICT (MSIT), Republic of Korea.

Institutional Review Board Statement: This study was conducted in accordance with the Declaration of Helsinki and approved by the Institutional Review Board of Seoul St. Mary's Hospital (KC23RISI0601) on 11 August 2023.

Informed Consent Statement: Patient consent was waived due to retrospective study design.

Data Availability Statement: Original data will be made available upon reasonable request.

Conflicts of Interest: The authors declare no conflicts of interest. The funders had no role in the design of the study, in the collection, analysis, or interpretation of data, in the writing of the manuscript, or in the decision to publish the results.

References

1. Le, H.V.; Wick, J.B.; Van, B.W.; Klineberg, E.O. Ossification of the Posterior Longitudinal Ligament: Pathophysiology, Diagnosis, and Management. *J. Am. Acad. Orthop. Surg.* **2022**, *30*, 820–830. [CrossRef] [PubMed]
2. Kim, T.J.; Bae, K.W.; Uhm, W.S.; Kim, T.H.; Joo, K.B.; Jun, J.B. Prevalence of ossification of the posterior longitudinal ligament of the cervical spine. *Jt. Bone Spine* **2008**, *75*, 471–474. [CrossRef] [PubMed]
3. Matsunaga, S.; Sakou, T. Ossification of the posterior longitudinal ligament of the cervical spine: Etiology and natural history. *Spine* **2012**, *37*, E309–E314. [CrossRef]
4. Emery, S.E. Cervical spondylotic myelopathy: Diagnosis and treatment. *J. Am. Acad. Orthop. Surg.* **2001**, *9*, 376–388. [CrossRef]
5. Ikuta, M.; Kaito, T.; Fujimori, T.; Kitahara, T.; Furuichi, T.; Bun, M.; Hirai, H.; Ukon, Y.; Kanie, Y.; Takenaka, S.; et al. Review of Basic Research about Ossification of the Spinal Ligaments Focusing on Animal Models. *J. Clin. Med.* **2023**, *12*, 1958. [CrossRef] [PubMed]
6. Kwok, S.S.S.; Cheung, J.P.Y. Surgical decision-making for ossification of the posterior longitudinal ligament versus other types of degenerative cervical myelopathy: Anterior versus posterior approaches. *BMC Musculoskelet. Disord.* **2020**, *21*, 823. [CrossRef]
7. Park, S.; Lee, D.H.; Lee, C.S.; Hwang, C.J.; Yang, J.J.; Cho, J.H. Anterior Decompression and Fusion for the Treatment of Cervical Myelopathy Caused by Ossification of the Posterior Longitudinal Ligament: A Narrative Review. *Asian Spine J.* **2023**, *17*, 582–594. [CrossRef]

8. Chiba, K.; Ogawa, Y.; Ishii, K.; Takaishi, H.; Nakamura, M.; Maruiwa, H.; Matsumoto, M.; Toyama, Y. Long-term results of expansive open-door laminoplasty for cervical myelopathy--average 14-year follow-up study. *Spine* **2006**, *31*, 2998–3005. [CrossRef]
9. Kim, N.; Cho, S.; Kim, T.H.; Oh, J.K.; Moon, S.H.; Kim, S.W. Comparison of Midline Splitting versus Unilateral Open Door Laminoplasty and Its Impact on Patient Outcomes. *Clin. Orthop. Surg.* **2023**, *15*, 444–453. [CrossRef]
10. Dong, F.; Shen, C.; Jiang, S.; Zhang, R.; Song, P.; Yu, Y.; Wang, S.; Li, X.; Zhao, G.; Ding, C. Measurement of volume-occupying rate of cervical spinal canal and its role in cervical spondylotic myelopathy. *Eur. Spine J.* **2013**, *22*, 1152–1157. [CrossRef]
11. Park, J.H.; Roh, S.W.; Rhim, S.C.; Jeon, S.R. Long-term outcomes of 2 cervical laminoplasty methods: Midline splitting versus unilateral single door. *J. Spinal Disord. Tech.* **2012**, *25*, E224–E229. [CrossRef]
12. Hejrati, N.; Pedro, K.; Alvi, M.A.; Quddusi, A.; Fehlings, M.G. Degenerative cervical myelopathy: Where have we been? Where are we now? Where are we going? *Acta Neurochir.* **2023**, *165*, 1105–1119. [CrossRef] [PubMed]
13. Takeuchi, K.; Yokoyama, T.; Aburakawa, S.; Saito, A.; Numasawa, T.; Iwasaki, T.; Itabashi, T.; Okada, A.; Ito, J.; Ueyama, K.; et al. Axial symptoms after cervical laminoplasty with C3 laminectomy compared with conventional C3-C7 laminoplasty: A modified laminoplasty preserving the semispinalis cervicis inserted into axis. *Spine* **2005**, *30*, 2544–2549. [CrossRef] [PubMed]
14. Lee, D.H.; Cho, J.H.; Hwang, C.J.; Lee, C.S.; Cho, S.K.; Ha, J.K. Can C3 Laminectomy Reduce Interlaminar Bony Fusion and Preserve the Range of Motion After Cervical Laminoplasty? *Spine* **2016**, *41*, 1884–1890. [CrossRef] [PubMed]
15. Yu, W.; Zhang, F.; Chen, Y.; Wang, X.; Chen, D.; Zheng, J.; Meng, X.; Huang, Q.; Yang, X.; Yin, M.; et al. Efficacy and safety of laminoplasty combined with C3 laminectomy for patients with multilevel degenerative cervical myelopathy: A systematic review and meta-analysis. *Eur. Spine J.* **2024**, *33*, 3915–3932. [CrossRef]
16. Cho, J.H.; Ha, J.K.; Kim, D.G.; Song, K.Y.; Kim, Y.T.; Hwang, C.J.; Lee, C.S.; Lee, D.H. Does preoperative T1 slope affect radiological and functional outcomes after cervical laminoplasty? *Spine* **2014**, *39*, E1575–E1581. [CrossRef]
17. Yonenobu, K.; Abumi, K.; Nagata, K.; Taketomi, E.; Ueyama, K. Interobserver and intraobserver reliability of the japanese orthopaedic association scoring system for evaluation of cervical compression myelopathy. *Spine* **2001**, *26*, 1890–1894, discussion 1895. [CrossRef]
18. Vernon, H. The Neck Disability Index: State-of-the-art, 1991–2008. *J. Manip. Physiol. Ther.* **2008**, *31*, 491–502. [CrossRef]
19. Fehlings, M.G.; Wilson, J.R.; Kopjar, B.; Yoon, S.T.; Arnold, P.M.; Massicotte, E.M.; Vaccaro, A.R.; Brodke, D.S.; Shaffrey, C.I.; Smith, J.S.; et al. Efficacy and safety of surgical decompression in patients with cervical spondylotic myelopathy: Results of the AOSpine North America prospective multi-center study. *J. Bone Jt. Surg. Am.* **2013**, *95*, 1651–1658. [CrossRef]
20. Head, J.; Rymarczuk, G.; Stricsek, G.; Velagapudi, L.; Maulucci, C.; Hoelscher, C.; Harrop, J. Ossification of the Posterior Longitudinal Ligament: Surgical Approaches and Associated Complications. *Neurospine* **2019**, *16*, 517–529. [CrossRef]
21. Ha, Y.; Shin, J.J. Comparison of clinical and radiological outcomes in cervical laminoplasty versus laminectomy with fusion in patients with ossification of the posterior longitudinal ligament. *Neurosurg. Rev.* **2020**, *43*, 1409–1421. [CrossRef] [PubMed]
22. Matsumoto, M.; Chiba, K.; Toyama, Y. Surgical treatment of ossification of the posterior longitudinal ligament and its outcomes: Posterior surgery by laminoplasty. *Spine* **2012**, *37*, E303–E308. [CrossRef]
23. Bernstein, D.N.; Prong, M.; Kurucan, E.; Jain, A.; Menga, E.N.; Riew, K.D.; Mesfin, A. National Trends and Complications in the Surgical Management of Ossification of the Posterior Longitudinal Ligament (OPLL). *Spine* **2019**, *44*, 1550–1557. [CrossRef]
24. Yamane, K.; Narita, W.; Takao, S.; Takeuchi, K. Exoscopic Minimally Invasive Open-Door Laminoplasty for Cervical Myelopathy: A Technical Note and Preliminary Analysis of Clinical Outcomes during the Acute Postoperative Period. *J. Clin. Med.* **2024**, *13*, 2173. [CrossRef]
25. Michael, K.W.; Neustein, T.M.; Rhee, J.M. Where should a laminoplasty start? The effect of the proximal level on post-laminoplasty loss of lordosis. *Spine J.* **2016**, *16*, 737–741. [CrossRef] [PubMed]
26. Sun, N.; Jiang, C.; Liu, Y. Surgical options for ossification of the posterior longitudinal ligament of the cervical spine: A narrative review. *J. Orthop. Surg. Res.* **2024**, *19*, 707. [CrossRef] [PubMed]
27. Sakai, K.; Yoshii, T.; Arai, Y.; Hirai, T.; Torigoe, I.; Inose, H.; Tomori, M.; Sakaki, K.; Matsukura, Y.; Okawa, A. Impact of preoperative cervical sagittal alignment for cervical myelopathy caused by ossification of the posterior longitudinal ligament on surgical treatment. *J. Orthop. Sci.* **2022**, *27*, 1208–1214. [CrossRef]
28. Inoue, T.; Maki, S.; Furuya, T.; Okimatsu, S.; Yunde, A.; Miura, M.; Shiratani, Y.; Nagashima, Y.; Maruyama, J.; Shiga, Y.; et al. Differences in Risk Factors for Decreased Cervical Lordosis after Multiple-Segment Laminoplasty for Cervical Spondylotic Myelopathy and Ossification of the Posterior Longitudinal Ligament: A Pilot Study. *Asian Spine J.* **2023**, *17*, 712–720. [CrossRef]
29. Lee, M.J.; Cassinelli, E.H.; Riew, K.D. Prevalence of cervical spine stenosis. Anatomic study in cadavers. *J. Bone Jt. Surg. Am.* **2007**, *89*, 376–380. [CrossRef]
30. Torg, J.S.; Pavlov, H.; Genuario, S.E.; Sennett, B.; Wisneski, R.J.; Robie, B.H.; Jahre, C. Neurapraxia of the cervical spinal cord with transient quadriplegia. *J. Bone Jt. Surg. Am.* **1986**, *68*, 1354–1370. [CrossRef]
31. Wang, H.; Zhang, L. Expansion of Spinal Canal with Lift-Open Laminoplasty: A New Method for Compression Cervical Myelopathy. *Orthop. Surg.* **2021**, *13*, 1673–1681. [CrossRef]
32. Furuya, T.; Sakai, K.; Yoshii, T.; Machino, M. Conservative Treatment and Surgical Indication of Cervical Ossification of the Posterior Longitudinal Ligament. *J. Clin. Med.* **2023**, *12*, 5719. [CrossRef] [PubMed]
33. Hosono, N.; Yonenobu, K.; Ono, K. Neck and shoulder pain after laminoplasty. A noticeable complication. *Spine* **1996**, *21*, 1969–1973. [PubMed]

34. Kawaguchi, Y.; Matsui, H.; Ishihara, H.; Gejo, R.; Yoshino, O. Axial symptoms after en bloc cervical laminoplasty. *J. Spinal Disord.* **1999**, *12*, 392–395. [CrossRef]
35. Sasaki, E.; Ono, A.; Yokoyama, T.; Wada, K.; Tanaka, T.; Kumagai, G.; Iwasaki, H.; Takahashi, I.; Umeda, T.; Nakaji, S.; et al. Prevalence and symptom of ossification of posterior longitudinal ligaments in the Japanese general population. *J. Orthop. Sci.* **2014**, *19*, 405–411. [CrossRef]
36. Koda, M.; Yoshii, T.; Egawa, S.; Sakai, K.; Kusano, K.; Nakagawa, Y.; Hirai, T.; Wada, K.; Katsumi, K.; Kimura, A.; et al. Neurological improvement is associated with neck pain attenuation after surgery for cervical ossification of the posterior longitudinal ligament. *Sci. Rep.* **2021**, *11*, 11910. [CrossRef] [PubMed]
37. Mesfin, A.; Park, M.S.; Piyaskulkaew, C.; Chuntarapas, T.; Song, K.S.; Kim, H.J.; Riew, K.D. Neck Pain following Laminoplasty. *Glob. Spine J.* **2015**, *5*, 17–22. [CrossRef]
38. Stephens, B.F.; Rhee, J.M.; Neustein, T.M.; Arceo, R. Laminoplasty Does not Lead to Worsening Axial Neck Pain in the Properly Selected Patient With Cervical Myelopathy: A Comparison With Laminectomy and Fusion. *Spine* **2017**, *42*, 1844–1850. [CrossRef]
39. Chen, G.; Wei, F.; Shi, L.; Li, J.; Wang, X.; Wang, M.; Wu, H.; Xu, Z.; Liu, X.; Liu, S. Inadequate spinal cord expansion in intraoperative ultrasound after decompression may predict neurological recovery of degenerative cervical myelopathy. *Eur. Radiol.* **2021**, *31*, 8478–8487. [CrossRef]
40. Pandita, N.; Gupta, S.; Raina, P.; Srivastava, A.; Hakak, A.Y.; Singh, O.; Darokhan, M.A.; Butt, M.F. Neurological Recovery Pattern in Cervical Spondylotic Myelopathy after Anterior Surgery: A Prospective Study with Literature Review. *Asian Spine J.* **2019**, *13*, 423–431. [CrossRef]
41. Cheung, W.Y.; Arvinte, D.; Wong, Y.W.; Luk, K.D.; Cheung, K.M. Neurological recovery after surgical decompression in patients with cervical spondylotic myelopathy—A prospective study. *Int. Orthop.* **2008**, *32*, 273–278. [CrossRef] [PubMed]

Journal of
Clinical Medicine

MDPI

Article

Two-Year Radiological Fusion Outcomes Following Biportal Endoscopic Transforaminal Lumbar Interbody Fusion Using Banana-Shaped Interbody Cages

Sang-Bum Kim, Dong-Hwan Kim, Daehee Choi and Ja-Yeong Yoon *

Department of Orthopedic Surgery, Chungnam National University Sejong Hospital, Sejong 30099, Republic of Korea; sangbumos@me.com (S.-B.K.); kidhw411@gmail.com (D.-H.K.)
* Correspondence: coffeesound2@gmail.com; Tel.: +82-44-995-5792; Fax: +82-44-995-5799

Abstract

Background: Biportal endoscopic transforaminal lumbar interbody fusion (BESS-TLIF) is an emerging minimally invasive technique. This study aimed to evaluate the two-year radiological fusion outcomes of single-level BESS-TLIF using a specific banana-shaped, porous titanium interbody cage. **Methods**: This retrospective study reviewed 51 patients who underwent the specified procedure. The primary endpoint was the radiological fusion rate, assessed by computed tomography (CT) over 24 months using a three-grade system. Factors influencing fusion, particularly bone graft composition (demineralized bone matrix [DBM] only vs. DBM with I-factor), were also analyzed. **Results**: The final complete fusion rate at two years was 96.1% (49/51; 95% Confidence Interval (CI), 86.5–99.5%). Bony fusion occurred predominantly in the posterior and intracage regions. The only significant factor influencing fusion was the bone graft material. The 'DBM with I-factor' group achieved complete fusion significantly faster than the 'DBM only' group (log-rank test, $p < 0.001$), with a higher final fusion rate (100% vs. 83.3%, $p = 0.045$). **Conclusions**: Single-level BESS-TLIF using a banana-shaped, porous titanium cage provides favourable two-year radiological fusion rates. The selective addition of I-factor as an osteoinductive supplement can significantly accelerate the time to achieve solid arthrodesis.

Keywords: endoscopic spinal surgery; transforaminal lumbar interbody fusion; radiological fusion; porous titanium cage; interbody fusion; minimally invasive spine surgery; I-factor

1. Introduction

Lumbar degenerative disease is one of the most common causes of low back pain and radiculopathy. For patients who fail to improve despite an adequate course of conservative treatment, spinal fusion has become an effective surgical option [1]. While traditional open transforaminal or posterior lumbar interbody fusion (TLIF/PLIF) has shown stable results, it is associated with significant paraspinal muscle injury, which can lead to increased post-operative pain and a prolonged recovery period. To overcome these drawbacks, minimally invasive spine surgery (MISS) techniques were developed, and more recently, biportal endoscopic spinal surgery (BESS) has emerged as an even more advanced minimally invasive approach. BESS-TLIF has been reported to have several clinical advantages, including minimal muscle damage and faster postoperative recovery [2]. However, the evidence regarding radiological fusion, one of the most critical criteria for the long-term success of BESS-TLIF, remains insufficient. Many existing studies have reported on relatively short-term follow-up periods of around 12 months or have relied on plain radiographs, which have limited accuracy for assessing bony fusion [3]. Furthermore, previous studies have often included heterogeneous patient cohorts with various types of interbody cages or multi-level fusions, making it difficult to evaluate the pure outcomes of a specific surgical procedure and implant combination [3,4].

In particular, recently developed 3D-printed porous titanium cages have been suggested to promote higher fusion rates by enhancing osseointegration compared to traditional materials like polyetheretherketone (PEEK) [5]. However, there is a lack of data on the long-term fusion patterns when these modern cages are used in BESS-TLIF procedures.

Therefore, the purpose of this study was to conduct a detailed analysis of the long-term, 24-month radiological fusion outcomes using computed tomography (CT), the gold standard for fusion assessment, in patients who underwent single-level BESS-TLIF with a single type of porous titanium cage (EIT Cellular Titanium TLIF Cage). We also aimed to evaluate the factors that may influence the fusion status at 24 months.

2. Materials and Methods

2.1. Patient Population

This retrospective study was approved by the Institutional Review Board of our institution (IRB No. 2025-07-005) and was conducted in accordance with the ethical principles of the Declaration of Helsinki. The requirement for written informed consent was waived due to the study's retrospective nature.

This study was designed to retrospectively evaluate patients who underwent primary single-level BESS-TLIF using the EIT Cellular Titanium TLIF Cage (DePuy Synthes, Johnson & Johnson; Tuttlingen, Germany) (Figure 1). We reviewed the medical records of patients who received this specific implant for degenerative lumbar disease. The inclusion criteria were: (1) a diagnosis of lumbar foraminal stenosis or degenerative spondylolisthesis of Meyerding grade I or less (representing low-grade instability); (2) persistent symptoms despite at least three months of conservative treatment; and (3) the availability of complete clinical and radiological data for a minimum of two years postoperatively.

Patients were excluded from the study if they had a history of previous surgery at the index level, required multi-level fusion, or underwent a hybrid surgical procedure combining different techniques. Patients who presented with other pathological conditions such as active infection, spinal tumours, metastatic disease, or acute fractures were also excluded. A total of 55 patients initially met these criteria. During the follow-up period, four patients (7.3%) developed significant cage subsidence (>3 mm), which was considered a procedural complication. As the resultant narrowing of the disc space also confounds the radiological assessment of bony fusion, these 4 patients were excluded from the primary per-protocol analysis of fusion grading. Therefore, a final cohort of 51 patients, comprising 22 males and 29 females, was included in the detailed radiological fusion analysis. All patients underwent follow-up CT scans at 3, 6, 12, and 24 months after surgery.

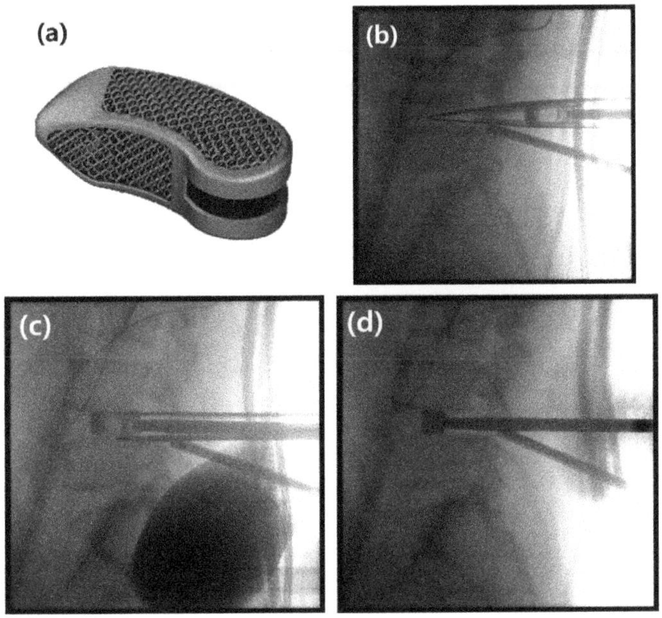

Figure 1. The banana-shaped EIT Cellular Titanium TLIF Cage and the intraoperative "insert-and-rotate" insertion technique. (**a**) Photograph of the EIT Cellular Titanium TLIF Cage, showing its porous, trabecular structure. (**b**) Intraoperative lateral C-arm image demonstrating the initial insertion of the cage into the posterior aspect of the disc space. (**c**) The "insert-and-rotate" maneuver is performed on the lateral view; the inserter handle is pivoted medially, which initiates the rotation of the cage. (**d**) Final lateral C-arm image confirming the cage has been rotated 90 degrees into its correct transverse position across the interbody space.

2.2. Surgical Procedures

All surgical procedures were performed under general anesthesia. Patients were positioned prone on a Jackson table, and the surgical field was prepared and draped in a standard sterile fashion for endoscopic spine surgery. The surgical approach was performed on the side with predominant radicular pain. In cases of bilateral symptoms, the left-sided approach was typically chosen to facilitate instrument handling for the right-handed surgeon.

Under C-arm fluoroscopic guidance, the operative disc level was identified. The pedicles of the superior and inferior vertebrae of the operative segment on the side of the surgical approach were then identified and marked on the skin. Two horizontal skin incisions, approximately 1.5 to 2.0 cm in length, were made directly over these pedicle markings. These incisions served as the entry portals for both the endoscopic procedure and the subsequent ipsilateral pedicle screw fixation.

Following the incisions, a sequential dilator was introduced to bluntly dissect the multifidus muscle, creating working channels down to the lamina. Initially, the upper incision served as the viewing portal and the lower as the working portal. An arthroscope was introduced through the upper portal, and a bipolar radiofrequency probe was inserted through the lower portal. This established the initial triangulation and allowed for soft tissue dissection and hemostasis. A clear surgical field was maintained throughout the procedure by ensuring a smooth and continuous outflow of saline irrigation.

Once a clear surgical field was established, an ipsilateral partial laminotomy was first performed and then extended via an undercutting technique to achieve bilateral decompression. Following this decompression, the ipsilateral inferior articular process (IAP) of the superior lamina was resected using an osteotome for autologous bone grafting (Figure 2a,b). Then, the superior articular process (SAP) of the inferior lamina was partially resected to fully expose the foraminal area (Figure 2c,d). This primary bony resection with the osteotome was performed while preserving the ligamentum flavum, which acted as a natural barrier to protect the dura and nerve roots. A high-speed burr was then used to remove any remaining sharp edges and meticulously shape a smooth and safe transforaminal pathway for the subsequent steps.

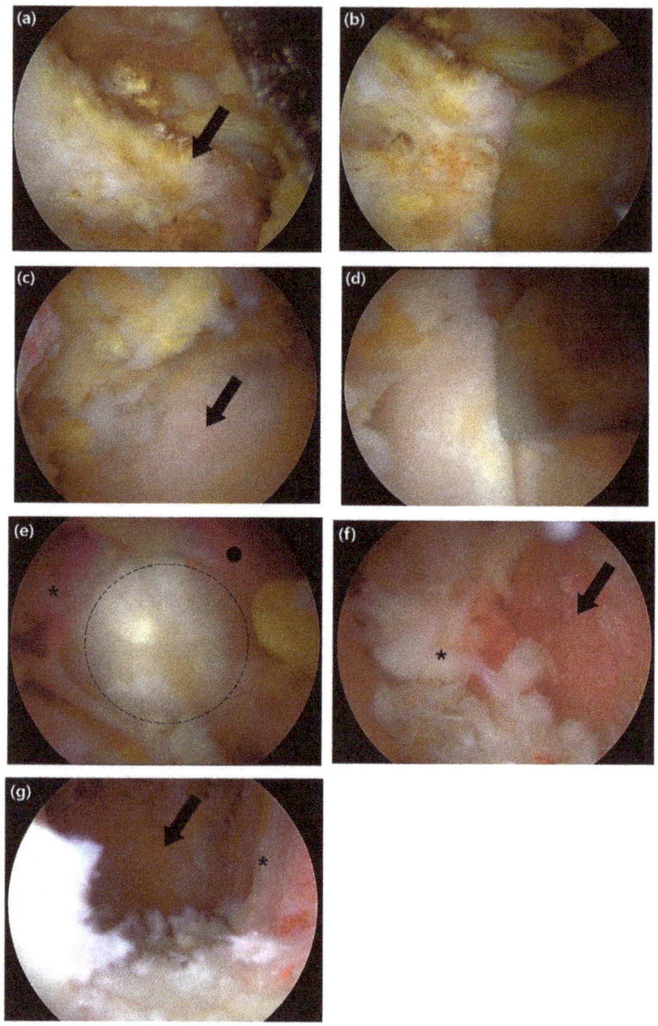

Figure 2. Intraoperative endoscopic views of the key steps for decompression and endplate preparation. (**a**) Endoscopic view showing the exposed inferior articular process (IAP) of the superior lamina (black arrow). (**b**) The IAP is resected using an osteotome. (**c**) After resection of the IAP, the superior articular process (SAP) of the inferior lamina is visualized (black arrow). (**d**) Resection of the SAP is performed with an osteotome to achieve foraminal decompression. (**e**) View after complete removal of the ligamentum flavum, showing the exposed annulus fibrosus. The exiting nerve root (asterisk), traversing nerve root (black circle), and the disc space (the dashed outline) are indicated. (**f**) The superior bony endplate of the inferior vertebra (black arrow) is revealed after meticulous stripping of the cartilaginous layer; a remnant disc fragment is marked with an asterisk. (**g**) Final view after endplate preparation, showing the prepared bony margin (asterisk) and the visualized anterior margin of the annulus (arrow), which confirms the anterior boundary of the disc space.

Following the completion of the bony work, the ligamentum flavum was completely removed to achieve full decompression. Using a curette and a rotating Kerrison punch, the ligament was first gently detached from the dura and excised on the ipsilateral side. The decompression was then extended to the contralateral side via a sublaminar approach. The ligament was removed either en bloc or in large fragments, ensuring the thorough decompression of the thecal sac and the traversing nerve root (Figure 2e).

Once neural decompression was completed, an annulotomy was performed using an annular knife (Figure 2f). A thorough discectomy was then carried out to create sufficient space for the interbody cage and bone graft. The nucleus pulposus was removed using a combination of curettes, pituitary forceps, and smooth-edged interbody disc reamers. Under magnified endoscopic vision, the cartilaginous endplates were then meticulously stripped from the underlying bone, which allowed for verification of complete residual disc removal and confirmation of endplate integrity (Figure 2g). This entire removal process was continued until the transverse fibres of the anterior longitudinal ligament (ALL) were clearly visualized, signifying the anterior boundary of the disc space.

Following endplate preparation, serial trials and interbody shapers were used to determine the optimal cage size that would ensure a press-fit and restore disc height. The saline irrigation was then temporarily paused to prevent graft washout. For interbody grafting, a composite of local autograft harvested during decompression and DBX Putty (demineralized bone matrix [DBM]; MTF Biologics; Edison, NJ, USA) was utilized. The local autograft provided essential osteogenic cells, while DBM served as an osteoconductive graft extender to supplement the often-limited autograft volume in MISS [6]. To further enhance the biological stimulus for fusion, an osteoinductive agent was considered. While bone morphogenetic protein-2 (BMP-2) is a potent option, its use within the interbody space has been associated with significant complications, such as ectopic bone formation, vertebral osteolysis, and inflammatory responses [5]. Therefore, I-factor bone graft (Cerapedix; Westminster, CO, USA), a synthetic peptide (P-15) with a favourable safety profile for interbody applications, was used as an osteoinductive supplement in this study [5,7,8]. Due to the additional cost, I-factor was administered only to those patients who provided specific informed consent. This material was delivered and compacted into the anterior portion of the disc space using a specialized funnel (Figure 3a–c).

The cage of the selected size was then packed with the remaining bone graft mixture. Throughout the insertion, the exiting and traversing nerve roots were protected under direct endoscopic visualization. The cage was inserted using an "insert-and-rotate" technique; it was first introduced into the posterior disc space, after which the inserter handle was pivoted medially. This maneuver allowed the banana-shaped cage to rotate into a transverse orientation as it was advanced across the disc space [9]. The cage was then gently impacted into its final position, and its placement was confirmed with C-arm fluoroscopy.

Posterior stabilization was then achieved with percutaneous pedicle screw fixation. Under fluoroscopic guidance, cannulated pedicle screws were inserted bilaterally; the contralateral screws were placed through separate incisions, while the ipsilateral screws were inserted through the established endoscopic portals. Rods were passed percutaneously, contoured to the desired lordosis, and the entire construct was secured (Figure 3d,e). After meticulous hemostasis was achieved with the radiofrequency probe, a drainage tube was placed at the surgical site. The fascia and skin incisions were then closed in a layered fashion.

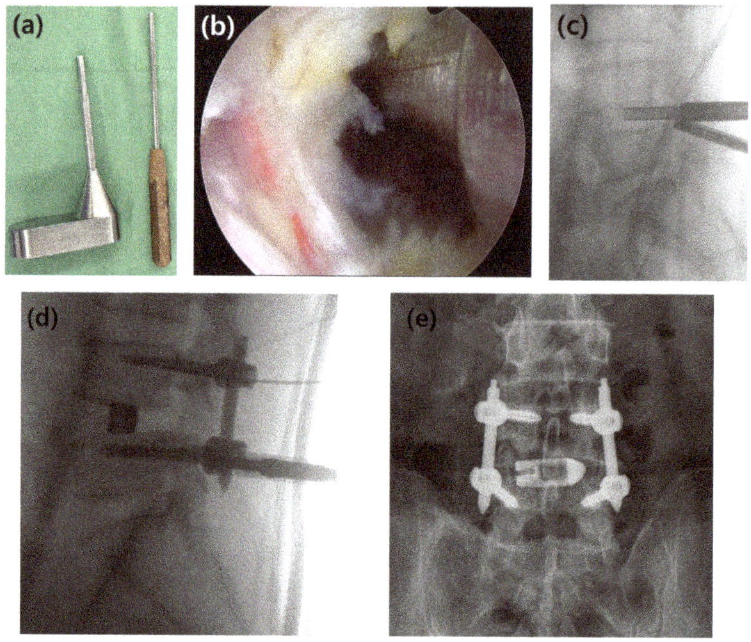

Figure 3. Surgical instruments and the procedure for interbody bone graft delivery. (**a**) The specialized bone graft funnel and the corresponding impactor used to deliver the graft material into the disc space. (**b**) Intraoperative endoscopic view showing the funnel correctly positioned at the entrance of the prepared disc space. (**c**) Lateral C-arm image confirming the position of the funnel and demonstrating the delivery of the bone graft material into the interbody space. (**d**) Intraoperative lateral C-arm image showing the insertion of percutaneous pedicle screws for posterior stabilization after cage placement. (**e**) Final anteroposterior radiograph showing the completed construct with the cage and pedicle screws.

2.3. Postoperative Management

Postoperatively, all patients were required to wear a thoracolumbar sacral orthosis (TLSO) for a period of six months to provide external stability. To further promote bony fusion, a 6-month course of teriparatide (Terrosa®; Gedeon Richter Plc.; Budapest, Hungary; 20 µg daily, subcutaneous injection) was administered. This 6-month duration was strategically chosen to maximize the therapeutic effect within teriparatide's peak "anabolic window," which is the initial phase when its bone-forming activity significantly exceeds bone resorption, while also maintaining cost-effectiveness for the patient [10,11].

2.4. Clinical and Radiological Assessment

2.4.1. Primary Endpoint: Radiological Fusion Assessment

The primary endpoint of this study was the radiological fusion rate, assessed using multi-planar reconstructed CT images obtained at 3, 6, 12, and 24 months postoperatively. To provide a detailed analysis, the location of new bone formation was classified based on its position relative to the cage. On sagittal plane images, the locations were defined as (A) anterior to the cage, (I) inside the cage, and (P) posterior to the cage. On coronal plane images, they were defined as (L) left of the cage, (I) inside the cage, and (R) right of the cage (Figure 4).

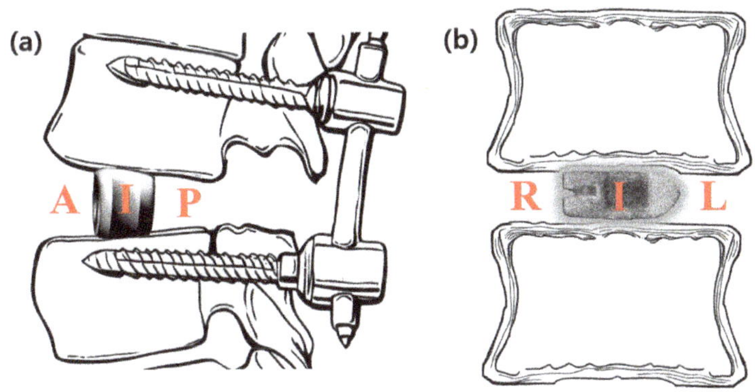

Figure 4. Schematic diagrams illustrating the classification of fusion location. The location of new bone formation was assessed relative to the interbody cage on multi-planar CT images. (**a**) On the sagittal plane, fusion was evaluated in three zones: anterior to the cage (A), inside the cage (I), and posterior to the cage (P). (**b**) On the coronal plane, fusion was evaluated in three zones: right of the cage (R), inside the cage (I), and left of the cage (L). The laterality (left/right) was determined based on the radiological orientation of the CT image.

The degree of fusion was evaluated using a simplified three-grade grading system. While the classification described by Bridwell et al. is a foundational standard, we adopted a more distinct definition for clarity, inspired by the methodology of a prior study on PLIF fusion rates [12]. Fusion was graded as follows: Grade 0 (Non-union) was defined as the complete absence of bone growth; Grade 1 (Partial Fusion) as the presence of bone growth without a continuous bone bridge connecting the superior and inferior vertebral bodies; and Grade 2 (Complete Fusion) as the formation of a continuous, solid bone bridge. For the final analysis, Grade 2 was considered a successful fusion (Figure 5).

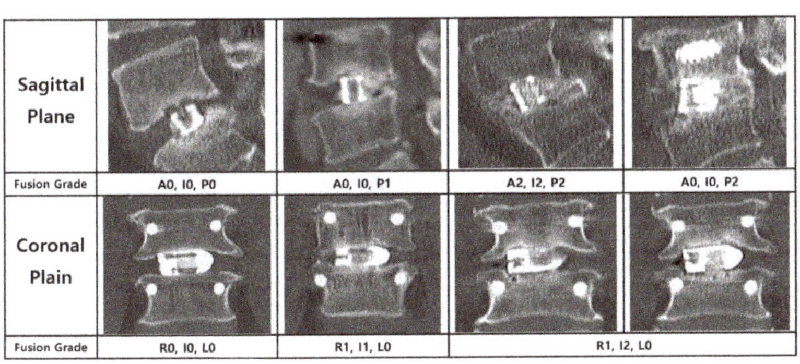

Figure 5. Radiological criteria and representative CT images for the three-grade fusion grading system. The figure illustrates the grading system used to assess bony fusion on multi-planar CT images, with representative examples provided for both the sagittal (left column) and coronal (right column) planes. Fusion was categorized into three grades: Grade 0 (Non-union) was defined as the complete absence of new bone formation; Grade 1 (Partial Fusion) as the presence of bone growth without a continuous bridging trabecular bone between the vertebral bodies; and Grade 2 (Complete Fusion) as the formation of a continuous, solid bone bridge. For the purpose of the final analysis in this study, only Grade 2 was considered a successful fusion.

2.4.2. Secondary Endpoints: Analysis of Factors Influencing Fusion

As a secondary analysis, we evaluated the influence of several variables on the radiological fusion outcome at 24 months. These variables included patient-related factors such as age and bone mineral density (BMD), and surgery-related factors such as implanted cage height, lordotic angle, and final cage position. The composition of the fusion materials, as previously described, was also analyzed as a factor, categorized into two groups: local autograft with DBM only, or with the addition of I-factor.

2.5. Statistical Analysis

All statistical analyses were performed using Python (version 3.9; Python Software Foundation; Wilmington, DE, USA) with the Pandas (version 1.5.3), SciPy (version 1.10.1), and Lifelines (version 0.27.8) libraries. Baseline characteristics were summarized using descriptive statistics (mean ± standard deviation (SD) or *n* [%]). The primary endpoint was the radiological fusion status (Grade 0, 1, or 2), assessed over 24 months. To identify factors influencing fusion, Fisher's exact test and the Kruskal–Wallis H test were used for univariable comparisons. Time-to-fusion events were analyzed using the Kaplan–Meier method with the log-rank test. The frequency of fusion at different anatomical locations was compared using Cochran's Q test with post hoc McNemar tests. A p-value < 0.05 was considered statistically significant.

3. Results

3.1. Baseline Demographic and Surgical Characteristics

The mean age of the cohort was 70.0 ± 9.7 years, with a mean BMD T-score of −1.7 ± 1.1 (Table 1). The study population consisted of 22 males (43.1%) and 29 females (56.9%). The most common surgical level was L4–5 (n = 27, 52.9%), followed by L5–S1 (n = 13, 25.5%). A bone graft mixture including I-factor was used in the majority of patients (n = 39, 76.5%). For the interbody cage, the most frequently used height was 12 mm (n = 20, 39.2%), and the most common lordotic angle was 8° (n = 38, 74.5%).

Table 1. Baseline Demographic and Surgical Characteristics (n = 51).

	All Patients (n = 51)
Age (years), mean (SD)	70.0 (9.7)
BMD, mean (SD)	−1.7 (1.1)
Sex, n (%)	
Male	22 (43.1%)
Female	29 (56.9%)
Fusion Material, n (%)	
DBM	12 (23.5%)
DBM with I-factor	39 (76.5%)
Surgical Level, n	
L1–2	1 (2.0%)
L2–3	2 (3.9%)
L3–4	8(15.7%)
L4–5	27 (52.9%)
L5–S1	13 (25.5%)
Cage Height (mm), n (%)	
9	1 (2.0%)
10	11 (21.6%)

Table 1. *Cont.*

	All Patients (n = 51)
11	11 (21.6%)
12	20 (39.2%)
13	8 (15.7%)
Cage Angle (°), n (%)	
8	38 (74.5%)
12	13 (25.5%)

Values are presented as mean (standard deviation) or n (%). SD: Standard Deviation; BMD: Bone Mineral Density; DBM: Demineralized Bone Matrix.

3.2. *Overall Fusion Rate Progression*

The overall radiological fusion status showed a clear progression towards solid union over the 24-month follow-up period (Figure 6). The rate of Complete Fusion (Grade 2) steadily increased from 19.6% at 3 months, to 49.0% at 6 months, 76.5% at 12 months, and ultimately reached 96.1% (49 of 51 patients; 95% CI, 86.5–99.5%) at the final follow-up. Notably, no cases of Non-union (Grade 0) were observed at or after the 12-month follow-up, leaving only two patients (3.9%) in a state of Partial Fusion at the study's conclusion.

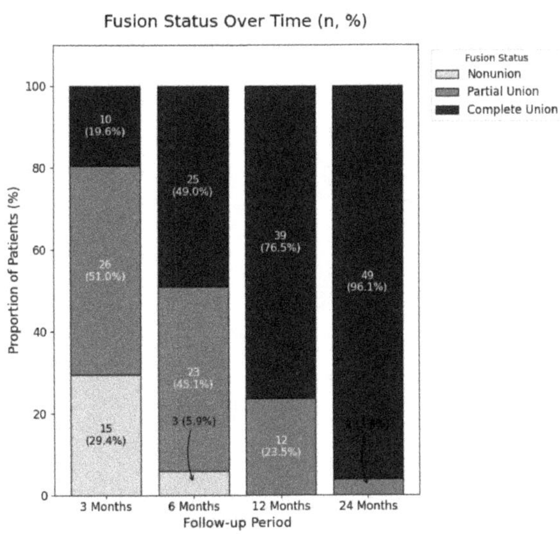

Figure 6. Progression of Radiological Fusion Status Over Time.

This 100% stacked bar chart illustrates the changes in fusion status at the 3, 6, 12, and 24-month follow-up points. The proportions of patients classified as non-union (Grade 0), partial fusion (Grade 1), and complete fusion (Grade 2) are represented by different shades. The numbers within each segment indicate the absolute number of patients (n) and the corresponding percentage (%). A clear, progressive increase in the rate of complete fusion is demonstrated, reaching 96.1% at the final follow-up.

3.3. *Analysis of Fusion Location at 24 Months*

The complete fusion rates at the 24-month follow-up were analyzed separately for the sagittal and coronal planes. In the sagittal plane, the complete fusion rate was highest in the posterior location (76.5%), followed by the intracage (62.7%) and anterior (31.4%) locations.

A Cochran's Q test confirmed a statistically significant difference among these three sites ($p < 0.0001$). Post hoc analysis revealed that fusion rates in the posterior and intracage locations were significantly higher than in the anterior location. In the coronal plane, the intracage location had the highest fusion rate (72.5%), compared to the left (29.4%) and right (21.6%) locations. This difference was also statistically significant ($p < 0.0001$, Cochran's Q test), with post hoc tests showing that the intracage fusion rate was significantly higher than both the left and right sides. These analyses statistically demonstrate that successful bony fusion occurred predominantly in the posterior region on sagittal view and within the intracage region on coronal view.

3.4. Factors Influencing Fusion Outcomes

An analysis was performed to identify factors associated with the final fusion status at 24 months (Table 2). No statistically significant association was found between the final fusion outcome (complete vs. partial Fusion) and patient-related factors, including mean age (69.8 vs. 75.0 years, $p = 0.679$) and BMD T-score (−1.7 vs. −2.1, $p = 0.561$). Similarly, various surgery-related factors—such as cage height, lordotic angle, insertion site, and final cage position—did not show a significant influence on the 24-month fusion rate (all $p > 0.05$).

Table 2. Analysis of Factors Associated with Fusion Status at 24 Months.

	Complete Fusion (n = 49)	Partial Fusion (n = 2)	p-Value
Age (years)	69.8 (9.7)	75.0 (11.3)	0.679
BMD (T-score)	−1.7 (1.1)	−2.1 (0.6)	0.561
Cage Height (mm)	11.5 (1.1)	10.5 (0.7)	0.171
Cage Angle (°)	9.0 (1.7)	10.0 (2.8)	0.422
Insertion Site			
Right	29 (59.2)	0 (0.0)	0.353
Left	20 (40.8)	2 (100.0)	
Cage Position			
Centre	23 (46.9)	1 (50.0)	
Anterior	22 (44.9)	1 (50.0)	0.981
Anterior–Posterior	2 (4.1)	0 (0.0)	
Posterior	2 (4.1)	0 (0.0)	
Fusion Material			
DBM only	10 (20.4)	2 (100.0)	
DBM with I-factor	39 (79.6)	0 (0.0)	0.045

Values are presented as mean (standard deviation) or n (%). Continuous variables were compared using the Kruskal–Wallis H test, and categorical variables were compared using Fisher's exact test. $p < 0.05$ was considered statistically significant. BMD: Bone Mineral Density; DBM: Demineralized Bone Matrix.

In contrast, the composition of the bone graft material was the only factor found to have a significant influence on the fusion outcome (Table 3). The 'DBM with I-factor' group demonstrated a significantly higher rate of achieving complete Fusion compared to the 'DBM only' group at all postoperative follow-up points: 3 months ($p < 0.001$), 6 months ($p = 0.002$), 12 months ($p = 0.022$), and at the final 24-month follow-up ($p = 0.045$). At the 24-month assessment, all 39 patients (100%) in the 'DBM with I-factor' group achieved complete Fusion, whereas 10 of the 12 patients (83.3%) in the 'DBM only' group achieved the same, with two patients remaining in a state of Partial Fusion.

Table 3. Comparison of Fusion Progression by Bone Graft Material.

Follow-Up	Fusion Status	DBM Only (n = 12)	DBM with I-Factor (n = 39)	p-Value
3 Months	Nonunion	11	4	<0.001
	Partial Union	1	25	
	Complete Union	0	10	
6 Months	Nonunion	2	1	0.002
	Partial Union	9	14	
	Complete Union	1	24	
12 Months	Nonunion	0	0	0.022
	Partial Union	6	6	
	Complete Union	6	33	
24 Months	Nonunion	0	0	0.045
	Partial Union	2	0	
	Complete Union	10	39	

Values are presented as n (%). p-values were obtained using Fisher's exact test to compare the distribution of fusion grades between the two groups at each time point. $p < 0.05$ was considered statistically significant. DBM: Demineralized Bone Matrix.

While comparisons at each individual follow-up point revealed higher fusion rates for the 'DBM with I-factor' group, to more comprehensively evaluate the overall progression of fusion over the entire follow-up period, a Kaplan–Meier analysis was performed (Figure 7). This analysis confirmed that the 'DBM with I-factor' group (n = 39) achieved complete Fusion at a significantly faster overall rate than the 'DBM only' group (n = 12). The difference between the survival curves was statistically significant (log-rank test, $p < 0.001$).

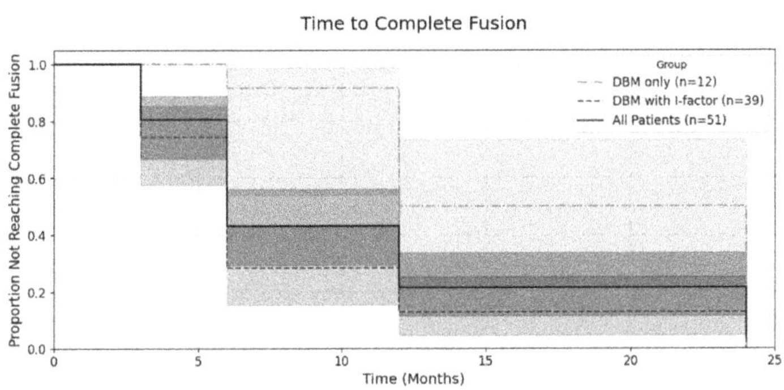

Figure 7. Kaplan–Meier curves for the time to complete fusion.

The plot shows the proportion of patients who had not yet achieved complete fusion over a 24-month follow-up period. The central lines represent the Kaplan–Meier estimates for each group: the solid line for all patients (n = 51), the dashed line for the DBM + I-factor group (n = 39), and the dash-dot line for the DBM only group (n = 12). Each corresponding shaded area represents the 95% confidence interval for that estimate. A log-rank test was used to compare the curves between the 'DBM only' and 'DBM with I-factor' groups, which showed a statistically significant difference ($p < 0.001$).

4. Discussions

The primary finding of this study is the high rate of radiological fusion following BESS-TLIF using the EIT Cellular Titanium cage. At the final 24-month follow-up, a complete fusion (Grade 2) rate of 96.1% was achieved. Our analysis also revealed that bony fusion occurred predominantly in the posterior and intracage regions, and that the addition of I-factor significantly accelerated the time to achieve solid fusion.

The 96.1% fusion rate in this study is consistent with the 95.2% pooled fusion rate for the BESS-TLIF technique reported in a recent meta-analysis [13]. Furthermore, this high fusion rate is comparable to the findings of a recent meta-analysis on conventional techniques, which reported fusion rates of 94.8% for MIS-TLIF and 93.9% for open TLIF [14]. This suggests that the BESS-TLIF technique, when combined with a porous titanium cage, can achieve a fusion success rate at least equivalent to that of more traditional and invasive approaches.

The high fusion rate in this study may also be attributable to the characteristics of the interbody cage. The banana-shaped design allows for a large footprint, maximizing contact with the biomechanically robust apophyseal ring of the vertebral endplate [15]. Moreover, the favourable outcomes in this study are likely attributable in large part to the characteristics of the interbody implant. The EIT cage is constructed from highly porous titanium, with a trabecular structure designed to mimic cancellous bone and facilitate osseointegration [16]. The clinical superiority of such materials over traditional PEEK is increasingly supported by high-level evidence; a recent meta-analysis confirmed that porous titanium cages are associated with significantly higher fusion rates and lower subsidence rates [17].

During our procedure, bone graft material was first placed into the prepared disc space, followed by the insertion of the interbody cage. This procedural sequence consequently leaves a relatively smaller volume of graft material in the posterior aspect of the segment. Despite this, a notable finding was that the rate of Complete Fusion in the posterior region (76.5%) was significantly higher than that in the anterior region. This finding is consistent with previous CT-based analyses of interbody fusion patterns, which have demonstrated that bone union tends to initiate at the posterior margin of the disc space [18]. Following stabilization with an interbody cage and pedicle screws, the posterior aspect of the disc space is subjected to significant compressive forces [19]. This concentrated mechanical stress is known to stimulate a robust bone formation response, which likely explains the observed fusion pattern [20].

Furthermore, the analysis of the coronal plane revealed another important fusion pattern: the rate of intracage fusion (72.5%) was significantly higher than the fusion rates in the lateral aspects of the disc space (29.4% on the left and 21.6% on the right). This finding is consistent with the biomechanical principles of interbody fusion. The interbody cage is designed to be the primary load-bearing structure, transmitting axial compressive forces through the centre of the vertebral endplates [21]. This creates an ideal mechanical environment for osteogenesis within and immediately around the cage, which also contains the most densely packed bone graft on an osteoconductive scaffold [22]. The lateral gutters, in contrast, are subjected to less direct compressive loading, which may explain the lower fusion rates observed in these areas [23].

The only factor found to have a statistically significant influence on fusion outcomes in this study was the composition of the bone graft material. The Kaplan–Meier analysis confirmed a significantly faster time to achieve solid fusion in the 'DBM with I-factor' group compared to the 'DBM only' group (log-rank test, $p < 0.001$). Furthermore, at the final 24-month follow-up, the Complete Fusion rate was 100% in the I-factor group versus 83.3% in the 'DBM only' group. This finding can be attributed to the different biological mechanisms of the graft materials. DBM primarily acts as an osteoconductive scaffold, providing a passive framework for bone growth. In contrast, I-factor is a synthetic peptide (P-15) that functions as an osteoinductive agent. Specifically, the P-15 peptide mimics the binding site of Type I collagen, which actively attracts osteoprogenitor cells and stimulates their attachment and proliferation to enhance the cascade of new bone formation [8]. While other potent osteoinductive agents, such as recombinant human bone morphogenetic protein-2 (rhBMP-2), are available, their use in MISS procedures has been linked to significant complications like ectopic bone formation and vertebral osteolysis, as noted in our methods [5,8]. Our results, which align with the known biological activity of P-15, suggest that the selective addition of this synthetic peptide, which offers a favourable safety profile, can be a valuable strategy to accelerate and ensure a higher probability of successful arthrodesis in BESS-TLIF procedures.

The present study has several distinct features. First, the study cohort was highly homogeneous. By including only patients who underwent single-level fusion with a single, specific type of interbody cage, we minimized the confounding effects of surgical and implant-related variables. This allows for a more direct assessment of the radiological outcomes of the BESS-TLIF procedure when performed under these standardized conditions. Second, our study utilized CT scans for fusion assessment up to a 24-month follow-up. The use of CT, which is considered the gold standard for evaluating bony fusion, at a long-term time point provides a more accurate and reliable assessment of fusion status compared to studies with shorter follow-up periods or those relying solely on plain radiographs.

This study has several limitations that should be acknowledged. First, its retrospective design is subject to inherent selection bias and potential inconsistencies in the collected data. Second, the relatively small sample size and the single-centre nature of the study may limit the generalizability of our findings to a broader patient population. Third, this was a single-arm study without a direct comparative control group, such as patients undergoing open TLIF or implantation with a different type of cage. Finally, our analysis focused exclusively on radiological outcomes, and a correlation with clinical results, such as pain and functional scores, was not performed. Therefore, the high radiological fusion rate reported here does not necessarily translate to a superior clinical outcome. Furthermore, it is important to note that four patients (7.3% of the initial cohort) were excluded from the final fusion analysis due to significant cage subsidence [6]. While these cases were excluded because severe subsidence confounds the accurate radiological assessment of fusion, subsidence itself can be considered a form of mechanical or biological failure. Therefore, the reported fusion rate of 96.1% should be interpreted with caution, as it represents a per-protocol outcome and may potentially overestimate the overall success rate of the procedure.

5. Conclusions

In conclusion, this study demonstrates that single-level BESS-TLIF using a banana-shaped, porous titanium cage can achieve a very high radiological fusion rate of 96.1% (95% CI, 86.5–99.5%) at the 24-month long-term follow-up. Successful bony fusion occurred predominantly in the posterior and intracage regions of the vertebral segment, suggesting the importance of a stable biomechanical environment. Furthermore, the addition of an osteoinductive biologic agent (I-factor) was found to significantly accelerate the time to achieve fusion. Therefore, the results of this study, with its strictly controlled variables, support that BESS-TLIF, when combined with a porous titanium implant of this specific design, is an effective minimally invasive treatment method capable of achieving reliable bony fusion.

Author Contributions: Conceptualization, S.-B.K. and J.-Y.Y.; Methodology, S.-B.K. and J.-Y.Y.; Software, D.C. and J.-Y.Y.; Validation, D.-H.K., D.C. and J.-Y.Y.; Formal Analysis, S.-B.K.

and J.-Y.Y.; Investigation, D.-H.K.; Resources, J.-Y.Y.; Data Curation, D.C., D.-H.K. and J.-Y.Y.; Writing—Original Draft Preparation, J.-Y.Y., S.-B.K. and D.-H.K.; Writing—Review & Editing, S.-B.K. and J.-Y.Y.; Visualization, J.-Y.Y.; Supervision, S.-B.K.; Project Administration, S.-B.K. All authors have read and agreed to the published version of the manuscript.

Funding: This research received no external funding.

Institutional Review Board Statement: The study was conducted in accordance with the Declaration of Helsinki, and ap-proved by the Institutional Review Board of Chungnam National University Sejong Hospital (IRB No. 2025-07-005, approved on [Date of Approval: 15 July 2025].

Informed Consent Statement: Informed consent was waived due to the retrospective nature of the study.

Data Availability Statement: The data presented in this study are available on request from the corresponding author. The data are not publicly available due to patient privacy and ethical restrictions.

Acknowledgments: The authors would like to thank research staff G. Choi and M. Jung for their valuable advice on the procedural aspects of data collection, and J. Kim, the head nurse of the operating room, for her support.

Conflicts of Interest: The authors declare no conflict of interest.

References

1. Reid, P.C.; Morr, S.; Kaiser, M.G. State of the union: A review of lumbar fusion indications and techniques for degenerative spine disease. *J. Neurosurg. Spine* **2019**, *31*, 1–14. [CrossRef]
2. Guo, H.; Song, Y.; Weng, R.; Tian, H.; Yuan, J.; Li, Y. Comparison of Clinical Outcomes and Complications Between Endoscopic and Minimally Invasive Transforaminal Lumbar Interbody Fusion for Lumbar Degenerative Diseases: A Systematic Review and Meta-analysis. *Glob. Spine J.* **2023**, *13*, 1394–1404. [CrossRef] [PubMed]
3. You, K.H.; Hyun, J.T.; Park, S.M.; Kang, M.S.; Cho, S.K.; Park, H.J. Comparison of clinical and radiologic outcomes between biportal endoscopic transforaminal lumbar interbody fusion and posterior lumbar interbody fusion. *Sci. Rep.* **2024**, *14*, 29652. [CrossRef] [PubMed]
4. Liawrungrueang, W.; Lee, H.-J.; Kim, S.B.; Park, S.-M.; Cholamjiak, W.; Park, H.-J. A Systematic Review of Biportal Endoscopic Spinal Surgery with Interbody Fusion. *Asian Spine J.* **2025**, *19*, 275–291. [CrossRef]
5. Hasan, S.; Al-Jamal, M.; Miller, A.; Higginbotham, D.O.; Cavazos, D.R.; Waheed, M.; Saleh, E.; McCarty, S.A. Efficacy and Outcome Measurement of iFactor/ABM/P-15 in Lumbar Spine Surgery: A Systematic Review. *Glob. Spine J.* **2023**, *14*, 1422–1433. [CrossRef]
6. Ha, D.H.; Oh, S.K.; Shim, D.M. Clinical Outcomes of a Zero Profile Implant for Single-Level Anterior Cervical Discectomy and Fusion. *J. Korean Soc. Spine Surg.* **2016**, *23*, 71–76. [CrossRef]
7. Kim, Y.H.; Ha, K.Y.; Kim, Y.S.; Kim, K.W.; Rhyu, K.W.; Park, J.B.; Shin, J.H.; Kim, Y.Y.; Lee, J.S.; Park, H.Y.; et al. Lumbar Interbody Fusion and Osteobiologics for Lumbar Fusion. *Asian Spine J.* **2022**, *16*, 1022–1033. [CrossRef]
8. Kim, Y.H.; Kim, K.W.; Rhyu, K.W.; Park, J.B.; Shin, J.H.; Kim, Y.Y.; Lee, J.S.; Ahn, J.H.; Ryu, J.H.; Park, H.Y.; et al. Bone Fusion Materials: Past, Present, and Future. *Asian Spine J.* **2025**, *19*, 490–500. [CrossRef]
9. Andresen, A.K.; Carreon, L.Y.; Overgaard, S.; Jacobsen, M.K.; Andersen, M.Ø. Safety and Reoperation Rates in Non-instrumented Lumbar Fusion Surgery: Secondary Report From a Randomized Controlled Trial of ABM/P-15 vs. Allograft With Minimum 5 years Follow-Up. *Glob. Spine J.* **2024**, *14*, 33–40. [CrossRef]
10. Pazianas, M. Anabolic Effects of PTH and the "Anabolic Window". *Trends Endocrinol. Metab.* **2015**, *26*, 111–113. [CrossRef]
11. Park, J.S.; Kim, H.J.; Park, S.J.; Kang, D.H.; Lee, C.S. A Comprehensive Review of Risk Factors and Prevention Strategies: How to Minimize Mechanical Complications in Corrective Surgery for Adult Spinal Deformity. *Asian Spine J.* **2025**, *19*, 463–475. [CrossRef]
12. Bridwell, K.H.; Lenke, L.G.; McEnery, K.W.; Baldus, C.; Blanke, K. Anterior fresh frozen structural allografts in the thoracic and lumbar spine. Do they work if combined with posterior fusion and instrumentation in adult patients with kyphosis or anterior column defects? *Spine* **1995**, *20*, 1410–1418. [CrossRef] [PubMed]
13. Lee, J.; Lee, D.H.; Jung, C.W.; Song, K.S. The Significance of Extra-Cage Bridging Bone via Radiographic Lumbar Interbody Fusion Criterion. *Glob. Spine J.* **2023**, *13*, 113–121. [CrossRef]
14. Luan, H.; Peng, C.; Liu, K.; Yang, H.; Tang, H. Comparing the efficacy of unilateral biportal endoscopic transforaminal lumbar interbody fusion and minimally invasive transforaminal lumbar interbody fusion in lumbar degenerative diseases: A systematic review and meta-analysis. *J. Orthop. Surg. Res.* **2023**, *18*, 888. [CrossRef]

15. Miller, L.E.; Bhattacharyya, S.; Pracyk, J. Minimally Invasive Versus Open Transforaminal Lumbar Interbody Fusion for Single-Level Degenerative Disease: A Systematic Review and Meta-Analysis of Randomized Controlled Trials. *World Neurosurg.* **2020**, *133*, 358–365.e4. [CrossRef] [PubMed]
16. Fushimi, K.; Miyagawa, T.; Iwai, C.; Nozawa, S.; Iinuma, N.; Tanaka, R.; Shirai, G.; Tanahashi, H.; Yokoi, T.; Akiyama, H. Transforaminal Lumbar Interbody Fusion with Double Banana Cages: Clinical Evaluations and Finite Element Model Analysis. *Global Spine J.* **2024**, *14*, 2031–2038. [CrossRef]
17. van den Brink, W.; Lamerigts, N. Complete Osseointegration of a Retrieved 3-D Printed Porous Titanium Cervical Cage. *Front. Surg.* **2020**, *7*, 526020. [CrossRef]
18. Zhai, W.; Liu, L.; Gao, Y.; Qin, S.; Han, P.; Xu, Y. Application of 3D-Printed Porous Titanium Interbody Fusion Cages versus Polyetheretherketone Cages in Anterior Cervical Discectomy and Fusion: A Systematic Review and Meta-Analysis Update. *Exp. Ther. Med.* **2024**, *28*, 290. [CrossRef]
19. Calek, A.K.; Cornaz, F.; Suter, M.; Fasser, M.R.; Baumgartner, S.; Sager, P.; Farshad, M.; Widmer, J. Load distribution on intervertebral cages with and without posterior instrumentation. *Spine J.* **2024**, *24*, 889–898. [CrossRef] [PubMed]
20. Segi, N.; Nakashima, H.; Ito, S.; Ouchida, J.; Yamauchi, I.; Matsumoto, T.; Kanbara, S.; Ito, K.; Imagama, S. Response to Letter to the Editor Regarding the Article Entitled "Trabecular Bone Remodeling After Posterior Lumbar Interbody Fusion: Comparison of the Osseointegration in Three-Dimensional Porous Titanium Cages and Polyether-Ether-Ketone Cages" by Segi et al. *Glob. Spine J.* **2025**, *15*, 2841–2843.
21. Polikeit, A.; Ferguson, S.J.; Nolte, L.P.; Orr, T.E. The importance of the endplate for interbody cages in the lumbar spine. *Eur. Spine J.* **2003**, *12*, 556–561. [CrossRef] [PubMed]
22. Kok, D.; Peeters, C.M.M.; Wapstra, F.H.; Bulstra, S.K.; Veldhuizen, A.G. Biomechanical evaluation of two minimal access interbody cage designs in a cadaveric model. *J. Exp. Orthop.* **2018**, *5*, 51. [CrossRef] [PubMed]
23. Cadman, J.; Sutterlin, C., 3rd; Dabirrahmani, D.; Appleyard, R. The importance of loading the periphery of the vertebral endplate. *J. Spine Surg.* **2016**, *2*, 178–184. [CrossRef] [PubMed]

MDPI AG
Grosspeteranlage 5
4052 Basel
Switzerland
Tel.: +41 61 683 77 34

Journal of Clinical Medicine Editorial Office
E-mail: jcm@mdpi.com
www.mdpi.com/journal/jcm

www.ingramcontent.com/pod-product-compliance
Lightning Source LLC
Chambersburg PA
CBHW040821250926
51850CB00007BA/1229
* 9 7 8 3 7 2 5 8 6 1 5 5 2 *